Advances in the One Health Approach

Integrating Human, Animal, and Environmental Health

nova
Medicine & Health
www.novapublishers.com
New York

Public Health in the 21st Century Series

Public Health Risks: Detection, Management and Control
Paulo Moreira, PhD (Editor)
ISBN: 979-8-89530-936-0
eBook ISBN: 979-8-90134-019-6

The Coronavirus Pandemic and the Challenges of Leadership: A Focus on the United States
Haroon A. Khan, PhD
ISBN: 979-8-89530-954-4
eBook ISBN: 979-8-89530-975-9

Health Promotion and Prevention: School-Age Children
Eda Kılınç İşleyen, PhD
ISBN: 979-8-89530-758-8
eBook ISBN: 979-8-89530-840-0

Machine Learning-Based Decision Support Systems for Diabetic Foot Ulcer Care
Mritunjay Rai, PhD,
Jay Kumar Pandey, PhD,
and Abhishek Kumar Saxena (Editor)
ISBN: 979-8-89530-542-3
eBook ISBN: 979-8-89530-779-3

The Evolution of Health Literacy: Empowering Patients Through Improved Education, 2nd Edition
Nitin Agarwal, MD,
David R. Hansberry, MD, PhD,
and Arpan V. Prabhu, MD (Editors)
ISBN: 979-8-89530-445-7
eBook ISBN: 979-8-89530-531-7

Triage in Radiation Accidents
Nural Öztürk, PhD,
and Sibel Karaca, PhD (Editors)
ISBN: 979-8-89530-415-0
eBook ISBN: 979-8-89530-451-8

Landscape of Pattern Learning Applied to Public Health and Social Sciences
Saurav Mallik, PhD,
Himanish Shekhar Das, PhD,
Hong Qin, PhD, Kangkana Bora, PhD,
and Koushik Mallick, PhD
ISBN: 979-8-89530-266-8
eBook ISBN: 979-8-89530-350-4

More information about this series can be found at

bitly

Maajid Mohi Ud Din Malik
Abhay Saraf
Harshal Tukaram Pandve
Quazi Syed Zahiruddin
Editors

Advances in the One Health Approach

Integrating Human, Animal, and Environmental Health

nova
Medicine & Health
www.novapublishers.com
New York

DOI: https://doi.org/10.52305/NOPH1608

Library of Congress Cataloging-in-Publication Data

Library of Congress Control Number: 2026935743
ISBN: 979-8-90134-202-2 (Hardcover)
ISBN: 979-8-90134-291-6 (eBook)

Published by Nova Science Publishers, Inc. † New York

This book is dedicated to all the healthcare professionals, veterinarians, environmental scientists, researchers, and educators who tirelessly work in the field of One Health and integrated health approaches. Your unwavering commitment to protecting human, animal, and environmental health, dedication to advancing interdisciplinary collaboration, and relentless pursuit of knowledge inspire us all.

We also dedicate this book to the communities and populations who are affected by emerging diseases, environmental health challenges, and zoonotic threats. Your resilience, trust in public health systems, and cooperation in prevention efforts motivate us to continuously strive for excellence in providing comprehensive and effective health protection.

To our families and loved ones, who have supported us throughout this journey, we dedicate this book with gratitude and love. Your unwavering support, understanding, and encouragement have been our pillars of strength.

Finally, we dedicate this book to the pursuit of knowledge and innovation in the field of One Health and integrated health sciences. May it inspire further advancements, cross-sector collaboration, and transformative discoveries that will shape the future of global health and improve the well-being of humans, animals, and the environment for generations to come.

Contents

Preface

Global health challenges remain among humanity's most complex and interconnected problems, affecting billions of individuals worldwide and representing significant burdens on healthcare systems, economies, and planetary well-being. As our understanding of health has evolved from compartmentalised medical models to integrated One Health frameworks, the role of collaborative, multisectoral approaches in health management has expanded dramatically, positioning interdisciplinary professionals as essential contributors to comprehensive, evidence-based health protection. This transformation in our approach to health has necessitated a corresponding evolution in how we educate and prepare health professionals to meet the multifaceted needs of populations facing emerging diseases, environmental degradation, and zoonotic threats across the entire spectrum of global health challenges.

The Inspiration for *Advances in the One Health Approach: Integrating Human, Animal, and Environmental Health* arose from our collective recognition that, while global health management has become increasingly sophisticated, a critical gap remained in comprehensive educational resources that could bridge the divide between theoretical understanding and practical implementation. Traditional approaches to health education often compartmentalise human medicine, veterinary science, and environmental health, failing to provide learners with the integrated, holistic perspective that modern health science demands. We recognised the urgent need for a resource that would not only present the fundamental science of One Health but also guide readers through the practical application of diverse, collaborative interventions, while acknowledging the complex interplay of biological, social, and environmental factors that influence health outcomes across species and ecosystems.

This book represents our commitment to providing public health students, practising professionals, veterinarians, environmental scientists, and other stakeholders with a comprehensive, evidence-based resource that spans the entire continuum of One Health implementation. From the foundational chapters that explore the historical evolution of One Health concepts and the interconnectedness of human, animal, and environmental health, to advanced discussions of emerging technologies such as integrated surveillance systems and digital health solutions, we have endeavoured to create a resource that is both academically rigorous and practically relevant. The content systematically progresses from basic concepts to specialised applications, ensuring that readers develop both the theoretical foundation and practical skills necessary to provide effective and collaborative health management.

What distinguishes this work from other texts in the field is our deliberate emphasis on integrating multiple sectoral approaches within a cohesive implementation framework. Rather than presenting human health surveillance, veterinary medicine, environmental monitoring, and policy development as separate entities, we have woven these approaches together to reflect the reality of modern One Health practice, where successful health outcomes require the skilful integration of multiple disciplines tailored to specific population and environmental needs. The inclusion of chapters on community engagement, research ethics, and cross-species transmission reflects our conviction that effective health management must address complex systems, not merely individual components.

Our approach to diverse populations and settings, including global health disparities and emergency response scenarios, acknowledges that One Health cannot be approached with a one-size-fits-all mentality. Similarly, our exploration of cultural and ethical considerations recognises that health is experienced and managed within complex social, economic, and environmental contexts that must be understood and respected by health professionals. The integration of case studies and practical applications throughout the text is designed to bridge the gap between theoretical knowledge and real-world decision-making, helping readers develop the critical thinking skills essential for effective One Health practice.

The inclusion of emerging technologies and digital health applications reflects our recognition that the field of integrated health is rapidly evolving, with new tools and approaches constantly expanding our surveillance and response capabilities. By exploring these innovations alongside traditional methods, we aim to prepare readers not only for current practice but also for the future of health management in an increasingly interconnected and environmentally challenged world.

As editors, we bring diverse perspectives and experiences to this work, united by our shared commitment to advancing the science and practice of One Health approaches. We have sought to create a resource that honours both the complexity of global health challenges and the sophistication of modern collaborative practice, while remaining accessible to learners at all levels of expertise. We hope that this book will serve not only as an educational tool but as a catalyst for continued innovation and improvement in how we approach the challenge of protecting human, animal, and environmental health, ultimately contributing to better outcomes and improved well-being for all living systems on our planet.

Dr. Maajid Mohi Ud Din Malik
Dr. Abhay Saraf
Dr. Harshal Tukaram Pandve
Dr. Quazi Syed Zahiruddin
Editors

Acknowledgments

We want to express our heartfelt gratitude to all those who have contributed to the creation and publication of *Advances in the One Health Approach: Integrating Human, Animal, and Environmental Health*. First and foremost, we would like to thank the contributors to this book, including experts in the fields of medicine, public health, veterinary science, environmental science, and allied health who have generously shared their knowledge, expertise, and valuable insights. Their contributions have played a crucial role in making this book a comprehensive and authoritative resource in the field of One Health.

We extend our sincere appreciation to our publisher for their support and belief in this project. Their dedication to disseminating cutting-edge research and facilitating knowledge sharing has been instrumental in bringing this book to fruition.

We would also like to acknowledge the reviewers who provided valuable feedback and constructive criticism during the review process. Their expertise and attention to detail have contributed significantly to the quality and accuracy of the content.

We are thankful to our families and loved ones for their unwavering support, understanding, and encouragement throughout the process of writing and editing this book. Their patience and belief in our work have been a constant source of motivation.

Lastly, we would like to express our most profound appreciation to the readers of *Advances in the One Health Approach: Integrating Human, Animal, and Environmental Health*. It is our sincere hope that this book proves to be an enlightening and informative resource, inspiring further research, collaboration, and advancements in the integrated approach to human, animal, and environmental health.

Acronyms

5G	Fifth Generation (wireless technology)
ACE2	Angiotensin-Converting Enzyme 2
ACPA	Anti-citrullinated protein antibody
ACL	Anterior Cruciate Ligament
ACT	Acceptance and Commitment Therapy
ADL	Activities of Daily Living
ADHD	Attention Deficit Hyperactivity Disorder
AI	Artificial Intelligence
AMF	Amplitude-Modulated Frequency
AMR	Antimicrobial Resistance
ANA	Antinuclear Antibodies
API	Application Programming Interface
APTA	American Physical Therapy Association
AROM	Active Range of Motion
AUDIT	Alcohol Use Disorders Identification Test
AUSCAN	Australian/Canadian hand OA Index
BAI	Beck Anxiety Inventory
BCT	Behavior change techniques
BDI-II	Beck Depression Inventory-II
BPI	Brief Pain Inventory
Bti	Bacillus thuringiensis israelensis
CBM	Cognitive Bias Modification
CBPR	Community-Based Participatory Research
CBT	Cognitive-Behavioral Therapy
CDC	Centers for Disease Control and Prevention
CDAI	Clinical Disease Activity Index
CEPI	Coalition for Epidemic Preparedness Innovations
CERC	Crisis and Emergency Risk Communication
CFS	Chronic Fatigue Syndrome
CIMT	Constraint-induced movement therapy
CITES	Convention on International Trade in Endangered Species
CME/CE	Continuing Medical Education/Continuing Education
CNS	Central Nervous System
COHFE	Competencies for One Health Field Epidemiology
COHERE	Checklist for One Health Epidemiological Reporting of Evidence
COMT	Catechol-O-Methyltransferase
COPM	Canadian Occupational Performance Measure

COVID-19	Coronavirus Disease 2019
CPM	Conditioned Pain Modulation
CPSP	Central Post-Stroke Pain
CRP	C-Reactive Protein
CRPS	Complex Regional Pain Syndrome
CSQ	Coping Strategies Questionnaire
CT	Computed Tomography
DALY	Disability-Adjusted Life Years
DAS28	Disease Activity Score
DASH	Disabilities of Arm, Shoulder and Hand
DAST	Drug Abuse Screening Test
DNA	Deoxyribonucleic Acid
DNIC	Diffuse noxious inhibitory controls
DVT	Deep Vein Thrombosis
ECG	Electrocardiogram
ECDC	European Centre for Disease Prevention and Control
EDA	Electrodermal activity
EEE	Eastern Equine Encephalitis
EEG	Electroencephalographic
EFSA	European Food Safety Authority
EIA	Exercise-Induced Analgesia
EID	Emerging Infectious Disease
EIDSS	Electronic Integrated Disease Surveillance System
EMAC	Emergency Management Assistance Compact
EMG	Electromyography
EMS	Electrical Muscle Stimulation
EPAs	Entrustable Professional Activities
ESBL	Extended-Spectrum Beta-Lactamases
ESR	Erythrocyte Sedimentation Rate
EU	European Union
FABQ	Fear-Avoidance Beliefs Questionnaire
FACIT-F	Functional Assessment of Chronic Illness Therapy-Fatigue
FAI	Femoroacetabular impingement
FAO	Food and Agriculture Organization
FDA	Food and Drug Administration
FEMA	Failure Mode and Effects Analysis
FES	Functional electrical stimulation
FITT	Frequency, Intensity, Time, Type
FLACC	Face, Legs, Activity, Cry, Consolability
FMS	Functional Movement Screen
GABA	Gamma-Aminobutyric Acid
GAD-7	Generalized Anxiety Disorder-7
GAPs	Good Agricultural Practices
GAVI	Global Alliance for Vaccines and Immunization
GDPR	General Data Protection Regulation
GIS	Geographic Information Systems

GISRS	Global Influenza Surveillance and Response System
GLASS	Global Antimicrobial Resistance and Use Surveillance System
GOARN	Global Outbreak Alert and Response Network
GOHF	Generalizable One Health Framework
GPHIN	Global Public Health Intelligence Network
GPS	Global Positioning System
GRADE	Grading of Recommendations Assessment, Development and Evaluation
GRRT	Global Rapid Response Team
GSR	Galvanic skin response
GTPS	Greater trochanteric pain syndrome
H1N1	Hemagglutinin Type 1 and Neuraminidase Type 1
H5N1	Hemagglutinin Type 5 and Neuraminidase Type 1
HACCP	Hazard Analysis and Critical Control Points
HAQ	Health Assessment Questionnaire
HCV	Hepatitis C Virus
HF	High Frequency
HIV	Human Immunodeficiency Virus
HPA	Hypothalamic-Pituitary-Adrenal
HRmax	Maximum Heart Rate
HRV	Heart rate variability
Hz	Hertz
IACUC	Institutional Animal Care and Use Committee
IASP	International Association for the Study of Pain
ICF	International Classification of Functioning, Disability and Health
ICS	Incident Command System
IES-R	Impact of Event Scale-Revised
IFC	Interferential Current Therapy
IHR	International Health Regulations
IL-1β	Interleukin-1 beta
IL-6	Interleukin-6
IMMPACT	Initiative on Methods, Measurement, and Pain Assessment in Clinical Trials
IMU	Inertial measurement unit
IoT	Internet of Things
IRB	Institutional Review Board
IRS	Indoor Residual Spraying
ISCIP	International SCI Pain Classification
ISI	Insomnia Severity Index
ISO	International Organization for Standardization
IT	Information technology
IT band	Iliotibial Band
IVM	Integrated Vector Management
kdr	Knockdown Resistance
KNGF	Royal Dutch Society for Physical Therapy
LAMP	Loop-mediated Isothermal Amplification

LF	Low Frequency
LGBTQ+	Lesbian, Gay, Bisexual, Transgender, Queer/Questioning, Plus
LIMS	Laboratory Information Management Systems
LISA	Local Indicators of Spatial Association
LLINS	Long-Lasting Insecticidal Nets
LLLT	Low-Level Laser Therapy
LWD	Long-wave Diathermy
MBCT	Mindfulness-Based Cognitive Therapy
MBSR	Mindfulness-Based Stress Reduction
MCID	Minimal clinically important differences
MERS	Middle East Respiratory Syndrome
MERS-CoV	Middle East Respiratory Syndrome Coronavirus
MET	Muscle Energy Technique
MFR	Myofascial Release
MHz	Megahertz
MinION	Portable DNA/RNA Sequencer
ML	Machine Learning
MMT	Manual Muscle Testing
MPS	Myofascial Pain Syndrome
MRI	Magnetic Resonance Imaging
MRSA	Methicillin-Resistant Staphylococcus Aureus
MSc	Master of Science
MW	Microwaves
MWD	Microwave Diathermy
NGO	Non-Governmental Organization
NICE	National Institute for Health and Care Excellence
NIH	National Institutes of Health
NIOSH	National Institute for Occupational Safety and Health
NLP	Natural Language Processing
NMDA	N-methyl-D-aspartate
NMES	Neuromuscular Electrical Stimulation
NPRS	Numerical Pain Rating Scale
NRS	Numerical Rating Scale
NSAID	Nonsteroidal anti-inflammatory drugs
OA	Osteoarthritis
OHHLEP	One Health High-Level Expert Panel
OPD	Outpatient Department
OPRM1	Opioid Receptor Mu 1
OSHA	Occupational Safety and Health Administration
PAR	Participatory Action Research
PASS	Pain Anxiety Symptoms Scale
PBM	Photobiomodulation
PCL-5	PTSD Checklist for DSM-5
PCR	Polymerase Chain Reaction
PCS	Pain Catastrophizing Scale
PD1/PD2	Provisional Diagnosis 1/2

PEDro	Physiotherapy Evidence Database
PEG	Pain intensity, Enjoyment of life, General activity
PEPFAR	President's Emergency Plan for AIDS Relief
PFGE	Pulsed-Field Gel Electrophoresis
PHQ-9	Patient Health Questionnaire-9
PMR	Progressive muscle relaxation
PPA	Physiotherapy Pain Association
PPE	Personal Protective Equipment
PPG	Photoplethysmography
PQRST	Provocation/Palliation, Quality, Region/Radiation, Severity, Timing
PRISM	Pain Recovery and Integrative Systems Model
PRM	Pattern Recognition Model
PROM	Passive Range of Motion
PRSS	Pain-Related Self-Statements Scale
PSQI	Pittsburgh Sleep Quality Index
PTSD	Post-Traumatic Stress Disorder
qPCR	Quantitative Polymerase Chain Reaction
QoL	Quality of Life
QST	Quantitative Sensory Testing
QUADAS	Quality Assessment of Diagnostic Accuracy Studies
RA	Rheumatoid arthritis
REBA	Rapid Entire Body Assessment
RespiMART	Respiratory Viruses Surveillance Platform
RF	Rheumatoid factor
RNA	Ribonucleic Acid
ROI	Return on investment
ROM	Range of Motion
RPA	Recombinase Polymerase Amplification
RPE	Rating of Perceived Exertion
RSI	Repetitive Strain Injuries
rTMS	repetitive Transcranial Magnetic Stimulation
RULA	Rapid Upper Limb Assessment
SARS	Severe Acute Respiratory Syndrome
SARS-CoV	Severe Acute Respiratory Syndrome Coronavirus
SARS-CoV-2	Severe Acute Respiratory Syndrome Coronavirus 2
SCI	Spinal cord injury
SCN9A	Sodium Voltage-Gated Channel Alpha Subunit 9
SDG	Sustainable Development Goal
SDGs	Sustainable Development Goals
SF-36	Short Form 36
SIGs	Special Interest Groups
SIR	Susceptible-Infected-Recovered
SIT	Sterile Insect Technique
SLMTA	Strengthening Laboratory Management Toward Accreditation
SMART	Specific, Measurable, Achievable, Relevant, Time-bound
STEC	Shiga Toxin-Producing E. coli

SUDS	Subjective Units of Distress
SVI	Social Vulnerability Index
SW	Short Waves
SWD	Shortwave Diathermy
TB	Tuberculosis
TCM	Traditional Chinese Medicine
TENS	Transcutaneous Electrical Nerve Stimulation
TNF-α	Tumor necrosis factor-alpha
TP	Trigger Point
TrP	Trigger Points
TRP	Transient Receptor Potential
TSK	Tampa Scale for Kinesiophobia
UNEP	United Nations Environment Programme
VAS	Visual Analog Scale
VMO	Vastus Medialis Obliquus
VR	Virtual Reality
VTE	Venous Thromboembolism
W/cm^2	Watts per Square Centimeter
WALT	World Association of Laser Therapy
WHO	World Health Organization
WNV	West Nile Virus
WOAH	World Organisation for Animal Health
WOMAC	Western Ontario and McMaster Universities Osteoarthritis Index

Chapter 1

The One Health Paradigm: Connecting Human, Animal, and Environmental Health

Maajid Mohi Ud Din Malik[1,*], PhD
and Harshal Tukaram Pandve[2], MD
[1]Department of Radiology and Imaging Technology, Dr. D. Y. Patil School of Allied Health Sciences, Dr. D. Y. Patil Vidyapeeth, Pune (Deemed to be University), Sant Tukaram Nagar, Pimpri, Pune, India
[2]Community Medicine (PSM), Pimpri Chinchwad Municipal Corporation's Postgraduate Medical Institute and Yashwantrao Chavan Memorial Hospital, Pimpri, Pune, India

Abstract

The One Health approach represents a transformative paradigm that recognises the interconnected nature of human, animal, and environmental health systems. This chapter explores the historical foundations of One Health, tracing its conceptual origins from Rudolf Virchow's pioneering work in the 19th century to modern applications in addressing complex global health challenges. The chapter examines how the COVID-19 pandemic has underscored the critical importance of integrated health approaches, demonstrating that diseases do not respect traditional sectoral boundaries. By analysing case studies including COVID-19, Ebola outbreaks, and climate-related health impacts, we illustrate how One Health principles can enhance surveillance systems, improve emergency response coordination, and promote sustainable development. The chapter concludes that moving beyond traditional siloed approaches toward integrated One Health strategies is essential for achieving Sustainable Development Goal 3 (Good Health and Well-being) and building resilient health systems capable of addressing 21st-century challenges. The evidence presented demonstrates that One Health is not merely a theoretical concept but a practical necessity for effective disease prevention, pandemic preparedness, and global health security.

Keywords: One Health, Rudolf Virchow, global health security, zoonotic diseases, pandemic preparedness, interdisciplinary collaboration, sustainable development, SDG 3, health systems integration, environmental Health

* Corresponding Author's Email: maajid.malik@dpu.edu.in

In: Advances in the One Health Approach
Editors: Maajid Mohi Ud Din Malik, Abhay Saraf, Harshal Tukaram Pandve et al.
ISBN: 979-8-90134-202-2

Introduction

In an increasingly interconnected world where human, animal, and environmental health challenges transcend traditional boundaries, the One Health approach has emerged as a fundamental paradigm for addressing complex health threats. The concept acknowledges that the health and well-being of humans, animals, and ecosystems are intricately linked, necessitating collaborative, multisectoral approaches to achieve optimal health outcomes for all (World Health Organisation, 2023). This paradigm shift represents more than an academic concept; it embodies a practical necessity for confronting 21st-century health challenges that cannot be effectively addressed through traditional, siloed approaches.

The One Health framework acknowledges that approximately 60% of all infectious diseases affecting humans are of zoonotic origin, meaning they are transmitted between animals and people. In comparison, 75% of emerging infectious diseases are also zoonotic (Wakimoto et al., 2021). This statistic alone underscores the crucial importance of understanding and managing the complex interactions between human and animal populations, as well as the environmental factors that influence the emergence and transmission of diseases. The COVID-19 pandemic has served as a stark reminder of how quickly zoonotic pathogens can spread globally, causing unprecedented disruptions to health, social, and economic systems.

The urgency of adopting One Health approaches has been further amplified by mounting evidence that human activities are the primary driving force behind new, emerging, and re-emerging diseases (World Bank, 2022). Factors such as deforestation, urbanisation, agricultural intensification, climate change, and global trade have created new pathways for pathogen spillover from wildlife to domestic animals and humans. These anthropogenic changes have fundamentally altered the ecological relationships between pathogens, their hosts, and the environment, necessitating integrated approaches that consider the health of all three domains simultaneously.

1.1. Historical Evolution of the One Health Concept

The intellectual foundations of One Health can be traced back to ancient civilisations that recognised connections between human and animal health. However, the modern scientific basis for this approach emerged during the 19th century through the groundbreaking work of several pioneering physicians and scientists. The historical evolution of One Health represents a journey from intuitive understanding to evidence-based practice, marked by key individuals who challenged the prevailing medical orthodoxy of their time.

The earliest formal articulation of One Health principles is attributed to Rudolf Virchow (1821-1902), the German physician and pathologist who fundamentally transformed our understanding of disease causation. Virchow's famous observation that "between animal and human medicine there are no dividing lines—nor should there be" laid the conceptual groundwork for what would eventually become the One Health movement (Tawde et al., 2024). His work extended far beyond this philosophical statement, as he conducted groundbreaking research on the life cycle of Trichinella spiralis, demonstrating how parasites could move between animal and human hosts, which led to the implementation of meat inspection laws in Germany.

Building upon Virchow's foundation, Canadian physician William Osler (1849-1919) advanced the One Health concept through his comparative pathology work at McGill University, where he taught both medical and veterinary students. Osler's integrative approach to education demonstrated the practical benefits of cross-disciplinary learning and collaboration, establishing precedents that continue to influence medical and veterinary education today. His publication, "The Relation of Animals to Man," exemplified the scholarly pursuit of understanding the connections between human and animal health.

The modern One Health movement gained significant momentum in the 20th century through the work of Calvin Schwabe, who coined the term "One Medicine" in 1964 while serving as chair of the Department of Epidemiology and Preventive Medicine at the University of California, Davis School of Veterinary Medicine (Lebov et al., 2017). Schwabe's contributions were particularly significant because he provided a scientific framework for integrating veterinary and human medicine to address public health challenges more effectively.

The establishment of the Veterinary Public Health division at the Communicable Diseases Centre (now CDC) in 1947 by James Steele marked another crucial milestone in the evolution of One Health practice. This initiative demonstrated how government institutions could operationalise One Health principles by creating formal structures for collaboration between human and animal health professionals (Lee & Brumme, 2013). The division's focus on zoonotic diseases such as bovine tuberculosis, brucellosis, rabies, and salmonellosis established essential precedents for surveillance and control programs that integrated human and animal health expertise.

The transition from "One Medicine" to "One Health" reflected a broader recognition that environmental factors play crucial roles in health outcomes (Table 1.1). This evolution was influenced by a growing awareness of ecological health concepts and the understanding that environmental degradation could have a direct impact on both human and animal Health. The inclusion of environmental Health as a third pillar of One Health represented a fundamental expansion of the concept, acknowledging that sustainable health outcomes require consideration of ecosystem health and ecological determinants of disease (Zinsstag et al., 2011).

Table 1.1. Evolution of One Health terminology and key contributors

Time Period	Key Figure(s)	Contribution	Terminology Used
1850s-1900s	Rudolf Virchow	Coined the term "zoonosis" and established connections between human and animal medicine	"Between animal and human medicine, there are no dividing lines"
1870s-1910s	William Osler	Comparative pathology, integrated teaching	"Relation of Animals to Man"
1940s-1970s	James Steele, Calvin Schwabe	Veterinary Public Health formalised the One Medicine concept	"One Medicine"
1990s-2000s	Multiple contributors	Environmental health integration	"One Health"
2010s-Present	Global organisations	Institutionalisation and policy integration	"One Health approach," "Tripartite/Quadripartite"

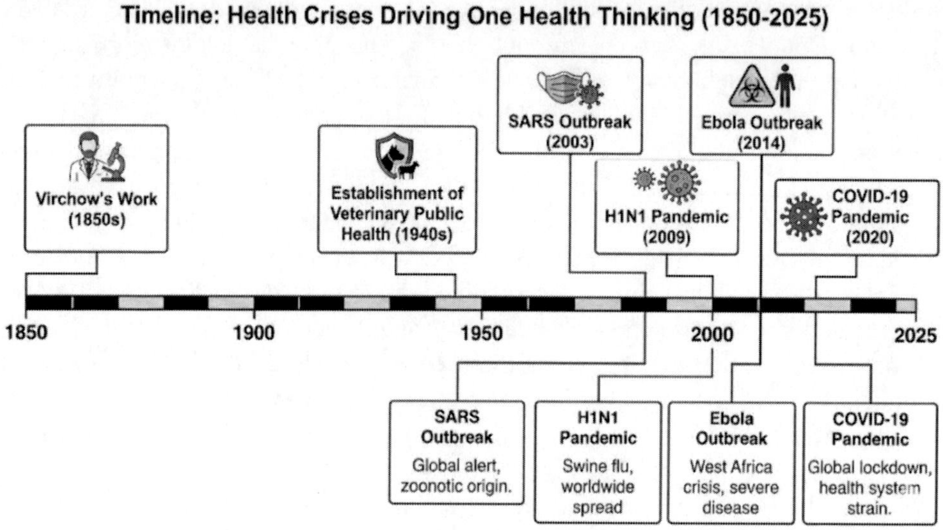

Figure 1. Timeline of one health development and major global health events.

Figure 1 illustrates a horizontal timeline spanning from 1850 to 2025, with key One Health milestones displayed above the timeline and primary disease outbreaks/health events listed below. Key milestones include Virchow's work (1850s), the establishment of veterinary public Health (1940s), the SARS outbreak (2003), the H1N1 pandemic (2009), the Ebola outbreak (2014), and the COVID-19 pandemic (2020). The timeline illustrates how health crises have driven the evolution of One Health thinking.

1.2. Interconnectedness of Human, Animal, and Environmental Health

The interconnectedness of human, animal, and environmental health systems represents the core principle underlying the One Health approach. This interconnectedness manifests through multiple pathways and mechanisms, demonstrating how health outcomes in one domain directly influence those in others. Understanding these connections is essential for developing effective interventions and policies that can address health challenges holistically.

Figure 2 shows A Venn diagram showing three overlapping circles representing Human Health, Animal Health, and Environmental Health. The central overlap area, labelled "One Health," showcases examples of shared challenges, including zoonotic diseases, antimicrobial resistance, and food safety. Each circle contains sector-specific elements, with arrows indicating bi-directional influences between all sectors.

Zoonotic disease transmission represents the most direct manifestation of the interconnections between human and animal health. Pathogens such as influenza viruses, coronaviruses, and bacterial agents like Salmonella species routinely cross species boundaries, often with environmental factors facilitating or inhibiting transmission. The emergence of SARS-CoV-2, the virus causing COVID-19, exemplifies how a pathogen can spill over from wildlife reservoirs, potentially through intermediate hosts, to cause a global pandemic affecting human populations (Daszak et al., 2022). The subsequent transmission of SARS-CoV-2 from humans back to various animal species, including mink, cats, and white-tailed deer, demonstrates the bidirectional nature of these health connections.

Environmental factors play a critical role in determining health outcomes across species boundaries. Climate change, for instance, affects disease transmission patterns by altering the geographic distribution of vector species, changing seasonal transmission dynamics, and creating new environmental conditions that favour pathogen survival and replication. The expansion of dengue fever into previously temperate regions exemplifies how ecological changes can directly impact human Health through altered disease ecology. Similarly, deforestation and habitat fragmentation increase contact between wildlife, domestic animals, and human populations, creating new opportunities for pathogen spillover events.

Agricultural systems provide another crucial interface where human, animal, and environmental Health intersect. Intensive livestock production can contribute to the development of antimicrobial resistance when antibiotics are used for growth promotion or disease prevention. Resistant bacteria can then spread through food chains, environmental contamination, and direct contact, ultimately affecting human health outcomes. The use of antimicrobials in agriculture also has ecological consequences, as drug residues and resistant bacteria can contaminate soil and water systems, creating environmental reservoirs of resistance genes.

Food safety represents a particularly complex area where all three health domains converge. Foodborne pathogens can originate from animal sources, be influenced by environmental conditions during production and processing, and ultimately affect human Health. The emergence of new food safety challenges, such as those associated with global food trade and shifting consumption patterns, necessitates integrated approaches that encompass the entire farm-to-fork continuum.

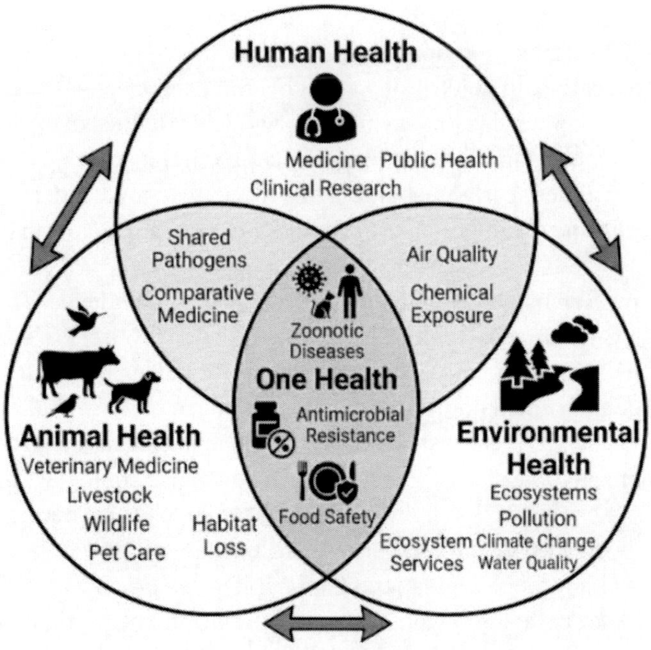

Figure 2. The one health framework - interconnections between human, animal, and environmental health.

Water systems serve as another critical interface connecting human, animal, and environmental health. Contaminated water sources can harbour pathogens that affect multiple species, while pollution from human and agricultural activities can degrade water quality with consequences for both human and wildlife Health. The concept of watershed Health exemplifies how environmental management decisions can have cascading effects on human and animal populations dependent on these resources.

The psychological and social dimensions of human-animal relationships also contribute to the interconnectedness of health outcomes. Companion animals can provide significant mental health benefits for humans while potentially serving as sources of zoonotic disease transmission. Working animals support human livelihoods and food security in many parts of the world, illustrating the direct impact of animal health on human economic and nutritional well-being.

1.3. Rudolf Virchow's Contributions and Modern Applications

Rudolf Virchow's contributions to the development of One Health principles extend far beyond his famous quote about the absence of dividing lines between human and animal medicine. His comprehensive approach to understanding disease causation, his pioneering work in cellular pathology, and his recognition of social determinants of Health established foundational principles that continue to guide modern One Health practice. Virchow's legacy exemplifies how individual scientific contributions can have a profound and lasting impact on entire fields of study and practice.

Virchow's investigation of a typhus epidemic in Upper Silesia in 1848 exemplified his integrated approach to health challenges. Rather than focusing solely on the biological aspects of the disease, Virchow examined the social, economic, and environmental factors that contributed to the emergence and spread of the epidemic. His report concluded that poor hygiene, lack of education, malnutrition, and governmental neglect were primary factors responsible for the epidemic, leading to his famous declaration that "medicine is a social science, and politics is nothing more than medicine on a grand scale" (Brown & Fee, 2006). This analysis demonstrated early recognition of what we now understand as the social determinants of Health and the importance of addressing upstream factors that influence disease emergence.

His research on Trichinella spiralis provided concrete evidence of zoonotic disease transmission, leading to practical public health interventions. Virchow's description of the parasite's life cycle in swine and its transmission to humans through consumption of undercooked pork demonstrated how understanding pathogen biology could inform prevention strategies. His advocacy for meat inspection programs represented an early example of One Health policy implementation, showing how scientific evidence could be translated into public health practice. The meat inspection laws that resulted from his work became models for food safety regulations worldwide and established precedents for government involvement in protecting public Health through regulation of animal-derived products.

Virchow's cellular pathology work established fundamental principles about disease causation that remain relevant to modern One Health practice. His recognition that disease processes involve cellular dysfunction provided a unifying framework for understanding pathology across species boundaries. This understanding facilitated comparative medicine approaches that recognise similarities in disease processes between humans and animals, enabling knowledge transfer and collaborative research efforts.

Modern applications of Virchow's principles are evident in contemporary One Health initiatives worldwide. The Global Health Security Agenda, launched in 2014, embodies Virchow's recognition that health challenges require coordinated responses that address social, economic, and political factors in addition to biological ones. The agenda's emphasis on strengthening surveillance systems, laboratory capacity, and emergency response capabilities across human and animal health sectors reflects the integrated approach that Virchow advocated.

Current antimicrobial resistance initiatives demonstrate how Virchow's systems thinking approach applies to modern health challenges. The World Health Organisation's Global Action Plan on Antimicrobial Resistance recognises that addressing resistance requires coordinated action across human medicine, veterinary medicine, agriculture, and environmental management. This comprehensive approach reflects Virchow's understanding that effective interventions must address all factors contributing to health problems, not just immediate biological causes.

Climate change and health initiatives also exemplify modern applications of Virchow's social medicine principles. Recognition that climate change affects Health through multiple pathways, including direct temperature effects, air quality impacts, food security implications, and social disruption, requires the kind of comprehensive analysis that Virchow pioneered. Modern climate-health adaptation strategies that integrate environmental monitoring, health surveillance, and social interventions reflect his understanding of the complex factors that influence population health outcomes.

The COVID-19 pandemic response has highlighted both the relevance of Virchow's principles and the consequences of ignoring them. Countries that implemented comprehensive responses addressing social, economic, and environmental factors alongside biomedical interventions generally achieved better outcomes than those focusing solely on clinical care. The recognition that vaccine equity, social support systems, and economic assistance were essential components of pandemic response demonstrates the continued relevance of Virchow's social medicine approach.

1.4. Global Health Challenges Requiring Integrated Approaches

Contemporary global health challenges have grown increasingly complex, requiring integrated approaches that transcend traditional disciplinary and sectoral boundaries. These challenges demonstrate the inadequacy of fragmented responses and underscore the need for One Health approaches to achieve sustainable solutions. The interconnected nature of modern health threats demands coordinated action across multiple sectors and levels of governance.

Emerging infectious diseases represent perhaps the most visible category of health challenges requiring One Health approaches. Since 2000, the world has witnessed several hundred emerging contagious disease outbreaks annually, with diseases such as SARS, avian influenza, MERS-CoV, Ebola, Zika, and COVID-19 demonstrating the potential for rapid global spread and significant health, social, and economic impacts (Ryu et al., 2017; World

Bank, 2022). The zoonotic origins of most emerging infectious diseases necessitate surveillance and response systems that integrate expertise in human, animal, and environmental Health. The increasing frequency of emerging infectious disease events is driven by multiple interconnected factors, exemplifying the need for One Health approaches. Human encroachment into previously undisturbed wildlife habitats increases the likelihood of pathogen spillover from wildlife to human populations. Agricultural intensification and changing land use patterns create new interfaces between wildlife, domestic animals, and human communities. Global travel and trade networks facilitate the rapid dissemination of pathogens following spillover events. Climate change alters the geographic distribution of vector species and influences seasonal transmission patterns for many infectious diseases.

Antimicrobial resistance represents another critical global health challenge that inherently requires One Health approaches for effective management. The development and spread of resistant bacteria occur across human medicine, veterinary practice, agriculture, and environmental systems, with resistant organisms and resistance genes moving freely between these domains. Effective interventions must address antimicrobial use patterns in all sectors while recognising that resistance development in one industry can have consequences for all others. The economic implications of antimicrobial resistance, estimated to potentially cause $100 trillion in lost global production by 2050 if current trends continue, underscore the urgency of implementing coordinated response strategies.

Food safety and security challenges increasingly require integrated approaches as global food systems become more complex and interconnected. Foodborne disease outbreaks can originate from contamination at any point in the farm-to-fork continuum, requiring surveillance and control systems that span agricultural production, food processing, distribution, and retail sectors. Climate change impacts on agricultural productivity, changing consumption patterns, and growing global populations create additional pressures on food systems, affecting both food security and safety outcomes.

Environmental health challenges such as air pollution, water contamination, and chemical exposures affect human, animal, and ecosystem Health simultaneously. Urban air pollution, for example, contributes to respiratory disease in humans while also affecting wildlife populations and ecosystem functioning. Addressing these challenges requires integrated approaches that consider sources, pathways, and receptors across multiple domains while recognising that environmental health interventions can have co-benefits for human and animal health.

Climate change represents an overarching challenge that affects virtually all aspects of Health and requires comprehensive One Health responses. Climate-related health impacts encompass direct effects, such as heat-related illnesses and injuries from extreme weather events, as well as indirect effects mediated through changes in disease vector distribution, food and water security, air quality, and social disruption. Effective climate adaptation strategies must integrate health system strengthening, environmental management, social protection, and economic development interventions to achieve comprehensive resilience.

Non-communicable diseases, while traditionally viewed as primarily human health concerns, are increasingly requiring One Health approaches as our understanding of their causes expands. Environmental exposures, food system factors, and social determinants of Health all contribute to the development and outcomes of non-communicable diseases. The concept of syndemic non-communicable diseases recognises how multiple diseases and risk factors interact with social and environmental conditions to produce adverse health outcomes in populations.

Table 1.2. Key global health challenges requiring One Health approaches

Challenge	Human Health Impact	Animal Health Impact	Environmental Health Impact	One Health Intervention Examples
Emerging Infectious Diseases	Direct disease burden, pandemic potential	Wildlife and livestock diseases	Ecosystem disruption	Integrated surveillance, wildlife monitoring
Antimicrobial Resistance	Treatment failures, increased mortality	Reduced treatment options	Environmental contamination	Stewardship programs across sectors
Climate Change	Heat stress, vector-borne diseases	Habitat loss, temperature stress	Ecosystem changes	Adaptation strategies, emission reduction
Food Safety	Foodborne illness	Production losses	Agricultural pollution	Farm-to-fork approaches
Air Pollution	Respiratory disease	Wildlife health impacts	Ecosystem acidification	Emission controls, urban planning

Mental health challenges also demonstrate the need for integrated approaches that consider social, environmental, and animal-related factors. The human-animal bond can provide significant mental health benefits, while environmental factors, such as access to green spaces and air quality, can also influence mental health outcomes. Social determinants such as housing, employment, and social support systems affect mental Health while also influencing physical health outcomes. Table 1.2 lists key global health challenges that require a one-health approach.

1.5. Case Studies: COVID-19, Ebola, and Climate Change Impacts

The COVID-19 pandemic provides a compelling contemporary example of how global health challenges necessitate integrated One Health approaches for an effective response to these challenges. The pandemic's zoonotic origins, rapid global spread, and multifaceted impacts on Health, society, and economy demonstrate both the necessity of One Health thinking and the consequences of fragmented response approaches. Analysis of the COVID-19 response reveals crucial lessons for future pandemic preparedness and the implementation of One Health principles at scale.

The emergence of SARS-CoV-2 most likely resulted from spillover events at the human-animal interface, with mounting scientific evidence supporting zoonotic origins through wildlife farming and trade pathways (Keusch et al., 2022). The initial outbreak's association with a live animal market in Wuhan highlighted the risks associated with wildlife trade and consumption, particularly in urban settings where diverse animal species are brought into close contact with large human populations. This case demonstrates how human activities that disrupt natural ecosystems and bring together diverse species can create opportunities for pathogen spillover events.

The pandemic's progression illustrated the critical importance of integrated surveillance systems that monitor pathogen circulation in human, animal, and environmental compartments. Countries with robust One Health surveillance networks were better positioned to detect and respond to SARS-CoV-2 transmission in animal populations, including outbreaks in mink farms, zoo animals, and companion animals. The development of standardised One Health investigation protocols by the Centres for Disease Control and Prevention (CDC) and other agencies demonstrated how rapid implementation of integrated approaches could enhance understanding of pathogen transmission dynamics (CDC, 2024).

COVID-19's impacts extended far beyond immediate health effects, demonstrating the interconnected nature of health, social, and economic systems. Pandemic response measures such as lockdowns and travel restrictions had significant environmental co-benefits, including temporary reductions in air pollution and greenhouse gas emissions. However, these measures also created new ecological challenges, including increased waste generation from personal protective equipment and changes in consumption patterns that affected resource use.

The pandemic highlighted substantial health inequities that reflected underlying social determinants of Health. Populations with limited access to healthcare, adequate housing, and economic resources experienced disproportionate impacts from COVID-19, demonstrating how social factors influence health outcomes during health emergencies. Effective pandemic response required addressing these social determinants alongside biomedical interventions, illustrating the relevance of Virchow's social medicine principles to contemporary health challenges.

The Ebola outbreaks in West Africa (2014-2016) and subsequent outbreaks in the Democratic Republic of Congo provide additional examples of how emerging infectious diseases require One Health approaches for adequate control. The Ebola virus's natural reservoir in fruit bat populations and spillover to human populations through hunting, handling, and consumption of infected animals demonstrated the critical importance of understanding human-wildlife interfaces in disease emergence and transmission.

An effective Ebola outbreak response required integration of human health interventions with wildlife health monitoring and community engagement approaches that addressed cultural practices related to wildlife hunting and consumption. Traditional burial practices that involved direct contact with deceased individuals also required culturally sensitive interventions that balanced public health needs with community values and beliefs. The outbreak response demonstrated how successful disease control involves understanding and addressing social, cultural, and environmental factors alongside clinical interventions.

Climate change impacts on Health provide examples of how environmental changes affect human and animal Health through multiple interconnected pathways. Rising temperatures, changing precipitation patterns, and increased frequency of extreme weather events create complex challenges that require integrated adaptation strategies. Vector-borne disease distribution changes exemplify these complex relationships, as climate change affects vector biology, pathogen development rates, and transmission dynamics while also influencing human and animal exposure patterns.

The expansion of dengue fever into previously temperate regions demonstrates how climate change can alter disease distribution patterns with significant public health implications. Effective adaptation strategies require integrated approaches that combine vector control interventions with environmental management, urban planning, and health system strengthening activities. These strategies must also consider how climate adaptation measures in one sector might affect health outcomes in others, such as how water storage for drought resilience might create new breeding sites for disease vectors.

Heat-related health impacts provide another example of how climate change requires integrated health responses. Rising temperatures affect human Health directly through heat-related illness while also affecting air quality, food security, and water availability. Effective adaptation strategies must address urban planning, housing quality, energy systems, and social support networks while considering how these interventions affect both human and environmental health outcomes.

These case studies demonstrate that effective responses to contemporary health challenges require the kind of integrated thinking and collaborative action that define One Health approaches. They also highlight how failure to adopt comprehensive approaches can result in missed opportunities for prevention and more costly response requirements when health emergencies occur.

1.6. One Health vs. Traditional Siloed Approaches

The comparison between One Health and traditional siloed approaches reveals fundamental differences in how health challenges are conceptualised, addressed, and managed. Conventional methods, while often effective within their specific domains, frequently fail to address the interconnected nature of contemporary health challenges, leading to fragmented responses that may be inefficient, ineffective, or even counterproductive. Understanding these differences is crucial for appreciating the value proposition of One Health and identifying opportunities for implementation.

Traditional siloed approaches typically organise health-related activities according to disciplinary boundaries, with human Health, animal health, and environmental Health managed by separate institutions with distinct mandates, funding streams, and regulatory frameworks. This organisational structure reflects historical patterns of professional development and institutional specialisation that served important purposes in advancing knowledge and technical expertise within specific domains. However, these same structures can create barriers to coordination and collaboration when health challenges span multiple domains.

The institutional separation between human and animal health systems exemplifies these barriers. Human health agencies typically focus on disease prevention and treatment in human populations, while animal health agencies concentrate on livestock diseases, food safety, and veterinary public Health. This division can lead to duplicated surveillance systems, inconsistent disease reporting standards, and delayed recognition of zoonotic disease threats that require coordinated responses across both sectors.

Communication barriers represent another significant limitation of siloed approaches. Different health sectors often employ distinct technical vocabularies, reporting systems, and conceptual frameworks that can hinder the sharing of information and collaborative problem-solving. These communication challenges can delay the recognition and response to outbreaks, particularly for zoonotic diseases, where effective control requires rapid information exchange between human and animal health authorities.

Resource allocation patterns in siloed systems may also create inefficiencies and gaps in coverage. Human health systems typically receive substantially more funding than animal health systems in most countries, even though effective zoonotic disease control often requires interventions in animal populations. This funding imbalance can result in inadequate animal surveillance systems that fail to provide early warning of zoonotic disease threats, ultimately requiring more costly human health interventions when spillover events occur.

Regulatory frameworks designed around sectoral boundaries can create additional challenges for implementing comprehensive health interventions. Food safety regulation, for example, often involves multiple agencies with jurisdiction over different aspects of the food system, potentially creating regulatory gaps or conflicting requirements that impede effective oversight. Similarly, controlling antimicrobial resistance requires coordinated regulation across human medicine, veterinary practice, and agricultural use; however, traditional regulatory structures may not be well-equipped to implement such comprehensive approaches.

One Health approaches address these limitations by promoting integration across traditional boundaries while maintaining the technical expertise that exists within individual sectors. Rather than eliminating specialisation, One Health seeks to create collaborative frameworks that enable sectors to work together more effectively on shared challenges. This integration can take various forms, from informal coordination mechanisms to formal institutional restructuring.

Integrated surveillance systems represent one of the most tangible benefits of One Health approaches over traditional siloed systems. By combining human and animal disease surveillance data, integrated systems can provide earlier detection of zoonotic disease threats and a more comprehensive understanding of disease transmission dynamics. The Global Health Security Agenda's emphasis on developing surveillance systems that span human and animal health sectors reflects recognition of these benefits.

Joint response mechanisms represent another area where One Health approaches offer advantages over traditional siloed responses. During disease outbreaks, integrated response teams that include expertise from multiple sectors can develop more comprehensive response strategies and implement interventions more efficiently than separate sectoral responses. The establishment of One Health investigation protocols for SARS-CoV-2 demonstrated how such integrated approaches could enhance outbreak response capabilities.

Economic analyses consistently demonstrate that One Health approaches offer favourable cost-benefit ratios compared to traditional siloed approaches, particularly for disease prevention activities. The World Bank estimates that implementing One Health-guided prevention measures would cost $10.3-11.5 billion annually, compared to $30.1 billion annually for managing pandemic responses using traditional approaches (World Bank, 2022). These economic advantages stem from the preventive focus of One Health approaches and their ability to address health challenges at their source, rather than managing consequences after they occur.

Policy integration represents another area where One Health approaches offer advantages over fragmented policy development. Health challenges such as antimicrobial resistance and climate change require policy responses that span multiple sectors and levels of government. One Health approaches facilitate the development of comprehensive policies that address these complex challenges holistically rather than through disconnected sectoral policies that may work at cross-purposes.

Despite these advantages, implementing One Health approaches faces significant practical challenges that must be acknowledged and addressed. Institutional change is often slow and difficult, particularly when it requires modifying established organisational structures and professional relationships. Professional training programs that prepare workers for interdisciplinary collaboration require time and resources to develop and implement. Funding mechanisms that support collaborative work across traditional boundaries may require new approaches to budget allocation and performance measurement.

The transition from siloed to integrated approaches, therefore, requires sustained commitment and careful attention to implementation challenges. Successful examples of One Health implementation demonstrate that these challenges can be overcome through appropriate leadership, stakeholder engagement, and institutional support. Still, they also highlight the importance of realistic timelines and expectations for change processes. Table 1.3 shows a comparison of traditional siloed versus one-health approaches.

Table 1.3. Comparison of traditional siloed vs. One Health approaches

Aspect	Traditional Siloed Approach	One Health Approach
Organisational Structure	Separate human, animal, and environmental health agencies	Integrated coordination mechanisms
Surveillance Systems	Parallel, sector-specific systems	Integrated surveillance across sectors
Communication	Limited cross-sector communication	Regular information sharing and joint planning
Resource Allocation	Sector-specific funding streams	Coordinated resource allocation
Response Mechanisms	Separate sectoral responses	Joint response teams and protocols
Cost-effectiveness	Higher long-term costs due to reactive approaches	Lower costs through a prevention focus
Disease Recognition	Delayed recognition of cross-sector threats	Earlier detection of zoonotic threats

Conclusion

The One Health paradigm represents a fundamental shift toward recognising the interconnected nature of 21st-century health challenges. COVID-19 demonstrated both the necessity of integrated approaches and the consequences of fragmented responses, with comprehensive strategies addressing social, economic, and environmental factors achieving superior outcomes. As urbanisation intensifies, climate change accelerates, and human-animal interactions evolve, interconnected health challenges will become increasingly prominent. The alignment with Sustainable Development Goals demonstrates how integrated thinking supports broader development objectives while addressing specific health threats. Although realising One Health's full potential requires a sustained commitment to institutional change and capacity development, the evidence suggests that these investments are justified. One Health offers a vital framework for addressing evolving global health challenges proactively in our interconnected world.

Acknowledgments

The authors would like to extend our appreciation to those who offered helpful commentary during the drafting process of this manuscript. We also acknowledge the role Nova Science Publishers played in enabling the work described herein.

References

Brown, T. M., & Fee, E. (2006). Rudolf Carl Virchow: Medical scientist, social reformer, role model. *American Journal of Public Health*, 96(12), 2104-2105. https://doi.org/10.2105/AJPH.2005.078436.

Centers for Disease Control and Prevention. (2024). Federal One Health coordination. Retrieved from https://www.cdc.gov/one-health/php/about/federal-one-health-coordination-1.html.

Daszak, P., Olival, K. J., & Li, H. (2022). Pandemic origins and a One Health approach to preparedness and prevention: Solutions based on SARS-CoV-2 and other RNA viruses. *Proceedings of the National Academy of Sciences*, 119(42), e2202871119. https://doi.org/10.1073/pnas.2202871119.

Lebov, J., Grieger, K., Womack, D., Zaccaro, D., Whitehead, N., Kowalcyk, B., & MacDonald, P. D. (2017). A framework for One Health research. *One Health*, 3, 44-50. https://doi.org/10.1016/j.onehlt.2017.03.004.

Lee, K., & Brumme, Z. L. (2013). Operationalising the One Health approach: The global governance challenges. *Health Policy and Planning*, 28(7), 778-785. https://doi.org/10.1093/heapol/czs127.

Ryu, S., Kim, B. I., Lim, J. S., Tan, C. S., & Chun, B. C. (2017). One Health perspectives on emerging public health threats. *Journal of Preventive Medicine and Public Health*, 50(6), 411-414. https://doi.org/10.3961/jpmph.17.097.

Tawde, P. P., Choudhari, S. G., Syed, Z. Q., & Gaidhane, A. (2024). Rudolf Virchow: Integrating medicine and social reform for public Health. *Cureus*, 16(8), e68161. https://doi.org/10.7759/cureus.68161.

Wakimoto, M. D., Menezes, R. C., Pereira, S. A., Nery, T., Castro-Alves, J., Penetra, S. L., Ruckert, A., Labonté, R., & Veloso, V. G. (2021). Why preparation for the next pandemic needs One Health approach implementation in letter and spirit. *One Health*, 13, 100321. https://doi.org/10.1016/j.onehlt.2021.100321.

World Bank. (2022). Putting pandemics behind us: Investing in One Health to reduce risks of emerging infectious diseases. World Bank Group.

World Health Organization. (2023). One Health. Retrieved from https://www.who.int/news-room/fact-sheets/detail/one-health.

Zinsstag, J., Schelling, E., Waltner-Toews, D., & Tanner, M. (2011). From "one medicine" to "one health" and systemic approaches to Health and well-being. *Preventive Veterinary Medicine*, 101(3-4), 148-156. https://doi.org/10.1016/j.prevetmed.2010.07.003.

Zinsstag, J., Crump, L., Schelling, E., Hattendorf, J., Maidane, Y. O., Ali, K. O., Munyua, P., Atherstone, C., Rüegg, S. R., Breiman, R. F., Hülsebusch, C., Umutoni, A., Walzer, C., Melin, M., Bonfoh, B., Graf, J. A., Probst-Hensch, N., Nguiadem, C., Tall, A., Tte, V., ... Zinsstag, J. (2018). Climate change and One Health. *FEMS Microbiology Letters*, 365(11), fny085. https://doi.org/10.1093/femsle/fny085.

Chapter 2

Global Health in the One Health Framework

Quazi Syed Zahiruddin[1], PhD, MD
and Maajid Mohi Ud Din Malik[2,*], PhD
[1]Directorate of Research and Innovations, Datta Meghe Institute of Higher Education and Research (DMIHER), India
[2]Radiology and Imaging Technology, Dr. D. Y. Patil School of Allied Health Sciences, Dr. D. Y. Patil Vidyapeeth Pune (Deemed to be University), Sant Tukaram Nagar, Pimpri, Pune, India

Abstract

Global Health has evolved from a narrow focus on disease control to a comprehensive approach that recognises the interconnected determinants of Health across populations and ecosystems worldwide. This chapter examines how the One Health framework provides a critical lens for understanding and addressing global health challenges in the 21st century. The analysis reveals persistent health disparities that reflect systemic inequities in social, economic, and environmental conditions, with people in the countries with the lowest life expectancy living an average of 33 years shorter than those in the countries with the highest life expectancy. International organisations, particularly the World Health Organisation (WHO) and the Quadripartite collaboration (FAO, UNEP, WHO, and WOAH), have established frameworks for coordinated global health action; yet implementation challenges persist. The chapter demonstrates how Sustainable Development Goal 3 (Good Health and Well-being) serves as a central organising principle for global health efforts, while highlighting the cross-cutting nature of Health across all 17 SDGs. Cross-border health challenges, ranging from pandemic threats to antimicrobial resistance, underscore the need for coordinated global governance mechanisms. The evidence presented illustrates that achieving health equity and global health security requires integrated approaches that address the social determinants of Health, strengthen health systems, and foster genuine international cooperation. The One Health framework emerges as an essential strategy for navigating the complex landscape of global health challenges and opportunities.

Keywords: global health, health equity, health disparities, international organisations, quadripartite collaboration, sustainable development goals, SDG 3, cross-border health challenges, global health governance, social determinants of health, world health organisation

---

* Corresponding Author's Email: maajid.malik@dpu.edu.in

In: Advances in the One Health Approach
Editors: Maajid Mohi Ud Din Malik, Abhay Saraf, Harshal Tukaram Pandve et al.
ISBN: 979-8-90134-202-2

Introduction

Global health has emerged as a defining challenge of the 21st century, encompassing the complex interactions between Health, development, security, and equity on a planetary scale. Unlike traditional approaches that focused primarily on controlling infectious diseases or providing medical care in developing countries, contemporary global health recognises that health outcomes are fundamentally shaped by social, economic, environmental, and political determinants that operate across local, national, and international levels (Pungartnik et al., 2023). The COVID-19 pandemic served as a stark reminder that health threats know no borders and that global health security depends on the strength of the weakest link in the international health system.

The integration of global health within the One Health framework represents a paradigmatic shift toward recognising the interconnected nature of human, animal, and environmental Health at a worldwide scale. This integration acknowledges that many of the most pressing global health challenges, from emerging infectious diseases to antimicrobial resistance, require collaborative approaches that transcend traditional sectoral boundaries and national jurisdictions. The World Health Organisation's definition of One Health as "an integrated, unifying approach that aims to sustainably balance and optimise the health of people, animals and ecosystems" provides a foundation for understanding how global health challenges must be addressed through coordinated, multisectoral action (World Health Organisation, 2022).

Contemporary global health is characterised by both remarkable progress and persistent inequities. Since 2000, significant improvements have been achieved in reducing child mortality, expanding access to essential health services, and controlling major infectious diseases such as HIV/AIDS, malaria, and tuberculosis. However, these gains have been unevenly distributed, with substantial disparities remaining between and within countries. The World Health Organisation's latest data reveal that health inequities can result in life expectancy differences of up to 33 years between the highest- and lowest-performing countries, reflecting the profound impact of social determinants on health outcomes (World Health Organisation, 2025).

The complexity of contemporary global health challenges requires sophisticated governance mechanisms that can coordinate action across multiple sectors, organisations, and levels of government. International organisations, particularly those comprising the Quadripartite collaboration, have developed increasingly sophisticated frameworks for global health cooperation. However, translating global commitments into effective local action remains a persistent challenge, particularly in contexts characterised by weak health systems, limited resources, and competing development priorities.

2.1. Defining Global Health within One Health Context

The conceptualisation of global Health has undergone significant evolution since the mid-20th century, transitioning from narrowly focused international health initiatives to comprehensive approaches that recognise Health as a worldwide public good requiring collective action across sectors and borders. Within the One Health framework, global Health encompasses not only human health outcomes but also the complex interactions between human, animal, and environmental health systems that influence health outcomes at local, national, and international scales. This expanded understanding recognises that effective global health interventions must address the fundamental drivers of health outcomes, including social, economic, environmental, and political determinants that operate across species boundaries.

The integration of One Health principles into global health thinking has been driven by recognition that many contemporary health challenges are inherently transboundary and multisectoral in nature. Emerging infectious diseases, antimicrobial resistance, climate change impacts on Health, and food safety challenges all require approaches that consider the complex interactions between human activities, animal populations, and environmental systems. The COVID-19 pandemic exemplified these interconnections, demonstrating how a pathogen originating from animal populations could rapidly spread globally through human networks while creating cascading impacts on social, economic, and environmental systems worldwide.

Contemporary definitions of global health within the One Health framework emphasise several key characteristics that distinguish it from earlier international health approaches. First, global health recognises Health as a shared responsibility requiring collective action across nations, sectors, and levels of governance. This perspective acknowledges that health outcomes in one location can have implications for populations worldwide, necessitating coordinated responses that transcend national boundaries. Second, global Health emphasises equity as a fundamental principle, recognising that disparities in health outcomes reflect underlying inequities in social, economic, and political systems that must be addressed through comprehensive interventions.

The scope of global Health within the One Health framework extends beyond traditional biomedical approaches to encompass what the World Health Organisation terms the "health in all policies" approach. This perspective recognises that health outcomes are influenced by policy decisions across sectors, including agriculture, education, housing, transportation, and environmental management. Effective global health action, therefore, requires coordination not only among health professionals but also among diverse stakeholders whose activities influence the determinants of Health across species and ecosystems.

The evolution of global health concepts from traditional international Health to contemporary One Health-integrated approaches reflects this growing understanding of health complexity (Table 2.1). This progression demonstrates how the field has moved from narrowly focused disease control efforts to comprehensive approaches that recognise the interconnected determinants of Health across species and ecosystems.

Table 2.1. Evolution of global health concepts and approaches

Time Period	Dominant Concept	Key Characteristics	Main Focus Areas	One Health Integration
1940s-1960s	International Health	Bilateral assistance, disease control	Tropical diseases, maternal-child Health	Minimal
1970s-1990s	International Health	Multilateral cooperation, primary healthcare	Essential services, health systems	Limited
2000s-2010s	Global Health	Shared challenges, global governance	MDGs, disease-specific initiatives	Emerging
2010s-Present	Global Health in One Health	Integrated approaches, planetary Health	SDGs, health security, equity	Central

Global health governance within the One Health framework requires new forms of institutional arrangements that can facilitate coordination across traditional organisational boundaries. The establishment of the Quadripartite collaboration among the Food and Agriculture Organisation (FAO), the United Nations Environment Programme (UNEP), the World Health Organisation (WHO), and the World Organisation for Animal Health (WOAH) represents an evolution toward more integrated global health governance structures. This collaboration recognises that effective responses to global health challenges require coordination among organisations with expertise in human Health, animal health, environmental Health, and food systems.

The measurement and monitoring of global health outcomes within the One Health framework present significant methodological challenges. Traditional health indicators, which focus primarily on human health outcomes, may not capture the full scope of One Health impacts, necessitating the development of new metrics that can assess the health of human, animal, and environmental systems simultaneously. The Sustainable Development Goals represent an attempt to develop such integrated measurement frameworks, with SDG 3 focusing specifically on Health and well-being while recognising the interconnections between Health and other development objectives.

The financing of global Health within the One Health framework also requires innovative approaches that can support interventions across traditional sectoral boundaries. Traditional health financing mechanisms may not be well-suited to supporting interventions that benefit multiple health systems, including human, animal, and environmental health. The development of new financing mechanisms that can capture the full range of One Health benefits represents an important area for innovation in global health policy and practice.

2.2. Health Disparities Across Regions and Populations

Health disparities represent one of the most persistent challenges in contemporary global Health, reflecting deep-seated inequities in the social, economic, and environmental conditions that determine health outcomes across populations and geographic regions. The World Health Organisation's recent World Report on Social Determinants of Health Equity reveals that these disparities can result in dramatic differences in life expectancy, with people in countries with the lowest life expectancy living an average of 33 years shorter than those in countries with the highest life expectancy (World Health Organisation, 2025). These disparities are not random occurrences but reflect systematic differences in how societies allocate resources and opportunities, reinforced by political choices and institutional arrangements that perpetuate inequitable health outcomes.

Figure 3 shows a world map illustrating variations in life expectancy across countries, with colour coding ranging from light gray (lowest) to dark gray (highest). The accompanying charts illustrate correlations between life expectancy and key social determinants, including education levels, income inequality, access to clean water, and environmental quality. The figure illustrates how health outcomes cluster geographically and correlate with social determinants of Health.

Within-country health disparities often mirror or exceed between-country inequality, highlighting the importance of addressing inequities at multiple scales simultaneously. Data from the WHO Health Inequality Data Repository demonstrates that children born in the poorest families are 13 times more likely to die before age five compared to children born in the wealthiest families within the same country. These disparities reflect the complex ways in which social determinants of Health operate at local levels, creating systematic differences in exposure to health risks and access to health-promoting resources.

Gender-based health disparities represent a particularly pervasive form of health inequity, with women and girls facing systematic disadvantages that affect health outcomes throughout their lives. Maternal mortality data illustrate these disparities starkly, with low- and lower-middle-income countries accounting for 94% of all maternal deaths despite significant progress in reducing maternal mortality globally. Indigenous women face particularly severe disadvantages, with maternal death rates up to three times higher than those of non-indigenous women in many high-income countries. These disparities reflect the intersection of gender inequities with other forms of social disadvantage, including racism, poverty, and geographic isolation.

Environmental health disparities increasingly drive global health inequities as climate change and environmental degradation disproportionately affect the world's most vulnerable populations. Air pollution causes approximately 7 million premature deaths annually, with the burden concentrated among populations in low- and middle-income countries and marginalised communities within high-income countries. Climate change is projected to push an additional 68-135 million people into extreme poverty by 2030, creating new forms of health vulnerability while exacerbating existing inequities.

The systematic nature of these disparities becomes apparent when examining how different population groups experience varying levels of health vulnerability and access to health-promoting resources (Table 2.2). These disparities reflect the complex interplay of social, economic, environmental, and political factors that determine health outcomes across different communities and regions.

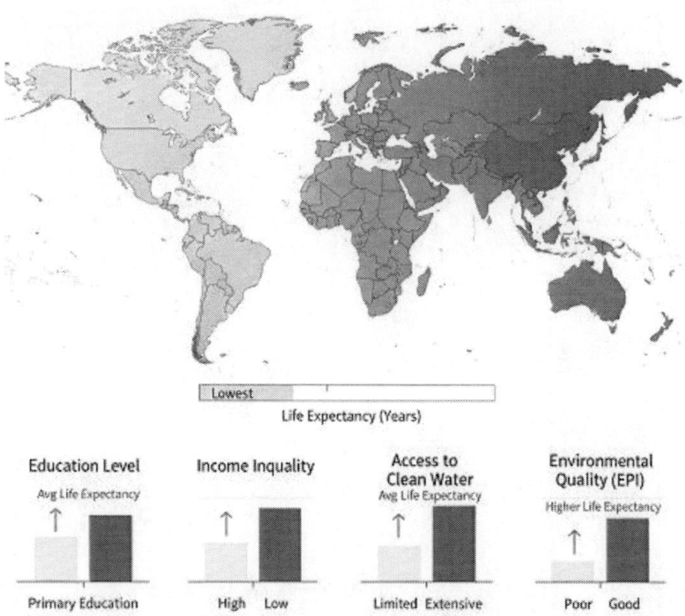

Figure 3. Global health disparities - Life expectancy and social determinants.

Table 2.2. Key global health disparities by population group

Population Group	Health Disparity Examples	Contributing Factors	One Health Implications
Low-income populations	13x higher under-5 mortality rates	Limited healthcare access, poor living conditions	Greater exposure to zoonoses and environmental hazards
Rural populations	Higher maternal mortality, limited specialist care	Geographic isolation, transportation barriers	Closer human-animal interfaces, agricultural exposures
Indigenous populations	Lower life expectancy, higher chronic disease rates	Historical marginalisation, cultural barriers	Traditional ecological knowledge, land use conflicts
Women and girls	Higher vulnerability to certain diseases, limited reproductive rights	Gender inequalities, cultural practices	Different exposure patterns, caregiving responsibilities
Elderly populations	Higher burden of non-communicable diseases	Age-related vulnerabilities, social isolation	Increased susceptibility to zoonoses, medication access
Persons with disabilities	Barriers to healthcare access, higher mortality	Physical and social barriers, discrimination	Modified risk profiles, accommodation needs

The COVID-19 pandemic revealed and exacerbated existing health disparities while creating new forms of health inequity. Populations with limited access to healthcare, adequate housing, and economic resources experienced disproportionate impacts from the pandemic, while containment measures often imposed greater hardships on already disadvantaged groups. The unequal global distribution of COVID-19 vaccines highlighted how global health inequities can undermine collective efforts to address shared health threats, with low-income countries receiving significantly fewer vaccines per capita than high-income countries throughout much of the pandemic response.

Migration and displacement create additional layers of health disparity that have become increasingly prominent in global health considerations. The number of forcibly displaced people has tripled from 2008 to 2024, reaching 122 million, with significant health consequences for these populations. Migrants and refugees often face service inequalities, discrimination, and loss of family support systems that negatively impact both physical and mental Health. In host countries, displaced populations usually lack access to essential health services while facing increased exposure to communicable diseases and other health risks.

The debt burden facing many low- and middle-income countries creates structural constraints that perpetuate health disparities by limiting governments' ability to invest in the social determinants of health. The total value of interest payments made by the world's 75 poorest countries has quadrupled over the past decade, pulling resources away from investments in health, education, and social protection systems. This dynamic creates a vicious cycle where countries with the most significant health needs have the least capacity to address the fundamental drivers of health outcomes.

Addressing global health disparities within the One Health framework requires comprehensive approaches that address the social determinants of Health while recognising the interconnected nature of human, animal, and environmental health outcomes. This perspective acknowledges that health disparities often reflect broader patterns of social and ecological injustice that affect multiple species and ecosystems simultaneously. Effective interventions must therefore address not only immediate health needs but also the underlying conditions that create and maintain health disparities across populations and regions.

2.3. International Organisations and Their Roles

The landscape of international health organisations has evolved significantly to embrace One Health principles, with major multilateral institutions developing increasingly sophisticated mechanisms for coordinating action across human, animal, and environmental health sectors. The World Health Organisation (WHO) serves as the central coordinating authority for international health work, directing and coordinating health activities within the United Nations system while providing leadership on global health matters (World Health Organisation, 2024). With 194 member states and a two-year budget exceeding $6 billion, the WHO's influence extends across all aspects of global health policy and practice.

The Quadripartite collaboration represents the most comprehensive example of international organisational coordination around One Health principles. This partnership brings together four major UN agencies: the Food and Agriculture Organisation (FAO), the United Nations Environment Programme (UNEP), the World Health Organisation (WHO), and the

World Organisation for Animal Health (WOAH, formerly OIE). The collaboration was formalised through a Memorandum of Understanding signed in 2022, transforming the previous Tripartite partnership to include environmental expertise through UNEP's participation (UNEP, 2022).

The One Health Joint Plan of Action (2022-2026), developed by the Quadripartite organisations, provides a comprehensive framework for implementing integrated approaches to health challenges at the human-animal-ecosystem interface. The plan encompasses six priority areas: capacity building, risk assessment and surveillance, preparedness and response, zoonotic disease control, food safety, and antimicrobial resistance. Three pathways for change guide implementation: governance mechanisms, organisational development, and data systems. The plan represents an unprecedented level of coordination among international organisations with complementary mandates and expertise (UNEP, 2022).

Figure 4 illustrates an organisational chart that shows the Quadripartite collaboration at the centre, with the WHO, FAO, WOAH, and UNEP as the core partners. Radiating outward are other key organisations (World Bank, Gates Foundation, EU, CDC, etc.), with connecting lines indicating relationships and types of collaboration. The chart includes symbols indicating different kinds of partnerships (funding, technical, policy) and shows both global and regional organisational structures.

The World Health Organisation's leadership in global health extends beyond the Quadripartite collaboration to encompass a wide range of health initiatives and partnerships. WHO's role as the custodian agency for 20 of the 27 indicators associated with Sustainable Development Goal 3 reflects its central position in monitoring and reporting on global health progress. The organisation's technical work spans health system strengthening, disease surveillance and response, health policy development, and standard-setting across all areas of public health practice.

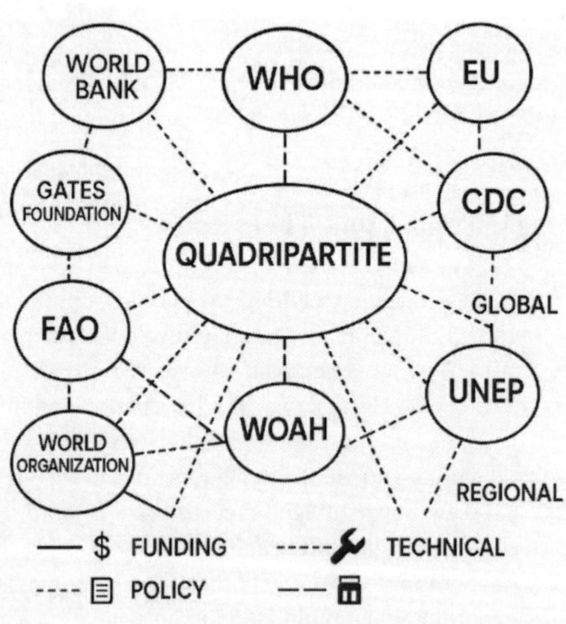

Figure 4. International Organisations in One Health - Roles and relationships.

The Food and Agriculture Organisation provides critical expertise in animal health, food safety, and agricultural systems that significantly impact human health outcomes. FAO's work in zoonotic disease surveillance, antimicrobial resistance monitoring in food systems, and food safety standards provides a solid foundation for implementing One Health. The organisation's extensive field presence and relationships with agricultural sectors worldwide position it as a crucial partner in translating One Health principles into practice at national and local levels.

The World Organisation for animal health plays a unique role in the global health architecture as the only international organisation with a mandate explicitly focused on animal health and welfare. WOAH's work in developing animal health standards, coordinating surveillance for animal diseases, and supporting veterinary services worldwide provides critical infrastructure for the implementation of One Health. The organisation's recent initiatives include developing competency frameworks for One Health field epidemiology and creating performance indicators for veterinary services that incorporate One Health principles (WOAH, 2024).

The United Nations Environment Programme's participation in the Quadripartite brings essential environmental health expertise to global One Health coordination. UNEP's work on environmental monitoring, pollution control, biodiversity conservation, and climate change provide crucial context for understanding the ecological factors that influence health outcomes. The organisation's leadership in sustainable development and environmental governance offers critical linkages between health objectives and broader environmental and development goals.

Beyond the Quadripartite organisations, numerous other international institutions contribute to global Health within the One Health framework. The World Bank's health portfolio exceeds $15 billion and includes significant investments in pandemic preparedness, strengthening health systems, and building One Health capacity. The Bank's recent report, "Putting Pandemics Behind Us," advocates for investing $10-11 billion annually in One Health approaches to prevent future pandemics, compared to the $30 billion annually required to manage pandemic responses.

The diverse roles and contributions of key international organisations in One Health implementation demonstrate the complexity of global health governance while highlighting opportunities for enhanced coordination and collaboration (Table 2.3). This organisational landscape reflects both the specialisation required for technical expertise and the integration needed for effective One Health approaches.

Table 2.3. Key international organisations and their One Health roles

Organisation	Primary Mandate	One Health Contributions	Key Initiatives	Member Countries
WHO	Global health leadership	Human health coordination, policy development	Health security, SDG 3 monitoring	194
FAO	Agriculture and food security	Animal health, food safety, and antimicrobial resistance	Zoonoses control, food systems	194
WOAH	Animal health and welfare	Animal disease surveillance, veterinary services	Animal health standards, epidemiology training	182
UNEP	Environmental protection	Environmental Health, pollution control	Climate-health nexus, chemicals management	193
World Bank	Development financing	Health system financing, pandemic preparedness	One Health investment strategies	189

Regional organisations play crucial roles in translating global One Health commitments into regional and national action. The African Union's African Centres for Disease Control and Prevention has developed a continental One Health strategy. At the same time, the European Union has integrated One Health principles into its health security and research policies. Regional development banks, such as the Asian Development Bank and the Inter-American Development Bank, are increasingly incorporating One Health considerations into their health and agriculture financing decisions.

Private foundations and non-governmental organisations also contribute significantly to global Health within the One Health framework. The Bill and Melinda Gates Foundation, with annual health spending exceeding $3 billion, has increasingly emphasised integrated approaches to health challenges. International NGOs, such as EcoHealth Alliance and the Wildlife Conservation Society, work at the intersection of conservation and Health to implement One Health approaches in field settings.

The governance challenges facing international health organisations in implementing One Health approaches reflect broader challenges in global governance. Coordination across organisations with different mandates, constituencies, and operating procedures requires sustained political commitment and innovative institutional arrangements. The success of the Quadripartite collaboration in developing joint plans and coordinating activities demonstrates the potential for international cooperation while also highlighting the complexity of translating agreements into practical action.

2.4. Sustainable Development Goals and One Health Alignment

The Sustainable Development Goals (SDGs), adopted by all United Nations member states in 2015, provide the most comprehensive framework for addressing global development challenges while recognising the interconnected nature of social, economic, and environmental objectives. SDG 3, "Ensure healthy lives and promote well-being for all at all ages," serves as the primary health goal, reflecting the understanding that health outcomes are influenced by progress across all 17 Sustainable Development Goals (SDGs). This interconnected approach aligns closely with One Health principles, which recognise that optimal health outcomes require coordinated action across human, animal, and environmental health domains (United Nations, 2015).

The integration of One Health principles throughout the SDG framework reflects recognition that contemporary development challenges require approaches that transcend traditional sectoral boundaries. SDG 2 (Zero Hunger) directly connects to One Health through its emphasis on sustainable agriculture, nutrition, and food safety. SDG 6 (Clean Water and Sanitation) addresses environmental health determinants while recognising connections to zoonotic disease transmission and antimicrobial resistance. SDG 13 (Climate Action) encompasses the health co-benefits of climate mitigation and adaptation while acknowledging the health impacts of environmental change.

SDG 3 encompasses 13 specific targets that address major health priorities, including maternal and child mortality, communicable diseases, non-communicable diseases, mental Health, substance abuse, road safety, sexual and reproductive Health, universal health coverage, environmental health risks, tobacco control, research and development, health financing, and health security. Achieving these targets requires coordinated action across multiple sectors and levels of governance, underscoring the need for One Health approaches to address global health challenges.

The target framework for SDG 3 demonstrates clear connections to One Health priorities. Target 3.3, which aims to "end the epidemics of AIDS, tuberculosis, malaria and neglected tropical diseases and combat hepatitis, waterborne diseases and other communicable diseases," directly addresses zoonotic and vector-borne diseases that require integrated human-animal-environmental approaches. Target 3.d, which seeks to "strengthen the capacity of all countries, particularly developing countries, for early warning, risk reduction and management of national and global health risks," explicitly calls for the kind of integrated surveillance and response systems that characterise One Health approaches.

The interconnections between various SDGs and One Health principles become particularly evident when examining specific targets across different goals (Table 2.4). These connections demonstrate how health outcomes are influenced by progress across multiple development domains and how One Health approaches can contribute to achieving various SDG objectives simultaneously.

The measurement and monitoring of SDG progress have revealed both significant achievements and persistent challenges, highlighting the need for One Health approaches. Global progress on SDG 3 has been mixed, with substantial improvements in some areas offset by stagnation or regression in others. Child mortality has declined significantly, with 133 countries meeting the target for under-5 mortality as of 2023. However, progress on other targets, including maternal mortality and non-communicable diseases, remains insufficient to meet the 2030 goals.

The COVID-19 pandemic significantly disrupted progress toward SDG 3 and other health-related targets, demonstrating the vulnerability of development gains to global health emergencies. Childhood vaccination rates declined substantially during the pandemic, while cases of tuberculosis and malaria increased compared to pre-pandemic levels. The pandemic's broader impacts on education, poverty, and economic development created cascading effects across multiple SDGs, illustrating the interconnected nature of development challenges.

One Health approaches offer significant potential for accelerating progress toward multiple SDGs simultaneously by addressing shared underlying determinants. Investments in integrated surveillance systems can contribute to achieving SDG 3 (Health), SDG 2 (Food Security), and SDG 15 (Terrestrial Ecosystems) by providing early warnings of threats across human, animal, and environmental health domains. Antimicrobial resistance interventions that span human medicine, veterinary practice, and agriculture can contribute to multiple health and development objectives while addressing a shared threat to public Health.

The financing requirements for achieving the SDGs highlight the economic rationale for One Health approaches. The estimated $2.5 trillion annual financing gap for achieving the SDGs reflects the challenge of mobilising resources for development objectives. One Health approaches can potentially reduce these financing requirements by addressing multiple objectives through integrated interventions while preventing costly crisis responses through proactive management of health risks.

Climate change poses fundamental challenges to SDG achievement while also creating opportunities for One Health approaches that generate co-benefits across health and environmental objectives. Climate mitigation efforts that reduce air pollution can generate immediate health benefits while contributing to long-term ecological goals. Ecosystem-based adaptation strategies can enhance resilience to climate impacts while protecting biodiversity and supporting sustainable development.

The "Leave No One Behind" principle, which underpins the SDGs, aligns closely with One Health commitments to health equity and inclusive development. This principle requires particular attention to the needs of marginalised populations who often face the most significant exposure to health risks at the human-animal-environment interface. Indigenous peoples, rural communities, and populations dependent on natural resources may be disproportionately affected by environmental health threats while having limited access to health services and social protection systems.

National implementation of the SDGs has increasingly incorporated One Health principles as countries recognise the interconnected nature of development challenges. Voluntary National Reviews submitted by countries to the UN High-Level Political Forum demonstrate growing awareness of cross-sectoral linkages and the need for integrated approaches to development planning. However, institutional arrangements for implementing integrated approaches often lag policy commitments, highlighting the need for continued capacity building and institutional innovation.

2.5. Cross-Border Health Challenges

Cross-border health challenges represent some of the most complex and urgent issues in contemporary global Health, requiring coordinated responses that transcend national boundaries and traditional sectoral approaches. These challenges are inherently suited to One Health approaches because they involve complex interactions between human, animal, and environmental health systems that operate across geographic and political boundaries. The COVID-19 pandemic provided a stark illustration of how rapidly health threats can spread globally, but numerous other cross-border health challenges require sustained international attention and coordination.

Emerging infectious diseases represent the most visible category of cross-border health challenges, with new pathogens regularly identified and existing diseases expanding into new geographic areas. Since 2000, the world has experienced numerous disease outbreaks that have crossed international boundaries, including SARS (2003), H1N1 influenza (2009), MERS-CoV (2012-present), Ebola (2014-2016, 2018-2020), Zika (2015-2016), and COVID-19 (2019-present). The zoonotic origins of most emerging infectious diseases highlight the importance of surveillance systems that monitor pathogen circulation in wildlife, domestic animals, and human populations simultaneously.

The factors driving the emergence and spread of infectious diseases across borders are themselves transnational in scope and require coordinated responses. International travel and trade networks facilitate the rapid dissemination of pathogens, with air travel enabling the global spread of infectious diseases within hours or days of initial transmission. Climate change alters the geographic distribution of disease vectors and influences seasonal transmission patterns, creating new areas of risk that may cross national boundaries. Deforestation and habitat fragmentation increase contact between human populations and wildlife reservoirs of potential pathogens, often in border regions where surveillance capacity may be limited.

Table 2.4. SDG targets with direct One Health relevance

SDG Goal	Target	One Health Connection	Implementation Examples
SDG 2	End hunger, achieve food security	Food safety, zoonoses, antimicrobial resistance	Integrated food systems approaches
SDG 3	Ensure healthy lives and well-being	Direct health outcomes across species	Zoonoses control, health systems strengthening
SDG 6	Clean water and sanitation	Waterborne diseases, environmental Health	Watershed management, water quality monitoring
SDG 11	Sustainable cities	Urban Health, human-animal interfaces	Urban planning, waste management
SDG 13	Climate action	Climate-health nexus, ecosystem health	Adaptation strategies, emission reduction
SDG 14	Life below water	Aquatic animal health, marine ecosystems	Sustainable fisheries, pollution control
SDG 15	Life on land	Wildlife health, biodiversity conservation	Habitat protection, wildlife management

Table 2.5. Major cross-border health challenges and response mechanisms

Challenge	Primary Transmission Routes	Affected Sectors	International Response Mechanisms
Emerging infectious diseases	Travel, trade, vectors, wildlife	Human, animal, environmental	IHR, WHO emergencies, research networks
Antimicrobial resistance	Healthcare, food trade, environment	Human medicine, veterinary medicine, and agriculture	Global action plans, surveillance networks
Air pollution	Atmospheric transport	Environmental, Human Health	Regional agreements, monitoring networks
Food safety	Global food trade	Agriculture, Public Health	Codex standards, trade agreements
Vector-borne diseases	Climate change, trade	Human, animal, environmental	Vector control programs, surveillance
Zoonoses	Animal trade, migration	Veterinary, Public Health	Joint surveillance, capacity building

Antimicrobial resistance represents perhaps the most complex cross-border health challenge, as it involves the global circulation of resistant organisms and resistance genes through multiple pathways, including human travel, animal trade, and environmental contamination. The use of antimicrobials in one country can contribute to the development of resistance globally. At the same time, resistant organisms can spread through food trade, migration, and shared environmental resources, such as water systems. Effective responses to antimicrobial resistance, therefore, require coordination across human medicine, veterinary practice, agriculture, and environmental management sectors at international scales.

The diversity and complexity of cross-border health challenges require sophisticated response mechanisms that can address the multiple pathways through which health threats cross national boundaries (Table 2.5). These challenges highlight why traditional approaches, which focus on single sectors or diseases, are insufficient for addressing contemporary global health threats.

Climate change creates new categories of cross-border health challenges while exacerbating existing ones. Rising temperatures and changing precipitation patterns impact the distribution of disease vectors, potentially expanding the geographic range of vector-borne diseases, including malaria, dengue, and chikungunya. Sea level rise and extreme weather events can create displacement and migration, facilitating disease transmission while overwhelming health systems in receiving areas. Air pollution generated in one country can impact health outcomes in neighbouring countries through atmospheric transport, necessitating regional cooperation for adequate control.

Food safety represents a growing cross-border health challenge as global food trade expands and supply chains become increasingly complex. Contaminated food products can rapidly spread foodborne pathogens across multiple countries, as demonstrated by numerous international food safety incidents involving products such as melamine-contaminated milk powder, E. coli-contaminated vegetables, and Salmonella-contaminated spices. The complexity of modern food supply chains makes outbreak investigation and source attribution increasingly complex, requiring new forms of international cooperation and information sharing.

The governance of cross-border health challenges requires sophisticated institutional arrangements that can coordinate action across multiple countries, sectors, and organisations. The International Health Regulations (2005) provide the primary legal framework for managing cross-border health threats, requiring countries to develop core capacities for disease surveillance, reporting, and response. However, the COVID-19 pandemic revealed significant gaps in IHR implementation and highlighted the need for stronger international coordination mechanisms.

Regional organisations play a crucial role in managing cross-border health challenges by facilitating coordination among neighbouring countries that may share similar disease risks or transmission pathways. The African Union's African Centres for Disease Control and Prevention, the European Centre for Disease Prevention and Control, and similar regional institutions provide platforms for information sharing, joint surveillance, and coordinated response activities. These regional approaches can be efficient for addressing cross-border health challenges that affect specific geographic areas.

Border areas present challenges for managing cross-border health threats because they often have limited health system capacity while facing higher exposure to international disease transmission. Border communities usually have extensive social and economic connections across international boundaries, creating pathways for disease transmission that national surveillance systems may overlook. Mobile populations, including migrant workers, refugees, and nomadic groups, may face vulnerability to cross-border health threats while having limited access to health services.

The digitalisation of health information systems offers new opportunities for managing cross-border health challenges through real-time information sharing and coordination. Digital health platforms can facilitate the rapid reporting of disease outbreaks, the sharing of surveillance data, and the coordination of response activities across international boundaries. However, digital health initiatives also raise important questions about data sovereignty, privacy protection, and equitable access to digital health technologies.

Trade policies and agreements increasingly incorporate health considerations as recognition grows that trade and Health are closely interconnected. Sanitary and phytosanitary measures in trade agreements can serve as important mechanisms for preventing cross-border transmission of diseases while also potentially creating barriers to trade and development. The development of trade policies that support both economic growth and health objectives requires careful attention to scientific evidence and international cooperation.

2.6. Global Health Governance and Policy Frameworks

Global health governance encompasses the complex web of formal and informal institutions, rules, and processes through which collective decisions are made about health challenges that transcend national boundaries. Within the One Health framework, global health governance must address the inherent complexity of coordinating action across multiple sectors (human, animal, and environmental), levels of government (local, national, and international), and types of actors (public, private, and civil society). The evolution of global health governance reflects a growing recognition that effective responses to 21st-century health challenges require more integrated, multi-stakeholder, and participatory approaches than traditional state-centred international cooperation.

The World Health Organisation serves as the primary institutional anchor for global health governance, with its constitution establishing WHO's role as "the directing and coordinating authority on international health work." However, the contemporary global health governance landscape extends far beyond the WHO to include numerous international organisations, regional bodies, private foundations, civil society organisations, and private sector actors. This pluralistic governance architecture offers advantages in terms of resources and expertise mobilisation, but also creates challenges in terms of coordination, accountability, and democratic legitimacy.

The Quadripartite collaboration represents an innovative approach to global health governance that addresses the need for coordination across sectors while preserving organisational autonomy and expertise. The collaboration's governance structure includes executive-level meetings among the Directors-General of the four organisations, supported by a rotating secretariat that facilitates coordination and communication between meetings. This structure enables high-level strategic coordination while delegating operational decisions to technical working groups and national-level implementation partners (WHO, 2024).

The development and implementation of the One Health Joint Plan of Action illustrate both the potential and limitations of contemporary global health governance mechanisms. The plan's development through a participatory process involving technical experts and stakeholders from multiple sectors demonstrates the potential for inclusive global health governance. However, implementation depends on voluntary action by member states and partner organisations, highlighting the challenges of translating global commitments into effective action at national and local levels.

The complexity of contemporary global health governance is reflected in the variety of mechanisms available for coordinating international action, each with distinct strengths and limitations for implementing One Health approaches (Table 2.6). Understanding these different governance mechanisms is essential for navigating the complex landscape of global health policy and identifying opportunities for enhanced coordination and effectiveness.

The International Health Regulations (2005) provide the primary legal framework for global health governance, establishing binding obligations for WHO member states to develop core capacities for disease surveillance, assessment, reporting, and response. However, the IHR were designed primarily with human infectious disease threats in mind and include limited provisions for the kind of integrated approaches across sectors that characterise One Health. Recent discussions about IHR amendments have included proposals to strengthen One Health provisions; however, negotiations have been complicated by disagreements over state sovereignty, financing, and equity concerns.

Regional governance mechanisms play increasingly important roles in global health governance by providing platforms for coordination among countries with shared geographic, cultural, or economic characteristics. The African Union's health governance initiatives, including the Africa CDC and the African Medicines Agency, demonstrate how regional organisations can develop governance capacity that complements global mechanisms. Similarly, the European Union's health security policies and research programs demonstrate how regional integration can facilitate coordinated approaches to addressing health challenges.

The rise of global health partnerships represents a significant development in global health governance, bringing together public and private actors around specific disease or issue areas. Partnerships such as Gavi (vaccines), the Global Fund (HIV, TB, malaria), and CEPI (epidemic preparedness) have mobilised substantial resources and achieved significant health improvements. However, these partnerships have also raised questions about democratic accountability, priority setting, and coordination with national health systems and broader development objectives.

Private sector engagement in global health governance has expanded significantly, with pharmaceutical companies, technology firms, and other businesses playing increasingly prominent roles in shaping global health policies and programs. This engagement presents significant advantages in terms of innovation, resources, and implementation capacity, but also raises concerns about conflicts of interest, corporate influence on public policy, and equitable access to health technologies.

Civil society organisations serve crucial roles in global health governance by advocating for marginalised populations, holding governments and international organisations accountable, and providing services in areas where public sector capacity is limited. However, civil society participation in global health governance often faces constraints related to resources, capacity, and access to decision-making processes, particularly for organisations from low- and middle-income countries.

Table 2.6. Key global health governance mechanisms and their One Health integration

Governance Mechanism	Primary Function	One Health Integration	Strengths	Limitations
WHO World Health Assembly	Global health policy setting	Increasing OH resolutions	Universal membership, legitimacy	Consensus requirements, limited enforcement
Quadripartite Collaboration	Sectoral coordination	Core OH governance mechanism	Technical expertise, joint planning	Voluntary implementation, resource constraints
G7/G20 Health Summits	Political leadership	Growing OH emphasis	Political visibility, resource mobilisation	Limited membership, short-term focus
International Health Regulations	Health security governance	Limited OH provisions	Legal framework, compliance monitoring	Enforcement challenges, scope limitations
Regional Organisations	Regional coordination	Variable OH integration	Geographic focus, shared interests	Limited resources, capacity constraints

The governance of global health research and knowledge production represents an increasingly important dimension of global health governance. Questions about research priority setting, intellectual property rights, data sharing, and equitable access to research benefits have become central to discussions about global health governance. The COVID-19 pandemic highlighted these issues particularly starkly, with debates about vaccine intellectual property and equitable access to research benefits reflecting broader tensions about power and equity in global health governance.

Digital health technologies are creating new opportunities and challenges for global health governance. Digital platforms can facilitate the real-time sharing of information, coordination of response activities, and delivery of health services across international boundaries. However, digital health initiatives also raise important questions about data governance, privacy protection, and digital divides that may exacerbate existing health inequities.

The financing of global health governance represents a persistent challenge, with many governance mechanisms dependent on voluntary contributions from donor countries and philanthropic organisations. This financing model creates vulnerabilities related to sustainability, predictability, and the influence of major donors over governance priorities. The development of more sustainable and equitable financing mechanisms for global health governance represents an important area for continued innovation and reform.

Climate change is creating new challenges for global health governance, requiring coordination across health and environmental policy domains, while addressing long-term risks that may not align with traditional policy and electoral cycles. The integration of health considerations into climate governance mechanisms, such as the UN Framework Convention on Climate Change, represents an important area of institutional innovation that may provide models for other cross-sectoral governance challenges.

Conclusion

Integrating global health within the One Health framework represents both conceptual evolution and practical necessity for addressing 21st-century health challenges that transcend traditional boundaries. Persistent health disparities—with life expectancy differences reaching 33 years between countries—underscore that global health is fundamentally about equity and social justice, not inevitable consequences of geography. The Quadripartite collaboration and the One Health Joint Plan of Action demonstrate an unprecedented potential for coordination. At the same time, alignment with the Sustainable Development Goals enables integrated approaches that address shared determinants across multiple objectives. Cross-border challenges, such as antimicrobial resistance and climate change, illustrate the fundamental interconnectedness of health, with COVID-19 revealing both the consequences of inadequate governance and the potential for collaboration. Future success depends on addressing equity, sustainability, and inclusive participation in global governance, building foundations for healthier, more resilient, and equitable societies worldwide.

Acknowledgments

The authors would like to extend our appreciation to those who offered helpful commentary during the drafting process of this manuscript. We also acknowledge the role Nova Science Publishers played in enabling the work described herein.

References

Pungartnik, P. C., Abreu, A., dos Santos, C. V. B., Cavalcante, J. R., Faerstein, E., & Werneck, G. L. (2023). The interfaces between One Health and Global Health: A scoping review. *One Health*, 16, 100573. https://doi.org/10.1016/j.onehlt.2023.100573.

UNEP. (2022). UNEP joins alliance to implement One Health approach. Retrieved from https://www.unep.org/news-and-stories/press-release/unep-joins-alliance-implement-one-health-approach.

United Nations. (2015). Transforming our world: The 2030 Agenda for Sustainable Development. UN General Assembly Resolution A/RES/70/1.

World Health Organization. (2022). *One Health*. Retrieved from https://www.who.int/health-topics/one-health.

World Health Organization. (2024). Quadripartite partners organise High-Level One Health meeting in collaboration with Brazil's Ministry of Health at the G20 Summit. Retrieved from https://www.who.int/news/item/01-11-2024-quadripartite-partners-organize-high-level-one-health-meeting-in-collaboration-with-the-brazil-s-ministry-of-health-at-the-g20-summit.

World Health Organization. (2025). Health inequities are shortening lives by decades. Retrieved from https://www.who.int/news/item/06-05-2025-health-inequities-are-shortening-lives-by-decades.

World Organisation for Animal Health. (2024). WOAH's One Health initiatives in 2024. Retrieved from https://www.woah.org/en/woahs-one-health-initiatives-in-2024/.

Chapter 3

Research Ethics and Collaborative Frameworks in One Health

Abhay Saraf[1], MD
and Maajid Mohi Ud Din Malik[2,*], PhD
[1]Dr. D. Y. Patil School of Allied Health Sciences, Dr. D. Y. Patil Vidyapeeth· Pune (Deemed to be University), Sant Tukaram Nagar, Pimpri, Pune, India
[2]Deaprtment of Radiology and Imaging Technology, Dr. D. Y. Patil School of Allied Health Sciences, Dr. D. Y. Patil Vidyapeeth· Pune (Deemed to be University), Sant Tukaram Nagar, Pimpri, Pune, India

Abstract

The integration of human, animal, and environmental health research within the One Health framework presents unique ethical challenges that require innovative approaches to research governance and community engagement. This chapter examines the complex moral landscape of multidisciplinary One Health research, exploring how traditional research ethics frameworks must be adapted to address the interconnected nature of health challenges spanning species and ecosystems. The analysis reveals that informed consent processes must be reconceptualised to accommodate diverse stakeholders, including human communities, animal welfare considerations, and environmental stewardship responsibilities. Cultural sensitivity emerges as a critical factor in global health research, particularly when working with Indigenous communities whose traditional knowledge systems offer valuable insights into human-animal-environment relationships. Institutional Review Board processes require substantial adaptation to evaluate research that spans multiple disciplines and regulatory domains. At the same time, data sharing and intellectual property frameworks must strike a balance between scientific openness and the diverse interests of various stakeholders. Community-based participatory research principles offer essential guidance for ensuring that One Health research meets the needs and priorities of affected communities while maintaining scientific rigour. The evidence suggests that successful One Health research relies on collaborative frameworks that integrate ethical principles across disciplines, while fostering meaningful partnerships among researchers, communities, and policymakers. These frameworks contribute to achieving Sustainable Development Goal 3 (Good Health and Well-being) by ensuring that research practices promote equity, respect human dignity, and protect the rights of all stakeholders in the research enterprise.

---

* Corresponding Author's Email: maajid.malik@dpu.edu.in

In: Advances in the One Health Approach
Editors: Maajid Mohi Ud Din Malik, Abhay Saraf, Harshal Tukaram Pandve et al.
ISBN: 979-8-90134-202-2

Keywords: research ethics, One Health, multidisciplinary research, informed consent, cultural sensitivity, institutional review boards, data sharing, intellectual property, community-based participatory research, collaborative frameworks, Indigenous knowledge, SDG 3

Introduction

The emergence of One Health as a dominant paradigm in addressing complex global health challenges has fundamentally transformed approaches to research ethics and collaborative frameworks in health sciences. Unlike traditional research that operates within well-defined disciplinary boundaries, One Health research requires integration across human Health, veterinary medicine, environmental science, and social science domains, creating novel ethical challenges that existing frameworks were not designed to address. The interconnected nature of health challenges spanning species and ecosystems demands collaborative approaches that bring together diverse stakeholders with varying ethical traditions, cultural perspectives, and professional obligations.

Contemporary One Health research encompasses investigations ranging from zoonotic disease surveillance to antimicrobial resistance studies, the health impacts of climate change, and food safety systems. Each of these research areas involves multiple species, diverse human communities, and complex environmental systems, requiring ethical frameworks that can simultaneously protect human research participants, ensure animal welfare, safeguard ecological integrity, and respect cultural values and traditional knowledge systems. The COVID-19 pandemic has highlighted both the urgent need for such integrated research and the ethical complexities that arise when research must be conducted rapidly across multiple sectors and international boundaries.

Ethical challenges in One Health research are compounded by the interdisciplinary nature of research teams, which may include physicians, veterinarians, environmental scientists, social scientists, policy makers, and community representatives, each bringing distinct ethical training and professional obligations. The integration of these diverse perspectives requires collaborative frameworks that can facilitate meaningful dialogue across disciplinary boundaries while maintaining the highest standards of ethical conduct. Recent scholarship has begun to articulate the need for new ethical frameworks designed explicitly for One Health research, recognising that traditional approaches developed for single-species or single-discipline research may be inadequate for addressing the complexity of integrated health challenges (Curtis & Haldane, 2024).

The global nature of many One Health challenges necessitates research collaborations that span national boundaries and involve communities with diverse cultural backgrounds, economic circumstances, and political systems. These international collaborations raise additional ethical considerations related to research capacity building, benefit sharing, data sovereignty, and the protection of vulnerable populations. The development of ethical frameworks for One Health research must therefore address both the technical challenges of integrating research across disciplines and the social challenges of ensuring equitable partnerships across diverse communities and contexts.

3.1. Ethical Considerations in Multidisciplinary Research

The conduct of multidisciplinary research within the One Health framework presents unique ethical challenges that arise from the integration of research traditions, methodologies, and stakeholder communities that have historically operated independently of each other. Traditional research ethics frameworks, developed primarily for single-discipline investigations, must be adapted to address the complex interactions between human, animal, and environmental health research while maintaining the fundamental ethical principles of respect for persons, beneficence, and justice across all domains of inquiry.

One of the most significant ethical challenges in multidisciplinary One Health research is the variation in moral standards and oversight mechanisms that apply to research involving humans, animals, and environmental systems. Comprehensive ethical frameworks, including requirements for informed consent, institutional review board oversight, and strict protection of participant privacy and confidentiality, govern human subjects research. Animal research operates under distinct ethical frameworks that emphasise animal welfare, minimisation of harm, and scientific necessity, as evaluated by institutional animal care and use committees. Environmental research may involve considerations of ecosystem integrity, biodiversity protection, and sustainable resource use, but often lacks formal ethical oversight mechanisms comparable to those for human or animal research.

The integration of these different ethical frameworks within a single research program creates potential conflicts and gaps in oversight that must be carefully managed and addressed. For example, a One Health investigation of zoonotic disease emergence might involve human epidemiological studies, animal surveillance activities, and environmental sampling, each of which would traditionally be subject to different ethical review processes and standards. The challenge lies in developing coherent ethical approaches that can address all aspects of such integrated research while ensuring that moral standards in one domain do not inadvertently compromise ethical obligations in others.

Figure 5 shows a complex diagram featuring three overlapping circles representing Human Research Ethics, Animal Research Ethics, and Environmental Research Ethics. The centre intersection shows "Integrated One Health Ethics" with key principles like respect for all stakeholders, integrated consent processes, and holistic benefit-risk assessment. Around the edges are specific ethical considerations unique to each domain, with connecting arrows showing how they must be harmonised in One Health research.

The temporal dimensions of One Health research also create distinctive ethical challenges. While human subjects research typically involves clearly defined research periods with specific consent and withdrawal procedures, environmental and animal health research often requires long-term monitoring and intervention activities that span multiple years or even decades. The integration of research activities with different temporal requirements necessitates flexible ethical frameworks that can accommodate varying research timelines while maintaining consistent ethical standards throughout extended research programs.

Interdisciplinary research teams bring together professionals with different ethical training, professional codes of conduct, and institutional affiliations, potentially creating conflicts between professional obligations and research requirements. Physicians may have primary obligations to individual patients that could conflict with the objectives of population health research. At the same time, veterinarians may face tensions between animal welfare concerns and the necessities of research. Environmental scientists may prioritise ecosystem-level outcomes that differ from individual-focused ethical frameworks common in medical research. These potential conflicts require explicit discussion and resolution within research teams, often necessitating the development of project-specific ethical protocols that can accommodate diverse professional obligations and responsibilities.

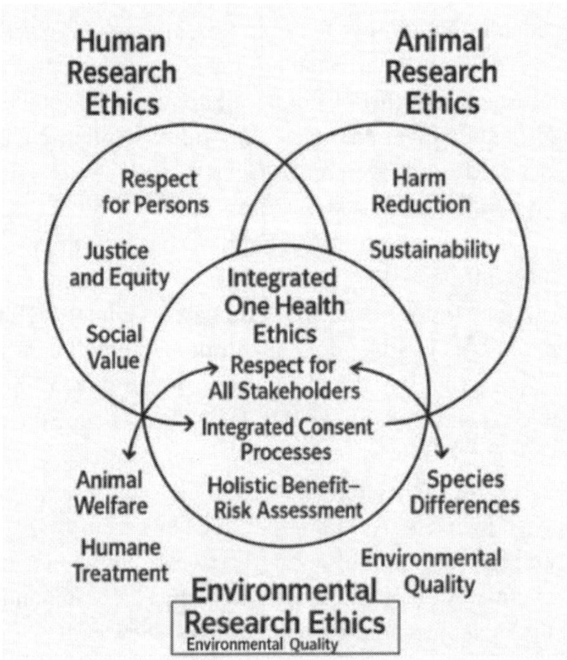

Figure 5. Ethical framework integration in One Health research.

The evaluation of risks and benefits in multidisciplinary One Health research requires consideration of outcomes across human, animal, and environmental domains, potentially involving trade-offs between benefits to one domain and risks to others. Traditional risk-benefit analysis frameworks developed for single-domain research may be inadequate for evaluating such complex trade-offs. For example, an intervention designed to reduce zoonotic disease transmission might provide benefits to human Health while imposing costs on animal welfare or environmental integrity. The ethical evaluation of such interventions requires frameworks that can weigh diverse types of outcomes and stakeholder interests.

Cultural and social considerations add additional layers of complexity to ethical frameworks for multidisciplinary One Health research. Many communities, particularly Indigenous populations, have an integrated understanding of human, animal, and environmental Health that differs from Western biomedical approaches to these domains. Research in such communities requires ethical frameworks that can respect and incorporate traditional knowledge systems while meeting contemporary ethical standards for research conduct. The integration of traditional knowledge with scientific research raises questions about intellectual property rights, benefit sharing, and appropriate acknowledgement of community contributions to research (Curtis & Haldane, 2024).

The global nature of many One Health research challenges necessitates international collaborations that must navigate different national and institutional ethical requirements.

Research conducted across multiple countries may be subject to varying ethical review processes, consent requirements, and data protection standards. The harmonisation of ethical requirements across international collaborations requires careful attention to ensuring that ethical standards meet the highest requirements in all participating jurisdictions while remaining practical for implementation across diverse contexts.

The integration of technology in One Health research raises additional ethical considerations regarding data collection, storage, and sharing across disciplines and institutions. Digital health technologies, environmental monitoring systems, and animal tracking devices generate vast amounts of data that may contain sensitive information about individuals, communities, and ecosystems. The ethical management of such data requires frameworks that can protect privacy and confidentiality across all domains while enabling the data integration necessary for effective One Health research.

3.2. Informed Consent Across Species and Communities

The principle of informed consent, fundamental to ethical research involving human participants, requires significant reconceptualisation within One Health research frameworks that encompass human communities, animal populations, and environmental systems. Traditional informed consent processes, designed for individual human research participants, must be adapted to address the complex stakeholder relationships and interconnected impacts that characterise One Health investigations. This adaptation requires innovative approaches that can simultaneously protect human autonomy, ensure animal welfare, and respect the interests of the community and the environment.

In human health research, informed consent traditionally involves individual participants making autonomous decisions about participating in research based on comprehensive information about the research's purposes, procedures, risks, and benefits. However, One Health research often involves community-level interventions or population-based studies where individual consent may be neither practical nor sufficient to address the full range of research impacts. For example, community-based vector control programs or environmental health interventions may affect entire populations regardless of individual participation decisions, necessitating community-level consent processes that complement individual consent procedures.

Community-based consent processes necessitate careful consideration of cultural values, decision-making structures, and power dynamics within communities. Many Indigenous communities have traditional governance structures and decision-making processes that must be respected and incorporated into research consent procedures. The development of culturally appropriate consent processes requires meaningful engagement with community leaders, elders, and other stakeholders to ensure that consent procedures align with community values and provide genuine opportunities for community self-determination regarding research participation (Ganjeh et al., 2025). Table 3.1 illustrates informed consent considerations across a single health domain.

Table 3.1. Informed consent considerations across One Health domains

Domain	Consent Approach	Key Considerations	Stakeholders Involved	Cultural Factors
Human Health	Individual and community consent	Autonomous decision-making, comprehension, voluntariness	Individuals, families, communities	Language, literacy, cultural values
Animal Health	Welfare assessment and owner consent	Animal welfare, owner rights, public health benefits	Animal owners, veterinarians, and communities	Relationship with animals, economic factors
Environmental Health	Stewardship consent and public engagement	Ecosystem integrity, intergenerational impacts, public goods	Land managers, communities, and future generations	Environmental values, traditional knowledge
Integrated One Health	Multistakeholder consent frameworks	Interconnected impacts, collective benefits, shared responsibilities	All stakeholders across domains	Holistic worldviews, systems thinking

The concept of consent must be expanded beyond individual human participants to address the welfare and interests of animal populations involved in One Health research. While animals cannot provide informed consent in the traditional sense, ethical animal research requires consideration of animal welfare, minimisation of harm, and scientific justification for animal involvement. In One Health research, animal welfare considerations may extend beyond individual research animals to include wild animal populations, domestic animals in research communities, and ecosystem-level impacts on animal habitats and food sources.

Animal research ethics in One Health contexts requires integration of veterinary ethics principles with public health considerations and community values regarding human-animal relationships. Many communities have cultural, economic, or spiritual relationships with animal populations that must be considered in research design and implementation. For example, research involving livestock in agricultural communities must consider both the economic impacts on animal owners and the cultural values related to animal husbandry and care. Similarly, research involving wildlife populations must consider ecosystem-level impacts and community relationships with wildlife.

Environmental dimensions of One Health research require consideration of consent-like processes related to environmental stewardship and intergenerational justice. While the environment cannot provide consent in a legal sense, ethical environmental research involves considering ecosystem integrity, sustainable resource use, and the impacts on future generations. Environmental stewardship principles suggest that research activities should minimise environmental harm and contribute to long-term environmental sustainability.

The integration of environmental considerations into consent processes may involve consultation with ecological stewardship organisations, indigenous communities with traditional environmental knowledge, and other stakeholders with interests in environmental protection. Such consultations can help ensure that research activities align with broader environmental values and contribute to sustainable environmental management practices.

Digital technologies increasingly used in One Health research create new challenges for informed consent processes, particularly regarding data collection, storage, and sharing across disciplines and institutions. Environmental monitoring systems, animal tracking devices, and human health monitoring technologies generate vast amounts of data that may contain sensitive information about individuals, communities, and ecosystems. The consent processes for such research must address data privacy, security, and sharing while enabling the data integration necessary for effective One Health research.

Cross-border One Health research presents additional challenges for informed consent processes, given the varying cultural contexts, legal requirements, and institutional standards across different countries and regions. International research collaborations must navigate different consent requirements while ensuring that ethical standards meet the highest requirements in all participating jurisdictions. This may require the development of flexible consent processes that can be adapted to different cultural and legal contexts while maintaining consistent ethical standards (Chattopadhyay et al., 2023).

The temporal dimensions of One Health research may necessitate dynamic consent processes that can adapt to changing research objectives, evolving community needs, and long-term monitoring requirements. Traditional consent processes assume relatively static research objectives and participant relationships, but One Health research may involve adaptive management approaches that respond to changing conditions and emerging health threats.

Dynamic consent frameworks that allow for ongoing negotiation and renegotiation of research relationships may be necessary to maintain ethical research conduct over extended time periods.

Health literacy and cultural competency considerations are crucial in One Health research consent processes, given the complexity of explaining interconnected health relationships and the diversity of communities that may be involved in research. Consent materials and processes must be developed to be accessible to participants with varying educational backgrounds, cultural contexts, and primary languages. This may require development of visual materials, community-based explanation processes, and culturally adapted consent procedures that can effectively communicate complex One Health concepts (Simonds et al., 2017).

3.3. Cultural Sensitivity in Global Health Research

Cultural sensitivity in One Health research encompasses the recognition, respect, and integration of diverse cultural perspectives, values, and knowledge systems that shape how different communities understand and experience the relationships between human, animal, and environmental Health. The global scope of One Health challenges necessitates research approaches that can engage meaningfully with cultural diversity while maintaining scientific rigour and ethical integrity. This requires moving beyond superficial cultural competency toward deeper cultural safety approaches that address power imbalances and structural inequalities that affect research relationships.

Indigenous communities worldwide possess sophisticated traditional knowledge systems that offer valuable insights into the interconnected nature of human, animal, and environmental health. These knowledge systems, developed over millennia of careful observation and interaction with local ecosystems, often embody holistic understandings of health that align closely with One Health principles. However, the integration of Indigenous knowledge into One Health research requires careful attention to cultural protocols, intellectual property rights, and power dynamics that have historically marginalised Indigenous perspectives in research contexts.

The concept of cultural safety, initially developed in New Zealand healthcare contexts, provides a more comprehensive framework for addressing cultural diversity in research than traditional cultural competency approaches. Cultural safety requires researchers and institutions to examine their own cultural assumptions, power positions, and institutional practices that may create barriers to meaningful participation by diverse communities. Rather than simply learning about other cultures, cultural safety requires the transformation of research practices and institutions to create environments where all participants feel respected, valued, and empowered (Curtis & Reid, 2019). Table 3.2 illustrates the distinction between cultural safety and cultural competency in health research.

The integration of traditional ecological knowledge into One Health research necessitates acknowledging that Indigenous communities are not merely sources of information, but instead knowledge holders with the right to control how their knowledge is utilised, shared, and attributed. This requires the development of research partnerships that respect Indigenous governance structures, provide meaningful opportunities for community control over research processes, and ensure that the benefits of research are shared with and benefit participating communities. Such partnerships often require long-term relationship building, cultural learning, and commitment to addressing community priorities alongside research objectives.

Table 3.2. Cultural safety vs. cultural competency in One Health research

Aspect	Cultural Competency	Cultural Safety
Focus	Learning about other cultures	Examining one's own culture and power
Goal	Becoming competent in other cultures	Creating safe spaces for all cultures
Power Analysis	Limited attention to power dynamics	Central focus on power relationships
Responsibility	Individual practitioner development	System-wide institutional change
Evaluation	Assessed by practitioners/institutions	Defined and evaluated by communities
Outcome Measures	Knowledge and skills acquisition	Community-defined safety and equity outcomes
Sustainability	Individual-focused, may not persist	Institutional change, more sustainable
One Health Relevance	May perpetuate existing hierarchies	Addresses structural barriers to participation

Language diversity represents a significant practical and ethical challenge in global One Health research. Effective communication about complex health relationships requires materials and processes that are accessible in local languages and culturally appropriate communication styles. This extends beyond translation to include adaptation of concepts, examples, and communication approaches that align with local cultural norms and understanding. The development of culturally and linguistically appropriate research materials requires significant investment and community partnership but is essential for meaningful participation and ethical research conduct.

Gender considerations add additional layers of complexity to cultural sensitivity in One Health research. Different cultures have varying norms regarding gender roles, women's participation in research, and decision-making authority within families and communities. One Health research that involves household-level interventions or community-based activities must carefully consider gender dynamics and ensure that research approaches do not inadvertently reinforce gender inequalities or exclude women from meaningful participation. This may require separate consultation processes for men and women, attention to gender-specific health concerns, and recognition of women's often extensive knowledge about health and environmental relationships.

Religious and spiritual considerations are often central to how communities understand Health and their relationships with animals and the environment. Many religious traditions have specific teachings regarding human-animal relationships, environmental stewardship, and health practices that must be considered in the design and implementation of One Health research. Research activities that conflict with religious beliefs or practices may not only be culturally insensitive but may also undermine research validity and community participation. Meaningful engagement with religious and spiritual leaders can help ensure that research approaches align with community values and beliefs.

Economic and social stratification within communities creates additional cultural considerations for One Health research. Research approaches that assume homogeneous community perspectives may miss essential differences in experiences, resources, and priorities among different community groups. Attention to social stratification is significant in One Health research because environmental and animal health challenges often disproportionately affect marginalised community members who may have different perspectives and priorities than community leaders or more privileged community members.

The globalisation of research creates challenges related to the imposition of Western research frameworks and ethical standards on communities with different cultural values and governance systems. While international ethical standards provide essential protections for research participants, their application must be sensitive to local cultural contexts and should not undermine local governance systems or cultural practices. This requires careful negotiation between international standards and regional cultural values, often necessitating adaptation of standard research procedures to accommodate cultural differences while maintaining ethical integrity.

Historical trauma related to colonisation, research exploitation, and cultural suppression affects many communities' willingness to participate in research and their trust in research institutions. One Health research in such communities requires acknowledging historical harms, engaging in transparent discussions about how current research differs from past exploitation, and demonstrating a genuine commitment to community benefit and control. This may require extended periods of relationship-building, community control over research priorities and methods, and explicit attention to addressing historical inequalities throughout the research process and its outcomes.

Cultural considerations extend beyond human communities to include cultural values related to animals and environmental relationships. Different cultures have varying perspectives on animal welfare, human-animal relationships, and environmental stewardship that must be considered in the design of One Health research. For example, research involving livestock in pastoral communities must consider cultural values related to animal husbandry, animal-human relationships, and the cultural significance of particular animal species. Similarly, environmental research must consider cultural values about land use, resource management, and spiritual relationships with natural environments (Richardson et al., 2021).

3.4. Institutional Review Board Processes for One Health Studies

Institutional Review Boards (IRBs) and their international equivalents serve as the primary gatekeepers for research ethics oversight; yet their traditional structures and review processes were designed primarily for single-discipline human subjects' research. The emergence of One Health research presents unprecedented challenges for IRB review systems, which must evaluate research protocols that span multiple species, disciplines, and regulatory frameworks. Adapting IRB processes for One Health research requires fundamental reconsideration of review criteria, expertise requirements, and coordination mechanisms to ensure comprehensive ethical oversight of complex, multidisciplinary research programs.

Traditional IRB review processes focus primarily on the protection of human subjects, evaluating research protocols according to federal regulations that emphasise informed consent, risk minimisation, and equitable subject selection. However, One Health research often involves integrated study designs where human, animal, and environmental components are interconnected in ways that make separate ethical review inappropriate or insufficient. For example, a zoonotic disease surveillance study might involve simultaneous human epidemiological investigation, animal sampling, and environmental monitoring, with each component informing and depending on the others.

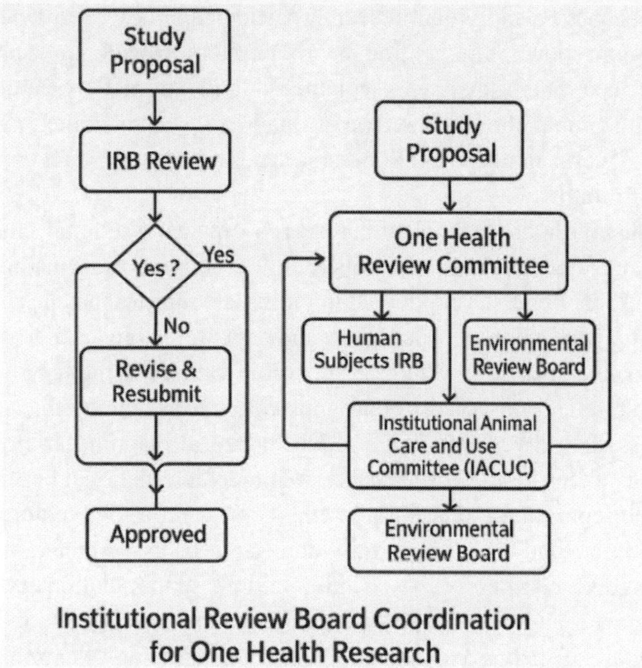

Figure 6. Institutional review board coordination for One Health research.

The evaluation of such integrated research requires IRB review processes that can assess the ethical implications of research across multiple domains while considering the interconnected nature of research activities. This necessitates expansion of traditional IRB expertise to include members with knowledge of veterinary ethics, environmental research ethics, and the specific challenges of interdisciplinary research. Some institutions have experimented with joint review processes involving multiple review boards, while others have developed specialised One Health IRBs with expanded membership and expertise.

Figure 6 shows a flowchart comparing the traditional single-IRB review process on the left with an integrated One Health review process on the right. The One Health process demonstrates coordination among the Human Subjects IRB, Institutional Animal Care and Use Committee (IACUC), Environmental Review Board, and Community Advisory Board, with central coordination through a One Health Review Committee. Decision points and feedback loops are shown throughout the process.

Coordination between different review boards presents significant logistical and substantive challenges. Traditional human subjects IRBs and Institutional Animal Care and Use Committees (IACUCs) operate under various regulatory frameworks, review criteria, and timelines, making coordination complex even when institutional commitment exists. Environmental research often lacks formal ethical review requirements altogether, creating gaps in oversight that must be addressed through institutional innovation. Some institutions have developed memoranda of understanding between review boards to facilitate coordination, while others have created overarching review committees specifically for multidisciplinary research.

The risk-benefit analysis conducted by IRBs must be expanded for One Health research to consider outcomes across multiple domains and stakeholder groups. Traditional risk-benefit analysis primarily focuses on individual research participants; however, One Health research may involve community-level interventions with population-wide impacts, environmental interventions with ecosystem-level consequences, and animal research with welfare implications for entire animal populations. The evaluation of such complex risk-benefit profiles requires review frameworks that can weigh diverse types of outcomes and consider impacts on multiple stakeholder groups.

International and multi-site One Health research creates additional challenges for IRB review due to varying regulatory requirements, cultural contexts, and institutional capacities across different locations. Research conducted in multiple countries may be subject to different ethical review requirements, consent procedures, and data protection standards. Some countries have well-developed ethical review systems comparable to those in the U.S., while others have limited ethical oversight capacity or different approaches to research ethics. Coordination of ethical review across such diverse contexts requires careful planning and often necessitates additional protections to ensure that ethical standards meet international best practices.

The evaluation of community consent and engagement processes requires expertise from the IRB that extends beyond traditional individual consent assessment. Many One Health research projects involve community-based interventions or population-level studies where community engagement and consent processes are as important as individual consent procedures. IRB review of such research requires an understanding of community governance structures, cultural decision-making processes, and appropriate community engagement approaches. This often necessitates community representation on IRBs or consultation with community advisory boards.

Data sharing and intellectual property considerations in One Health research create novel challenges for IRB review that extend beyond traditional confidentiality and privacy protections. One Health research often generates data that may be valuable to multiple disciplines, institutions, and stakeholders, requiring careful evaluation of data sharing agreements, intellectual property arrangements, and long-term data stewardship responsibilities. IRBs must evaluate whether proposed data-sharing arrangements adequately protect participant interests while enabling the collaborative data use necessary for effective One Health research.

The temporal dimensions of One Health research require IRB review processes that can accommodate adaptive research designs, long-term monitoring activities, and evolving research objectives. Traditional IRB review assumes relatively static research protocols with clearly defined endpoints. Still, One Health research often involves adaptive management approaches that must respond to changing conditions, emerging health threats, and evolving community needs. This requires the development of dynamic review processes that can provide ongoing oversight and approval for protocol modifications while maintaining ethical integrity (Grady, 2015).

Technology integration in One Health research creates new categories of risk and benefit that traditional IRB review processes may not be equipped to evaluate. Environmental monitoring systems, animal tracking devices, and digital health technologies generate new types of data with novel implications for privacy and security. The evaluation of such technologies requires expertise in digital privacy, cybersecurity, and the ethical implications of emerging technologies from the IRB. Many IRBs are still developing the capacity to evaluate such research, necessitating additional training and the development of expertise in this area.

The evaluation of traditional knowledge integration in One Health research requires an understanding of Indigenous research ethics, community governance structures, and appropriate protocols for working with traditional knowledge holders by the IRB. This extends beyond standard cultural competency to include understanding of Indigenous research methodologies, community-based participatory research approaches, and appropriate benefit-sharing arrangements. Some institutions have developed Indigenous research ethics boards or have incorporated Indigenous expertise into existing review structures.

Capacity-building and training requirements for IRB members and staff pose significant challenges for institutions seeking to develop One Health research review capabilities. Traditional IRB training focuses primarily on human subject's research regulations and may not adequately prepare reviewers for the complexity of multidisciplinary One Health research. Development of appropriate training programs requires coordination across disciplines and may necessitate partnerships with veterinary colleges, environmental science departments, and community organisations to provide comprehensive expertise.

3.5. Data Sharing and Intellectual Property Issues

Data sharing and intellectual property management in One Health research present complex challenges that arise from the integration of diverse data types, multiple stakeholder interests, and varying institutional and cultural approaches to knowledge ownership and sharing. The collaborative nature of One Health research generates valuable data assets that can benefit multiple disciplines, institutions, and communities. However, managing these assets requires careful attention to legal, ethical, and practical considerations that extend far beyond traditional academic data sharing arrangements.

One Health research typically generates diverse data types, including human health information, animal health data, environmental monitoring results, and traditional knowledge contributions from community partners. Each data type may be subject to different privacy protections, ownership rights, and sharing restrictions that must be carefully coordinated within integrated research programs. Human health data is typically subject to strict privacy protections under regulations such as HIPAA in the United States. In contrast, animal health data may be considered proprietary by animal owners or government agencies. Environmental data may be subject to national security considerations or traditional knowledge protections depending on the research context.

The integration of traditional knowledge into One Health research creates intellectual property challenges because such knowledge is often collectively held by communities rather than owned by individuals and may be considered sacred or culturally sensitive information that cannot be freely shared. Traditional knowledge systems frequently embody a sophisticated understanding of human-animal-environment relationships, developed over generations through careful observation and practice. The integration of such knowledge into scientific research requires respectful partnership approaches that recognise community rights to control how their knowledge is used and shared (Özdemir et al., 2022). Table 3.3 shows data types and sharing considerations in one Health.

Table 3.3. Data types and sharing considerations in One Health research

Data Type	Privacy/ Confidentiality Issues	Ownership Considerations	Sharing Restrictions	Technical Challenges
Human Health Data	HIPAA, individual privacy rights	Individual and institutional rights	IRB approval, consent requirements	De-identification, secure storage
Animal Health Data	Owner confidentiality, trade secrets	Owner and institutional rights	Veterinary-client privilege, commercial sensitivity	Species-specific data formats
Environmental Data	Location sensitivity, national security	Government and institutional rights	National security, endangered species	Spatial data complexity, sensor integration
Traditional Knowledge	Cultural protocols, sacredness	Community collective rights	Community consent, cultural protocols	Knowledge representation, context preservation
Genomic Data	Individual and family privacy	Complex ownership questions	International regulations, patent issues	Storage requirements, computational analysis
Integrated Datasets	Multiple overlapping protections	Multiple stakeholder claims	Complex approval processes	Interoperability, standardisation

International data sharing in One Health research must navigate varying national regulations, cultural expectations, and institutional policies regarding the transfer of cross-border data. The European Union's General Data Protection Regulation (GDPR), various national data sovereignty laws, and bilateral data-sharing agreements create a complex regulatory landscape that researchers must understand and comply with. Additionally, many countries have specific regulations regarding the export of biological samples and associated data that may apply to One Health research involving genetic or environmental data.

The commercialisation potential of One Health research creates additional intellectual property considerations that must be balanced against scientific openness and public health needs. Research findings that contribute to the development of diagnostic tools, therapeutics, or interventions may have significant commercial value, creating tensions between public access to research results and intellectual property protections that incentivise innovation and investment. These tensions are particularly acute in global health contexts where research may be conducted in low-income settings but commercialised by institutions in high-income countries.

Patent protection considerations in One Health research may involve complex questions about the patentability of naturally occurring phenomena, traditional knowledge, and research methods that integrate across disciplines. While naturally occurring, genetic sequences are generally not patentable, diagnostic methods, therapeutic interventions, and research tools developed through One Health research may be eligible for patent protection. The evaluation of patent protection requires careful consideration of prior art, including traditional knowledge that may have anticipated research findings. It must comply with varying national patent laws and international patent agreements.

Data sovereignty considerations are critical when One Health research involves Indigenous communities or is conducted in countries with strong national data protection policies. Data sovereignty refers to the right of nations and communities to control data that relates to their citizens, resources, or territories. In the context of One Health research, this may include rights to control genetic data from local plant and animal species, traditional knowledge about local ecosystems, and health data from community members. Respecting data sovereignty requires meaningful community engagement in decisions about data collection, storage, sharing, and use.

The development of data sharing agreements for One Health research necessitates careful consideration of balancing scientific openness with legitimate privacy, security, and ownership interests. Effective data sharing agreements must specify permitted uses of shared data, attribution requirements, obligations for data security and confidentiality, and procedures for resolving disputes about data use. Such contracts may need to accommodate different institutional policies, national regulations, and community requirements, making their development complex and time-consuming.

Technology platforms for One Health data sharing must address interoperability challenges while maintaining appropriate security and access controls. One Health research often involves data collected using different methods, formats, and standards across disciplines, making data integration technically challenging. The development of shared data platforms requires careful attention to data standardisation, metadata requirements, and technical infrastructure that can support secure data sharing while maintaining usability for diverse research communities.

Benefit-sharing arrangements in One Health research must address how benefits from research will be distributed among the various contributors to research success, including academic institutions, community partners, government agencies, and private sector collaborators. Traditional academic benefit sharing through publication and citation may be insufficient to recognise the contributions of community knowledge holders, government data providers, and private sector partners. More comprehensive benefit-sharing arrangements may include financial benefits, capacity building opportunities, technology transfer, and priority access to research results and derived products.

Long-term data stewardship responsibilities in One Health research require consideration of how valuable data assets will be maintained, updated, and made accessible over extended time periods. Unlike research in single disciplines, One Health research may generate data that remains valuable for multiple decades and may need to be integrated with future research programs. This requires the development of a sustainable data management infrastructure, funding arrangements for long-term data maintenance, and governance structures that can make decisions about data access and use over extended periods.

The evaluation of data quality and provenance becomes particularly important in One Health research, where data integration across sources and disciplines is essential for research validity. Data sharing arrangements must include provisions for documenting data quality, collection methods, and any limitations or biases that may affect data interpretation. This is particularly important when traditional knowledge is integrated with scientific data, as different knowledge systems may have different standards for evidence and validation (Carroll et al., 2015).

3.6. Community-Based Participatory Research Principles

Community-Based Participatory Research (CBPR) principles provide essential frameworks for conducting ethical and practical One Health research by ensuring that research serves community needs and priorities while building local research capacity and promoting equitable partnerships between academic researchers and community stakeholders. The application of CBPR principles to One Health research necessitates adapting traditional community engagement approaches to address the complexity of research that spans multiple species, ecosystems, and stakeholder communities, while maintaining the fundamental commitments of CBPR to community ownership, collaborative decision-making, and mutual benefit.

The foundational principle of CBPR emphasises community ownership and control over research processes, from problem definition through implementation and dissemination of results. In One Health contexts, this principle requires careful consideration of how to define "community" when research may affect multiple human communities, animal populations, and environmental systems. Community definition may need to include not only human residents of a geographic area but also animal owners, ecological stewardship groups, traditional knowledge holders, and other stakeholders with interests in research outcomes.

Community engagement in One Health research necessitates acknowledging that different communities may possess varying levels of scientific literacy, employ distinct cultural approaches to knowledge production, and have diverse priorities regarding research outcomes. Effective community engagement requires the development of culturally appropriate communication strategies, investment in relationship building, and a commitment to addressing community priorities, even when these may not perfectly align with the researcher's interests.

This often requires an extended timeline for research development and implementation, allowing for meaningful community input and the development of partnerships.

Figure 7 illustrates a circular diagram depicting the CBPR process adapted for One Health research. The centre shows "Community-Researcher Partnership" surrounded by six interconnected phases: 1) Community Priority Setting, 2) Collaborative Research Design, 3) Capacity Building, 4) Data Collection & Analysis, 5) Action Planning, and 6) Evaluation & Dissemination. Each phase includes specific One Health considerations and shows feedback loops between all components.

Capacity building represents a central component of CBPR that takes on additional complexity in One Health research due to the interdisciplinary nature of research skills and knowledge required. Effective capacity building in One Health contexts may require development of community expertise in human Health, animal health, and environmental health domains, as well as an understanding of how these domains interact. This may involve training community members in data collection techniques, research ethics, and scientific communication, while also building the capacity of researchers in community engagement, cultural competency, and traditional knowledge systems.

The principle of mutual benefit in CBPR requires that research provide tangible benefits to participating communities while advancing scientific knowledge. In One Health research, mutual benefit may encompass multiple types of outcomes, including improved health services, enhanced environmental management, strengthened animal health programs, and increased community capacity to address integrated health challenges. The identification and achievement of mutual benefits requires ongoing dialogue between researchers and communities throughout the research process to ensure that research activities align with evolving community needs and priorities.

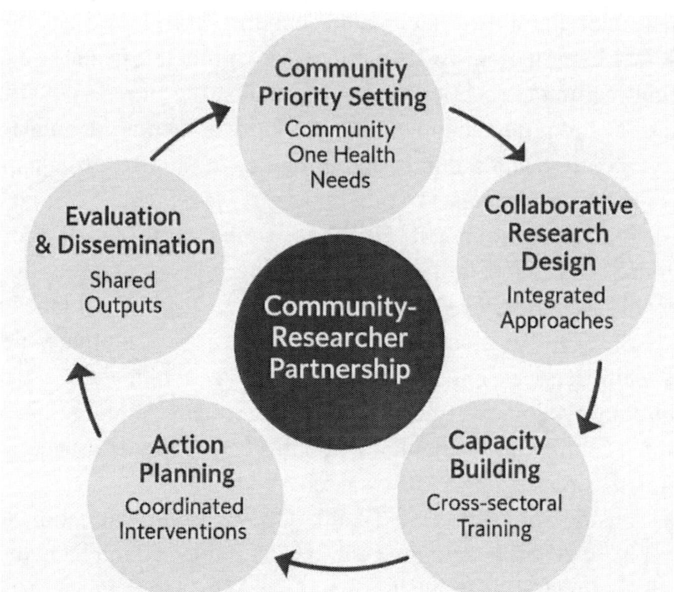

Figure 7. Community-based participatory research framework for One Health.

Collaborative decision-making in One Health CBPR requires the development of governance structures that can accommodate diverse stakeholders with different expertise, interests, and decision-making authorities. This may involve the creation of community advisory boards that include representatives from various community sectors, the establishment of research oversight committees with shared membership between researchers and the community, and the development of consensus-building processes to address complex decisions about research design, implementation, and dissemination.

The integration of traditional knowledge systems into One Health CBPR requires respectful recognition of Indigenous and local knowledge as valid and valuable ways of understanding human-animal-environment relationships. This goes beyond simply collecting traditional knowledge to incorporate community knowledge holders as full partners in research design, implementation, and interpretation. Effective traditional knowledge integration requires an understanding of local knowledge systems, recognition of appropriate protocols for accessing and utilising traditional knowledge, and a commitment to ensuring that research benefits flow back to the knowledge-holding communities.

Data ownership and sharing in One Health CBPR require careful attention to community rights to control information about their Health, environment, and traditional practices. CBPR principles emphasise community ownership of data generated through participatory research; however, implementing this principle in One Health contexts requires navigating complex legal and institutional frameworks regarding data ownership, intellectual property rights, and academic publication requirements. This may require development of innovative data sharing agreements that recognise community ownership while enabling scientific publication and broader research impact (Tapia et al., 2024).

Cultural safety considerations in One Health CBPR require attention to power dynamics, historical trauma, and structural inequalities that may affect community-researcher relationships. Many communities that would benefit from One Health research have experienced historical exploitation by researchers, government agencies, and other external institutions, creating legitimate scepticism about participating in research. Building trust and ensuring cultural safety requires acknowledging historical harms, demonstrating a genuine commitment to community benefit, and being willing to modify research approaches to align with community values and priorities.

Evaluation of CBPR outcomes in One Health research requires the development of success measures that capture both scientific advancements and community benefits across multiple domains. Traditional academic evaluation primarily focuses on publication output and scientific impact. Still, CBPR evaluation requires attention to community-defined outcomes, such as improved health services, enhanced local capacity, strengthened community networks, and increased community empowerment. The development of comprehensive evaluation frameworks requires community input to identify appropriate success measures and methodologies for assessing the impact of research.

Sustainability considerations in One Health CBPR require attention to how research partnerships and capacity-building activities will be maintained beyond the duration of specific research projects. Effective CBPR builds lasting community capacity and establishes ongoing alliances that can support continued research and action on community priorities. This requires investment in institutional relationships, training programs, and infrastructure that can support long-term collaboration between the community and researchers.

Scaling up CBPR approaches to address larger-scale One Health challenges requires careful attention to maintaining community partnership principles while expanding the research's impact. Many One Health challenges operate at regional, national, or global scales that may exceed the capacity of individual community partnerships. Scaling up CBPR approaches may require the development of networks of community partnerships, policy advocacy based on community priorities, and institutional changes that can support community engagement at larger scales.

Training and education requirements for researchers engaged in One Health CBPR extend beyond traditional research methods training to include community engagement skills, cultural competency, and understanding of power dynamics in research relationships. Many academic institutions provide limited training in CBPR approaches, necessitating additional professional development and mentorship opportunities for researchers seeking to conduct ethical and practical community-engaged research. This training should include attention to the specific challenges of conducting CBPR across multiple disciplines and stakeholder communities.

Conclusion

One Health research ethics represents a fundamental transformation that requires the integration of diverse ethical traditions to address interconnected health challenges spanning species, disciplines, and cultures. Traditional frameworks must be substantially adapted, particularly by reconceptualising informed consent to encompass human communities, animal welfare, and environmental stewardship through multistakeholder approaches. Cultural sensitivity—evolving toward cultural safety—addresses power imbalances and values Indigenous knowledge systems. Institutional Review Boards require adaptation for coordinated, multidisciplinary oversight, while data sharing frameworks must balance privacy protection, community rights, recognition of traditional knowledge, and scientific openness. Community-based participatory research principles provide valuable guidance but demand substantial investment in relationship building and capacity development. Future challenges from climate change and technological advancements require adaptive ethical frameworks that maintain core principles. Alignment with Sustainable Development Goals demonstrates that ethical research practices are both morally required and strategically crucial for achieving lasting impact and building collaborative partnerships essential for addressing complex global health issues.

Acknowledgments

The authors would like to extend our appreciation to those who offered helpful commentary during the drafting process of this manuscript. We also acknowledge the role Nova Science Publishers played in enabling the work described herein.

References

Carroll, S. R., Rodriguez-Lonebear, D., & Martinez, A. (2019). Indigenous data governance: Strategies from United States Native Nations. *Data Science Journal*, 18, 31. https://doi.org/10.5334/dsj-2019-031.

Chattopadhyay, S., Harper, I., Pinto, A. D., et al. (2023). Making research ethics work for global Health: Towards a more agile and collaborative approach. *BMJ Global Health*, 8(7), e011415. https://doi.org/10.1136/bmjgh-2022-011415.

Curtis, V., & Haldane, V. (2024). Can One Health policy help us expand an ethics of interconnection and interdependence? *AMA Journal of Ethics*, 26(2), E162-170. https://doi.org/10.1001/amajethics.2024.162.

Curtis, E., & Reid, P. (2019). Why cultural safety rather than cultural competency is required to achieve health equity: A literature review and recommended definition. *International Journal for Equity in Health*, 18, 174. https://doi.org/10.1186/s12939-019-1082-3.

Ganjeh, Y., Ngaruiya, C., Albee, B., Funaro, M. C., Bongomin, F., Greeno, R. V., Bothwell, L., & Ebbs, D. (2025). Community based participatory research in global Health: Time to provide appropriate ethics training for community researchers. *INQUIRY: The Journal of Health Care Organization, Provision, and Financing*, 62. https://doi.org/10.1177/00469580251350492.

Grady, C. (2015). Institutional review boards: Purpose and challenges. *Chest*, 148(5), 1148-1155. https://doi.org/10.1378/chest.15-0706.

Özdemir, V., Ho, C. W. L., & Kılıç, Ş. (2022). Operationalising "One Health" as "One Digital Health" through a global framework that emphasises fair and equitable sharing of benefits from the use of artificial intelligence and related digital technologies. *Frontiers in Public Health*, 10, 768977. https://doi.org/10.3389/fpubh.2022.768977.

Richardson, G. E., et al. (2021). Ethics, One Health approaches, and SDGs: Conference lessons for an emerging field. *Frontiers in Public Health*, 12, 1448409. https://doi.org/10.3389/fpubh.2024.1448409.

Rodriguez, J. (2024). One Health ethics and the ethics of zoonoses: A silent call for global action. *Veterinary Sciences*, 11(9), 394. https://doi.org/10.3390/vetsci11090394.

Simonds, V. W., Wallerstein, N., Duran, B., & Villegas, M. (2017). Health literacy and informed consent materials: Designed for documentation, not comprehension of health research. *Journal of Health Communication*, 22(8), 682-690. https://doi.org/10.1080/10810730.2017.1341568.

Tapia, J. L., Lopez, A., Turner, D. B., et al. (2024). The bench to community initiative: Community-based participatory research model for translating research discoveries into community solutions. *Frontiers in Public Health*, 12, 1394069. https://doi.org/10.3389/fpubh.2024.1394069.

Chapter 4

Integrated Surveillance Systems: Building Bridges Across Sectors

Purnachandra Kawdu Lamghare[1]
and Maajid Mohi Ud Din Malik[2,*], PhD
[1]Department of Radio-Diagnosis, Dr. D. Y. Patil Medical College, Hospital and Research Centre, Dr. D. Y. Patil Vidyapeeth, Pune (Deemed to be University), Sant Tukaram Nagar, Pimpri, Pune, India
[2]Department of Radiology and Imaging Technology, Dr. D.Y. Patil School of Allied Health Sciences, Dr. D. Y. Patil Vidyapeeth Pune (Deemed to be University), Sant Tukaram Nagar, Pimpri, Pune, India

Abstract

Integrated surveillance systems represent a transformative approach to global health security by bridging human, animal, and environmental health sectors through the One Health paradigm. This chapter examines the principles and implementation of integrated surveillance networks that enhance early detection, response capabilities, and prevention of infectious disease outbreaks. The evolution from siloed surveillance systems to interconnected platforms demonstrates significant advances in digital health technologies, artificial intelligence applications, and data integration methodologies. Through a comprehensive analysis of global influenza surveillance networks, particularly the WHO Global Influenza Surveillance and Response System (GISRS), this chapter illustrates successful models of international cooperation and real-time data sharing. Key challenges, including data interoperability, standardisation protocols, and cross-sectoral coordination, are addressed alongside technological solutions and policy frameworks. The integration of these systems contributes directly to achieving Sustainable Development Goal 3 (Good Health and Well-being) while supporting broader global health security objectives. Case studies demonstrate how integrated approaches improve surveillance sensitivity, reduce response times, and enhance pandemic preparedness through multi-sectoral collaboration and innovative early warning mechanisms.

Keywords: integrated surveillance systems, One Health approach, digital health surveillance, early warning systems, data interoperability, global influenza surveillance, GISRS, zoonotic disease surveillance, SDG 3 Good Health and Well-being, pandemic

* Corresponding Author's Email: maajid.malik@dpu.edu.in

In: Advances in the One Health Approach
Editors: Maajid Mohi Ud Din Malik, Abhay Saraf, Harshal Tukaram Pandve et al.
ISBN: 979-8-90134-202-2

preparedness, artificial intelligence in health surveillance, cross-sectoral coordination, health security

Introduction

The emergence of infectious diseases at the interface between human, animal, and environmental Health has fundamentally challenged traditional surveillance approaches that operate within isolated sectoral boundaries. Recent global health crises, including the COVID-19 pandemic, have highlighted the critical limitations of fragmented monitoring systems and underscored the urgent need for integrated surveillance networks that can simultaneously detect, assess, and respond to health threats across multiple domains. The recognition that approximately three-quarters of emerging infectious diseases originate from animal sources underscores the imperative for surveillance systems that bridge the traditional divide between human and veterinary health monitoring (WHO, 2023).

This chapter examines the evolution from conventional surveillance approaches toward integrated systems that embody the One Health paradigm, demonstrating how technological innovations, international cooperation frameworks, and policy coordination can enhance global health security. Through a detailed analysis of successful models, such as the Global Influenza Surveillance and Response System, an examination of digital health technologies, and an assessment of data integration challenges, this chapter provides comprehensive insights into building effective cross-sectoral surveillance networks. The discussion encompasses both the transformative potential of integrated approaches and the practical difficulties that must be addressed to achieve sustainable implementation across diverse healthcare contexts and resource settings.

4.1. Principles of Integrated Surveillance

Integrated surveillance systems emerge from recognising that health threats transcend traditional sectoral boundaries, requiring coordinated responses across multiple domains. This represents a paradigm shift from isolated disease monitoring to comprehensive systems that synthesise data from human, animal, environmental, and food safety sectors. Approximately 75% of emerging infectious diseases originate from animals, with pathogen spillover occurring at the interfaces between humans and ecosystems (WHO, 2023).

The foundational principle underlying integrated surveillance is the One Health approach, which recognises the interconnectedness of human, animal, and environmental health as inseparable components of the ecosystem. This holistic perspective enables earlier threat detection, more comprehensive risk characterisation, and more effective interventions than traditional approaches, achieved through harmonised data collection methods, standardised case definitions, uniform reporting protocols, and shared analytical frameworks.

Modern integrated surveillance operates on core principles that distinguish it from conventional approaches. Multi-sectoral data integration captures information from clinical networks, veterinary monitoring, environmental sensing, and community reporting, thereby detecting subtle patterns that are often missed by isolated systems. Real-time data sharing facilitates rapid information exchange through advanced digital platforms, enabling continuous streaming, automated analysis, and immediate alerts. Standardised data formats and interoperability protocols ensure information from different sectors can be combined within unified analytical frameworks.

Implementation requires substantial coordination between organisations with different mandates: human health systems focus on clinical cases and outbreak investigation, animal health emphasises disease freedom and trade facilitation, environmental systems prioritise ecosystem monitoring, and food safety focuses on contamination prevention and consumer protection.

4.2. Human, Animal, and Environmental Surveillance Networks

An integrated surveillance system architecture encompasses three harmonised primary domains for effective cross-sectoral monitoring. Human health surveillance networks form the foundation, building upon decades of experience in infectious disease monitoring through hierarchical structures that connect local facilities with district, regional, and national authorities across multiple administrative levels.

Contemporary human health systems have evolved beyond traditional passive reporting to incorporate active surveillance strategies, sentinel monitoring networks, and syndromic surveillance platforms. Syndromic surveillance represents a significant innovation, utilising indicators such as fever and respiratory symptoms to detect potential outbreaks before laboratory confirmation. These systems analyse emergency department visits, pharmacy sales, and absenteeism patterns in schools. The COVID-19 pandemic highlighted the critical importance of syndromic surveillance when traditional laboratory-based systems became overwhelmed (Ramos et al., 2024).

Animal health surveillance networks operate through different organisational structures, focusing on livestock populations and wildlife monitoring. Wildlife surveillance has emerged as crucial for detecting zoonotic pathogens. Cambodia's Wildlife Health Surveillance Network exemplifies this approach, where environmental stewards monitor wildlife health events to provide early warnings of avian influenza and other zoonotic threats (WHO, 2024).

Environmental surveillance networks provide essential information about ecosystem health, ecological contamination, and climate factors that influence disease transmission. These systems monitor air quality, water contamination, biodiversity indicators, and meteorological variables. Integration enables sophisticated risk assessment models accounting for ecological drivers. Remote sensing technologies enable continuous monitoring across large geographic areas, tracking changes in land use, deforestation, urbanisation, and climate variables that influence disease emergence.

The integration of human, animal, and environmental surveillance networks require sophisticated data management platforms that can accommodate diverse data types, reporting frequencies, and analytical requirements. RespiMART, developed by the World Health Organisation, exemplifies this approach by providing a central data platform that exchanges, harmonises, consolidates, and stores surveillance data on respiratory viruses, including influenza, SARS-CoV-2, and respiratory syncytial virus (WHO, 2024). This platform supports both FluNet for virological surveillance data and FluID for epidemiological surveillance data, demonstrating how integrated systems can accommodate different types of surveillance information within unified analytical frameworks. Table 4.1 shows a comparison of surveillance network characteristics.

4.3. Technology and Digital Health Solutions

The advancement of integrated surveillance systems depends critically on technological innovations that enable efficient data collection, transmission, analysis, and visualisation across multiple sectors and geographic scales. Digital health solutions have transformed surveillance capabilities by providing platforms for real-time data sharing, automated analysis, and coordinated response. These technologies address fundamental challenges in traditional surveillance systems, including delayed reporting, fragmented data management, and limited analytical capabilities.

Mobile health technologies have revolutionised data collection in resource-limited settings by enabling healthcare workers to report surveillance information directly from field locations using smartphones and tablet devices. These mobile platforms support standardised data entry forms, automated data validation, and immediate transmission to central databases, significantly reducing reporting delays and improving data quality. Mobile technologies also enable two-way communication between field workers and surveillance coordinators, facilitating real-time guidance, quality assurance, and response coordination.

Cloud computing platforms provide the necessary infrastructure to support large-scale surveillance operations, offering reliable data storage, processing capacity, and accessibility from multiple locations. Cloud-based surveillance systems can accommodate sudden increases in data volume during outbreak situations, provide redundant data storage to prevent information loss, and enable simultaneous access by multiple users across different organisations and geographic locations. These platforms also support automated backup procedures, data security protocols, and disaster recovery capabilities that are essential for maintaining surveillance operations during emergencies.

Artificial intelligence and machine learning technologies are increasingly integrated into surveillance systems to enhance pattern detection, automate alert generation, and support predictive modelling capabilities. Machine learning algorithms can identify subtle patterns in surveillance data that traditional analytical approaches might miss, detect anomalies that suggest emerging threats, and generate automated alerts when predefined thresholds are exceeded. Natural language processing technologies enable automated analysis of unstructured text data from social media, news reports, and informal communication channels, providing additional sources of surveillance information (McClymont et al., 2024).

The application of artificial intelligence in surveillance systems has demonstrated significant potential for enhancing early warning capabilities. Machine learning algorithms can identify subtle patterns in surveillance data that traditional analytical approaches might miss, detect anomalies that suggest emerging threats, and generate automated alerts when predefined thresholds are exceeded. Natural language processing technologies enable automated analysis of unstructured text data from social media, news reports, and informal communication channels, providing additional sources of surveillance information (McClymont et al., 2024).

Blockchain technologies offer promising solutions for ensuring data integrity, supporting secure information sharing, and maintaining audit trails in multi-organisational surveillance networks. Blockchain platforms can provide tamper-proof data storage, enable controlled access to sensitive surveillance information, and support automated execution of data sharing agreements between organisations. These capabilities are particularly valuable in international surveillance networks where trust, accountability, and data provenance are critical concerns.

Geographic information systems provide essential capabilities for spatial analysis, mapping, and visualisation of surveillance data across geographic scales. These systems enable identification of geographic clustering patterns, support risk mapping activities, and facilitate resource allocation decisions based on the spatial distribution of surveillance indicators. Advanced GIS platforms integrate real-time surveillance data with demographic, environmental, and infrastructure datasets to support comprehensive situational awareness and decision-making processes.

Data integration platforms represent perhaps the most critical technological component of integrated surveillance systems, providing the infrastructure necessary to combine data streams from multiple sectors, organisations, and geographic locations. These platforms must accommodate diverse data formats, harmonise different reporting standards, and provide analytical tools that can generate meaningful insights from complex, multi-dimensional datasets. The WHO's RespiMART platform demonstrates how successful data integration can support global surveillance networks by providing centralised data management, standardised reporting protocols, and analytical capabilities that serve multiple surveillance programs simultaneously. Table 4.2 shows digital health technologies in integrated surveillance.

4.4. Early Warning Systems and Alert Mechanisms

Early warning systems represent the operational culmination of integrated surveillance activities, transforming surveillance data into actionable intelligence that can trigger timely public health responses. These systems utilise sophisticated algorithms, threshold-based monitoring, and predictive modelling to detect emerging threats before they develop into major public health emergencies. The effectiveness of early warning systems depends critically on the quality and timeliness of surveillance data, the appropriateness of analytical methods, and the responsiveness of public health agencies to generated alerts.

Contemporary early warning systems operate through multiple complementary mechanisms that provide different types of information about potential health threats. Threshold-based monitoring systems continuously analyse surveillance indicators against predetermined benchmarks, generating alerts when reported cases, laboratory confirmations, or syndromic indicators exceed expected levels. These systems typically employ statistical models that account for seasonal patterns, secular trends, and reporting variations to distinguish genuine increases in disease activity from normal fluctuations in surveillance data.

Predictive modelling approaches utilise mathematical models to forecast disease trends based on current surveillance data, environmental conditions, and population characteristics. These models can provide advanced warning of potential outbreaks, estimate the magnitude and geographic extent of emerging threats, and assess the likely effectiveness of different intervention strategies.

Table 4.1. Comparison of surveillance network characteristics

Surveillance Domain	Primary Focus	Data Types	Reporting Frequency	Key Challenges
Human Health	Clinical cases, outbreaks, public health threats	Case reports, laboratory results, and syndromic indicators	Daily to weekly	Privacy protection, data quality, reporting compliance
Animal Health	Livestock disease, wildlife health, zoonotic risks	Veterinary diagnoses, production data, and mortality events	Weekly to monthly	Limited wildlife access, resource constraints, and farmer cooperation
Environmental Health	Ecosystem indicators, contamination, and climate factors	Sensor data, laboratory analyses, and remote sensing	Continuous to seasonal	Spatial coverage, sensor maintenance, data interpretation

Table 4.2. Digital health technologies in integrated surveillance

Technology Category	Applications	Advantages	Implementation Challenges
Mobile Health Platforms	Field data collection, real-time reporting	Reduced reporting delays, improved accessibility	Device management, network coverage, and user training
Artificial Intelligence	Pattern detection, automated alerts, predictive modelling	Enhanced sensitivity, reduced false positives	Algorithm validation, data quality requirements
Cloud Computing	Data storage, processing, and multi-user access	Scalability, reliability, cost-effectiveness	Security concerns, internet dependency
Blockchain	Data integrity, secure sharing, audit trails	Enhanced trust, tamper-proof records	Technical complexity, energy consumption
Geographic Information Systems	Spatial analysis, mapping, risk assessment	Geographic insights, visualisation capabilities	Data integration complexity, technical expertise requirements

Table 4.3. Data integration challenges and solutions

Challenge Category	Specific Issues	Potential Solutions	Implementation Requirements
Technical Interoperability	Diverse data formats, incompatible systems	Standardised APIs, standard data formats	Technical expertise, infrastructure investment
Semantic Interoperability	Inconsistent definitions, terminology conflicts	Data dictionaries, ontology development	Cross-sectoral collaboration, expert consensus
Organisational Interoperability	Different mandates, reporting structures	Memoranda of understanding, governance frameworks	Leadership commitment, policy alignment
Legal and Policy Barriers	Privacy regulations, data sharing restrictions	Data governance frameworks, consent mechanisms	Legal expertise, policy development
Resource Constraints	Limited funding, technical capacity	Shared infrastructure, international cooperation	Sustained funding commitments, capacity building

Machine learning approaches have shown promise for predictive modelling applications, as they can incorporate complex, non-linear relationships between surveillance indicators and disease outcomes that traditional statistical models cannot adequately capture.

Event-based surveillance systems monitor informal information sources, such as media reports, social media posts, and unofficial communications, to detect unusual health events that may not be captured through formal surveillance channels. These systems provide complementary information to indicator-based surveillance by identifying potential threats that have not yet been reported through formal systems. The integration of event-based and indicator-based surveillance creates comprehensive early warning capabilities that can detect threats through multiple pathways (Patel et al., 2024).

The implementation of early warning systems requires careful attention to the trade-offs between sensitivity and specificity that determine the system's ability to detect genuine threats while minimising false alarms. High-sensitivity systems detect most genuine threats but may generate numerous false alarms, which can overwhelm response capabilities and erode confidence in the system. High specificity systems minimise false alarms but may miss genuine threats, particularly those with unusual characteristics or those occurring in unexpected locations or populations.

Automated alert generation mechanisms utilise predefined algorithms to evaluate surveillance data and generate alerts when specified criteria are met. These systems can provide immediate notification of potential threats, enabling rapid response initiation. However, automated systems require careful calibration to ensure that generated alerts are actionable and relevant to public health priorities. Many successful early warning systems combine automated alert generation with human expert review to ensure that alerts are appropriately prioritised and context-specific information is incorporated into alert messages.

Communication systems represent a critical component of early warning infrastructure, ensuring that generated alerts reach relevant decision-makers and response personnel promptly. Modern alert systems utilise multiple communication channels, including e-mail, text messaging, mobile applications, and web-based dashboards, to ensure that alerts are received even if primary communication channels are disrupted. Alert messages must be clear, actionable, and contain sufficient information to enable appropriate response decisions.

The COVID-19 pandemic highlighted both the potential and limitations of early warning systems in detecting and responding to emerging health threats. While several surveillance systems detected unusual pneumonia cases in the early stages of the pandemic, delays in information sharing, limitations in laboratory capacity, and challenges in international coordination hindered the global response. These experiences have informed ongoing efforts to strengthen early warning capabilities through improved data sharing protocols, enhanced laboratory networks, and more robust international coordination mechanisms.

China's experience with artificial intelligence-based surveillance systems during dengue prevention and control demonstrates the potential of advanced early warning technologies. Modern integrated systems can successfully capture and integrate multi-channel surveillance data, utilise artificial intelligence models to trigger early warnings, and provide comprehensive tools for risk assessment and emergency response coordination. The system's ability to proactively capture and integrate heterogeneous surveillance data from multiple sources enables more timely and effective responses to emerging threats.

4.5. Data Integration and Interoperability Challenges

Successful implementation of integrated surveillance depends critically on addressing complex technical, organisational, and policy challenges related to data integration and interoperability. These challenges arise from fundamental differences in data structures, reporting standards, and organisational cultures across the human health, animal health, environmental health, and food safety sectors.

Technical interoperability challenges arise from diverse data formats, database structures, and analytical platforms. Human health systems utilise standardised classifications, such as the International Classification of Diseases, while animal health systems rely on different taxonomies optimised for veterinary applications. Data standardisation efforts focus on developing common data elements, standardised vocabularies, and harmonised reporting formats to ensure consistency and accuracy. The Fast Healthcare Interoperability Resources (FHIR) standard has emerged as a leading framework for health data exchange, providing standardised formats that are extendable across multiple sectors.

Semantic interoperability challenges involve ensuring data elements have consistent meanings across systems. Terms like "case," "outbreak," and "surveillance" may have different definitions across various sectors, necessitating comprehensive data dictionaries and standardised definitions.

Organisational interoperability challenges emerge from different mandates and reporting requirements. Human health agencies report to health ministries, which focus on population health, while animal health agencies report to agriculture ministries, emphasising food production and trade facilitation.

Legal frameworks governing data sharing vary significantly, with health data privacy regulations, agricultural data protection policies, and environmental data restrictions creating barriers. Resource constraints pose persistent challenges, particularly in resource-limited settings, necessitating higher upfront investments and ongoing operational expenses.

The European Union's antimicrobial resistance surveillance highlights both the potential and challenges of multi-sectoral integration, necessitating extensive agency coordination, laboratory method harmonisation, and innovative analytical approaches that accommodate diverse data sources (Delpy et al., 2024). Table 4.3 presents data integration challenges and their corresponding solutions.

4.6. Case Study: Influenza Surveillance Networks

The Global Influenza Surveillance and Response System (GISRS) represents one of the most successful examples of international integrated surveillance, demonstrating how coordinated global networks can provide effective early warning capabilities for pandemic threats. Established in 1952, GISRS has evolved from a network of influenza monitoring laboratories into a comprehensive surveillance system that monitors influenza viruses, provides recommendations for seasonal vaccine composition, and serves as a global alert mechanism for pandemic threats (McCauley & Hay, 2018).

GISRS operates through a network of 142 National Influenza Centres in 115 countries, supported by six WHO Collaborating Centres, four WHO Essential Regulatory Laboratories, and 13 WHO H5 Reference Laboratories. This network annually tests several million respiratory specimens to monitor the spread and evolution of influenza viruses, providing data that informs both seasonal vaccine development and pandemic preparedness activities. The system's success demonstrates the potential for international cooperation in surveillance while highlighting the technical and organisational challenges involved in maintaining global networks.

The technical infrastructure of GISRS centres on two primary databases: FluNet, for virological surveillance data, and FluID, for epidemiological surveillance data. These platforms enable participating laboratories to report surveillance findings in standardised formats, facilitating global analysis and comparison of influenza activity patterns. The recent expansion of GISRS to include monitoring of other respiratory viruses, including SARS-CoV-2 and respiratory syncytial virus, demonstrates the system's adaptability to emerging surveillance needs and its potential to serve as a model for integrated respiratory virus surveillance (WHO, 2025).

The operational success of GISRS depends on several key factors that provide lessons for other integrated surveillance initiatives. First, the system maintains clear governance structures that define roles and responsibilities for participating organisations while providing sufficient flexibility to accommodate different national contexts and capabilities. The WHO provides central coordination and technical support while allowing individual countries to adapt surveillance activities to their specific epidemiological situations and resource constraints.

Second, GISRS utilises standardised case definitions, laboratory methods, and reporting protocols that ensure data comparability across different laboratories and countries. These standards are regularly updated to incorporate new diagnostic technologies and evolving understanding of influenza epidemiology, demonstrating the importance of maintaining current technical standards while preserving historical data continuity.

Third, the system emphasises capacity building and technical support to ensure that participating laboratories can maintain quality standards and contribute meaningful data to the global network. This includes training programs, proficiency testing, quality assurance activities, and technical assistance for laboratory strengthening. The WHO's recent training initiatives for the genetic characterisation of influenza and SARS-CoV-2 in Africa exemplify these capacity-building efforts.

The COVID-19 pandemic provided a critical test of GISRS adaptability and demonstrated both the strengths and limitations of existing surveillance networks. GISRS laboratories rapidly adapted their procedures to include SARS-CoV-2 testing and reporting, enabling monitoring of COVID-19 alongside influenza surveillance activities. This adaptation was facilitated by existing laboratory capacity, established reporting relationships, and flexible data management platforms that could accommodate new data elements.

However, the pandemic also revealed challenges in maintaining influenza surveillance activities during periods when healthcare systems were overwhelmed with COVID-19 responses. Many countries reduced influenza testing activities to focus resources on COVID-19, creating gaps in influenza surveillance data during critical periods. This experience underscored the importance of maintaining core surveillance activities even during emergency responses and the necessity for surveillance systems that can simultaneously accommodate multiple pathogens.

The expansion of GISRS into an enhanced global surveillance system (e-GISRS) represents an evolution toward more comprehensive surveillance of respiratory viruses, incorporating lessons learned from the COVID-19 pandemic. This expanded system will monitor epidemic and pandemic threats from multiple respiratory viruses while maintaining the core functions that have made GISRS successful for influenza surveillance. The expansion includes enhanced integration with other surveillance networks, improved early warning capabilities, and strengthened laboratory networks that can support broader monitoring of respiratory viruses.

The leveraging of GISRS infrastructure for COVID-19 surveillance demonstrates how established surveillance networks can provide rapid response capabilities for emerging threats. Countries with strong influenza surveillance systems were better positioned to adapt to COVID-19 surveillance requirements, implement effective testing strategies, and contribute to global situational awareness efforts. This experience validates the investment in sustained surveillance capacity as a critical component of pandemic preparedness.

The success of GISRS provides essential insights for developing other integrated surveillance networks. The system's emphasis on standardised protocols, quality assurance, capacity building, and international cooperation has created a sustainable platform that has operated effectively for over 70 years. The recent expansion to include other respiratory viruses demonstrates how successful surveillance networks can evolve to address new challenges while maintaining their core functions and operational effectiveness.

Conclusion

Successful implementation of integrated surveillance depends critically on addressing complex technical, organisational, and policy challenges related to data integration and interoperability, which emerge from fundamental differences in data structures, reporting standards, and organisational cultures across sectors.

Technical interoperability challenges arise from diverse data formats and analytical platforms. Human health systems utilise the International Classification of Diseases, while animal health systems employ different taxonomies. The Fast Healthcare Interoperability Resources standard has emerged as a leading framework, providing standardised formats that are extendable across sectors.

Semantic interoperability challenges require ensuring data elements have consistent meanings, as terms like "case" and "outbreak" may have different sectoral definitions, necessitating comprehensive data dictionaries.

Organisational interoperability challenges arise from different mandates—health agencies report to health ministries focused on population health, while animal health agencies report to agriculture ministries that emphasise food production.

Legal frameworks governing data sharing vary significantly, creating barriers through health data privacy regulations and agricultural data protection policies. Resource constraints represent persistent challenges, particularly in resource-limited settings.

The European Union's antimicrobial resistance surveillance highlights both the potential and challenges, necessitating extensive coordination, laboratory harmonisation, and innovative analytical approaches (Delpy et al., 2024). Table 4.3 presents data integration challenges and corresponding solutions.

Acknowledgments

The authors would like to extend our appreciation to those who offered helpful commentary during the drafting process of this manuscript. We also acknowledge the role Nova Science Publishers played in enabling the work described herein.

References

Delpy, L., Astbury, C. C., Aenishaenslin, C., Häsler, B., Rushton, J., & Ravel, A. (2024). Integrated surveillance systems for antibiotic resistance in a One Health context: a scoping review. *BMC Public Health*, 24, 1717. https://doi.org/10.1186/s12889-024-19158-6.

McCauley, J. W., & Hay, A. J. (2018). The WHO Global Influenza Surveillance and Response System (GISRS)—A future perspective. *Influenza and Other Respiratory Viruses*, 12(5), 551-557. https://doi.org/10.1111/irv.12565.

McClymont, H., Lambert, S. B., Barr, I., Durrheim, D. N., Trent, M., & Dalton, C. B. (2024). Internet-based surveillance systems and infectious diseases prediction: An updated review of the last 10 years and lessons from the COVID-19 pandemic. *Journal of Epidemiology and Global Health*, 14, 645-657. https://doi.org/10.1007/s44197-024-00272-y.

Patel, A., Maruthananth, K., Matharu, N., Pinto, A. D., & Hosseini, B. (2024). Early warning systems for acute respiratory infections: scoping review of global evidence. *JMIR Public Health and Surveillance*, 10, e62641. https://doi.org/10.2196/62641.

Ramos, P. I. P., Marcilio, I., Bento, A. I., Penna, G. O., de Oliveira, J. F., Khouri, R., Andrade, R. F. S., Carreiro, R. P., Oliveira, V. A., Galvão, L. A. C., Landau, L., Barreto, M. L., van der Horst, K., & Barral-Netto, M. (2024). Combining digital and molecular approaches using Health and alternate data sources in a next-generation surveillance system for anticipating outbreaks of pandemic potential. *JMIR Public Health and Surveillance*, 10, e47673. https://doi.org/10.2196/47673.

Singh, S., Sharma, P., Pal, N., Sarma, D. K., Tiwari, R., & Kumar, M. (2024). Holistic one health surveillance framework: synergising environmental, animal, and human determinants for enhanced infectious disease management. *ACS Infectious Diseases*, 10, 808-826. https://doi.org/10.1021/acsinfecdis.3c00625.

World Health Organization. (2023). One Health. https://www.who.int/news-room/fact-sheets/detail/one-health.

World Health Organization. (2024). One Health in action: What wildlife health surveillance can tell us about pandemic prevention. https://www.who.int/westernpacific/newsroom/feature-stories/item/one-health-in-action--what-wildlife-health-surveillance-can-tell-us-about-pandemic-prevention.

World Health Organization. (2024). Global Influenza Surveillance and Response System (GISRS). https://www.who.int/initiatives/global-influenza-surveillance-and-response-system.

World Health Organization. (2025). Expanding the Global Influenza Surveillance and Response System to include other respiratory viruses with epidemic or pandemic potential. https://www.who.int/news/item/25-03-2025-expanding-the-global-influenza-surveillance-and-response-system-to-include-other-respiratory-viruses-with-epidemic-or-pandemic-potential.

Zhang, H., Wang, L., Lai, S., Li, Z., Sun, Q., & Zhang, P. (2017). Surveillance and early warning systems of infectious disease in China: From 2012 to 2014. *International Journal of Health Planning and Management*, 32(3), 329-338. https://doi.org/10.1002/hpm.2434.

Chapter 5

Emerging Infectious Diseases: Patterns, Predictions, and Preparedness

Pratap Bhan Kaushik[1] and Maajid Mohi Ud Din Malik[2,*], PhD

[1]Department of Community Medicine, Dr. D. Y. Patil Medical College, Hospital and Research Centre, Dr. D. Y. Patil Vidyapeeth, Pune (Deemed to be University)- Sant Tukaram Nagar, Pimpri, Pune, India
[2]Department of Radiology and Imaging Technology, Dr. D. Y. Patil School of Allied Health Sciences, Dr. D. Y. Patil Vidyapeeth· Pune (Deemed to be University), Sant Tukaram Nagar, Pimpri, Pune, India

Abstract

The 21st Century has witnessed an unprecedented surge in emerging infectious diseases (EIDs), from SARS in 2003 to the COVID-19 pandemic, highlighting critical vulnerabilities in global health security. This chapter examines the complex patterns of disease emergence, the multiple drivers contributing to increased EID frequency, and the evolving strategies for prediction and preparedness. Emerging infectious diseases are defined as infections that have newly appeared in a population or are rapidly increasing in incidence or geographic range, with approximately 75% originating from animal sources through zoonotic spillover events. Historical analysis reveals accelerating patterns of emergence driven by globalisation, urbanisation, climate change, land-use modifications, and increased human-animal interactions. Advanced predictive modelling approaches, including mathematical transmission models, risk assessment frameworks, and artificial intelligence applications, are transforming our ability to anticipate and respond to emerging threats. Case studies of SARS, MERS, COVID-19, and mpox demonstrate both the devastating potential of EIDs and the critical importance of rapid detection, coordinated international response, and sustained preparedness investments. Modern preparedness frameworks emphasise the One Health approach, integrating human, animal, and environmental health surveillance systems to enable early warning and coordinated response capabilities. These developments directly support Sustainable Development Goal 3 (Good Health and Well-being) by strengthening the resilience and pandemic preparedness capacities of health systems, which are essential for protecting global population health.

---

* Corresponding Author's Email: maajid.malik@dpu.edu.in

In: Advances in the One Health Approach
Editors: Maajid Mohi Ud Din Malik, Abhay Saraf, Harshal Tukaram Pandve et al.
ISBN: 979-8-90134-202-2

Keywords: emerging infectious diseases, zoonotic spillover, One Health approach, predictive modelling, risk assessment, SARS, MERS, COVID-19, Mpox, pandemic preparedness, global health security, SDG 3 Good Health and Well-being, surveillance systems, early warning systems

Introduction

The emergence of infectious diseases represents one of the most persistent and evolving threats to global health security in the modern era. While contagious diseases have shaped human history for millennia, the 21st Century has ushered in an unprecedented period of disease emergence characterised by increased frequency, geographic spread, and potential for pandemic development. The severe acute respiratory syndrome outbreak in 2003, the H1N1 influenza pandemic in 2009, the Middle East respiratory syndrome emergence in 2012, the Ebola epidemic in West Africa from 2013-2016, and most notably the COVID-19 pandemic beginning in 2019, have collectively demonstrated both the devastating potential of emerging infectious diseases and the critical importance of robust preparedness and response systems.

Understanding the patterns, drivers, and dynamics of disease emergence has become essential for protecting global health security and achieving sustainable development objectives. The complex interplay between pathogen evolution, environmental changes, human behaviour, and social systems creates conditions that facilitate the spillover of pathogens from animal reservoirs to human populations and their subsequent adaptation for human-to-human transmission. These emerging events are no longer isolated incidents but represent predictable consequences of anthropogenic environmental changes, globalisation processes, and increasing connectivity between previously separated ecological and social systems.

This chapter provides a comprehensive examination of emerging infectious diseases from both historical and contemporary perspectives, analysing the factors driving increased emergence frequency, exploring advanced approaches to prediction and risk assessment, and evaluating the preparedness frameworks necessary to mitigate future pandemic threats. Through detailed case studies and analysis of current surveillance and response systems, this chapter contributes to a broader understanding of how integrated health security approaches can strengthen global resilience against emerging infectious disease threats, while supporting the achievement of Sustainable Development Goal 3 and broader sustainable development objectives.

5.1. Defining Emerging and Re-Emerging Infectious Diseases

The conceptual framework for understanding emerging infectious diseases has evolved significantly, reflecting advances in scientific understanding and practical challenges of identifying novel health threats. Emerging infectious diseases are defined as those "that have newly appeared in a population or have existed but are rapidly increasing in incidence or geographic range" (Today's Clinical Lab, 2024), encompassing genuinely novel pathogens and previously known pathogens expanding into new populations or demonstrating altered characteristics.

Re-emerging infectious diseases refer to infections that were previously controlled but are experiencing resurgence due to environmental changes, infrastructure deterioration, social behaviours, or pathogen characteristics. The World Health Organisation's R&D Blueprint maintains a priority list, including known threats and "Disease X," which represents serious international epidemic potential from pathogens currently unknown to cause human disease (WHO, 2024).

Epidemiological characteristics defining emerging diseases include rapid incidence changes, geographic expansion through human travel and environmental changes, and zoonotic transmission, which represents spillover events from animal reservoirs (Woolhouse & Brierley, 2018). Temporal aspects are crucial—emergence events may occur as isolated spillovers, limited outbreaks, or successful establishment leading to endemic circulation or pandemic spread.

Contemporary understanding emphasises the One Health approach, recognising the interconnectedness of human, animal, and environmental health (Ryu et al., 2017). This perspective acknowledges that most emerging diseases originate in animal populations, requiring surveillance integration across domains for comprehensive monitoring of emergence risk.

5.2. Historical Patterns of Disease Emergence

The historical record reveals distinct patterns of infectious disease emergence that have accelerated dramatically in recent decades, reflecting fundamental changes in human-environment relationships. The 20th and 21st centuries have witnessed unprecedented acceleration in both frequency and global impact of emerging infectious diseases.

The early 21st century represents a particularly intensive period. The SARS outbreak in 2003 demonstrated how previously unknown coronaviruses could rapidly spread across international borders, infecting over 8,000 people across 30 countries with at least 774 deaths (Bell, 2004). The 2009 H1N1 influenza pandemic exhibited efficient human-to-human transmission, prompting the WHO to declare the first influenza pandemic of the 21st century.

The emergence of MERS-CoV in 2012 highlighted sporadic spillover events from dromedary camel reservoirs, which persisted with repeated emergence without achieving pandemic spread (CDC, 2019). The 2013-2016 West Africa Ebola epidemic represented the largest outbreak in history, demonstrating how emerging diseases could overwhelm resource-limited health systems.

The COVID-19 pandemic, which began in 2019, fundamentally altered the understanding of emerging infectious disease potential, with SARS-CoV-2 causing unprecedented global impacts (Zhou et al., 2020).

Analysis reveals concerning trends, including decreasing time intervals between major events, an expanded geographic scope, and increased pathogen diversity. Approximately 75% of emerging infectious diseases originate from animal sources, with spillover events typically occurring at the interfaces between human and wildlife habitats (Wang & Crameri, 2014).

Figure 8 illustrates the chronological progression of significant emerging infectious disease events from 2000 to 2024, demonstrating the accelerating frequency and global impact of disease emergence. The timeline shows major outbreaks including SARS (2003), H1N1 influenza pandemic (2009), MERS emergence (2012), Ebola epidemic in West Africa (2013-2016), Zika virus spread (2015-2016), and COVID-19 pandemic (2019-present), along with recent mpox outbreaks (2022-2024). Each event is mapped with its geographic origin, pathogen type, and scale of global spread, revealing patterns of increasing interconnectedness and rapid international dissemination. The figure demonstrates how the intervals between major emergence events have decreased over time, while the geographic scope and potential for pandemic spread have expanded, reflecting the combined effects of globalisation, environmental change, and enhanced surveillance capabilities that enable earlier detection of emerging threats.

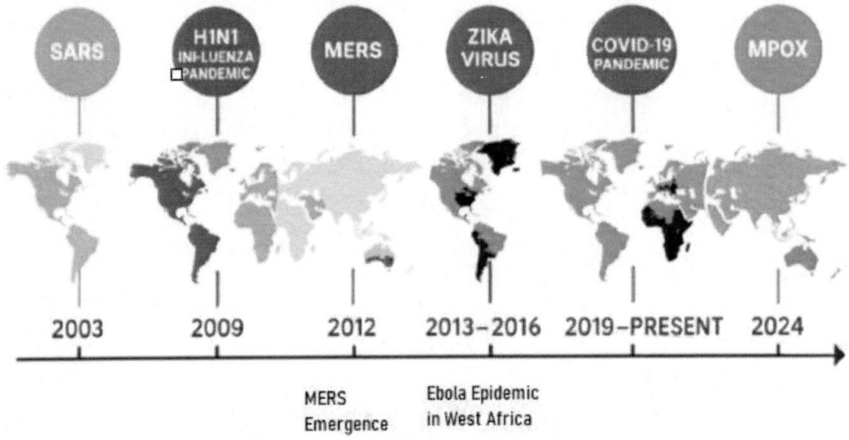

Figure 8. Timeline of major emerging infectious disease events in the 21st century.

Table 5.1 shows major emerging infectious disease events of the 21st century.

5.3. Factors Driving Disease Emergence in the 21st Century

The accelerating frequency and severity of emerging infectious disease events in the 21st Century reflect the convergence of multiple anthropogenic factors that have fundamentally altered the ecological and social conditions governing pathogen-host interactions. These drivers operate at multiple spatial and temporal scales, from local environmental modifications to global climate change, and their synergistic effects create unprecedented opportunities for pathogen spillover, adaptation, and spread. Understanding these drivers is essential for developing effective prevention strategies and anticipating future emergence risks.

Climate change represents one of the most pervasive and significant drivers of infectious disease emergence, operating through multiple mechanisms that affect pathogen survival, vector biology, host susceptibility, and human behaviour. Rising global temperatures have expanded the geographic ranges of many disease vectors, particularly arthropods such as mosquitoes and ticks, enabling the transmission of vector-borne diseases in previously unsuitable climatic zones (Baker et al., 2022). Changes in precipitation patterns, including both increased flooding and prolonged droughts, create new breeding habitats for disease vectors while also affecting water quality and availability, which in turn influence waterborne disease transmission.

Table 5.1. Major emerging infectious disease events of the 21st century

Disease	Year of Emergence	Pathogen Type	Geographic Origin	Primary Transmission Mode	Global Impact
SARS	2003	Coronavirus	China	Respiratory droplets, close contact	>8,000 cases, 774 deaths, 30 countries
H1N1 Influenza	2009	Influenza A virus	Mexico/USA	Respiratory droplets, airborne	>1.4 billion cases, 151,700-575,400 deaths
MERS	2012	Coronavirus	Saudi Arabia	Respiratory droplets, camel contact	>2,600 cases, >900 deaths, 27 countries
Ebola (West Africa)	2013-2016	Filovirus	Guinea	Direct contact with body fluids	>28,600 cases, >11,300 deaths, 10 countries
Zika	2015-2016	Flavivirus	Brazil	Mosquito-borne, sexual transmission	>1 million cases, congenital disabilities, 86 countries
COVID-19	2019-present	Coronavirus	China	Respiratory droplets, airborne	>700 million cases, >7 million deaths, global

Table 5.2. Key drivers of emerging infectious diseases in the 21st century

Driver Category	Specific Mechanisms	Examples of Impact	Geographic Scope
Climate Change	Temperature increase, precipitation changes, extreme weather	Vector range expansion, altered seasonality	Global
Globalisation	International travel, trade networks, and connectivity	Rapid pathogen dissemination, supply chain contamination	Global
Urbanisation	Population density, infrastructure deficits, and environmental modification	Enhanced transmission, vector breeding sites	Regional/Local
Land-use Change	Deforestation, agricultural expansion, and habitat fragmentation	Wildlife-human interface, spillover events	Regional/Local
Agricultural Intensification	Livestock concentration, antimicrobial use, monoculture	Pathogen evolution, resistance development	Regional
Demographic Changes	Population growth, ageing, and immunocompromised populations	Increased susceptibility, transmission potential	Global/Regional

The relationship between climate change and zoonotic disease emergence is particularly complex, involving alterations in wildlife host populations, pathogen survival in environmental reservoirs, and the frequency of human-wildlife contact events. Climate-induced habitat modifications force wildlife populations into new geographic areas, potentially bringing them into closer contact with human populations and domestic animals. Extreme weather events associated with climate change, such as hurricanes, floods, and droughts, can disrupt ecological balances and create opportunities for pathogen spillover through mechanisms such as forced wildlife displacement and environmental contamination.

Globalisation and increased international connectivity have transformed the potential for infectious disease spread from localised outbreaks to pandemic threats within unprecedented time scales. The dramatic expansion of global air travel, with flights more than doubling since 2000, enables infected individuals to reach virtually any location on Earth within 24-48 hours, often before symptoms of infection become apparent (Baker et al., 2022). The compressed timescale between initial exposure and global dissemination presents challenges for traditional public health responses, which rely on case identification, isolation, and contact tracing.

International trade networks have created additional pathways for pathogen dissemination through the movement of animals, animal products, food commodities, and other goods that may harbour infectious agents. The global food system, with its complex supply chains spanning multiple countries and continents, presents opportunities for foodborne pathogens to spread widely before contamination is detected. Similarly, the international trade in wildlife and wildlife products creates pathways for zoonotic pathogens to spread far from their natural reservoirs.

Urbanisation represents another major driver of emerging infectious disease risk, operating through mechanisms that affect both pathogen transmission dynamics and human susceptibility to infection. The rapid growth of urban populations, particularly in developing countries, often occurs without adequate infrastructure development, resulting in overcrowding, inadequate sanitation, and poor waste management that facilitate the transmission of pathogens. Urban environments also create novel ecological niches that can support disease vectors and reservoir species in proximity to dense human populations.

The urban heat island effect, combined with climate change, creates favourable conditions for the expansion of vector-borne diseases into metropolitan areas. Cities provide abundant breeding sites for mosquitoes and other arthropod vectors through features such as stagnant water in containers, stormwater systems, and urban wetlands. The concentration of susceptible human populations in urban areas facilitates efficient pathogen transmission once it occurs, potentially leading to rapid and explosive growth of outbreaks.

Land-use change and environmental modification are direct drivers of emerging infectious disease risk, as they affect wildlife habitats and human-wildlife interfaces. Deforestation, agricultural expansion, mining activities, and infrastructure development bring human populations into contact with previously isolated wildlife populations and their associated pathogens. These activities often create edge effects that concentrate wildlife populations in smaller habitat fragments, potentially increasing pathogen prevalence through stress-related immunosuppression and increased contact rates between hosts.

Agricultural intensification and livestock production systems have created new opportunities for pathogen evolution and spillover through several mechanisms. The concentration of genetically similar animals in high-density production systems creates ideal conditions for the rapid evolution and adaptation of pathogens. The use of antimicrobial agents in agricultural settings contributes to the development of antimicrobial resistance, potentially creating pathogens that are more difficult to treat if they spill over to human populations.

Demographic and social changes have altered human susceptibility to infectious diseases and the potential for disease spread within human populations. Population growth, ageing populations in developed countries, and the increasing prevalence of immunocompromising conditions such as HIV/AIDS and diabetes create larger pools of susceptible individuals. Changes in social behaviours, including patterns of sexual contact, recreational activities, and food consumption practices, can create new pathways for the transmission of emerging pathogens.

Socioeconomic factors, including poverty, inequality, and weak governance systems, contribute to the risk of emerging infectious diseases by limiting the capacity for effective prevention, detection, and response activities. Resource-limited settings often lack the surveillance infrastructure necessary to detect emerging threats early, the laboratory capacity to confirm diagnoses rapidly, or the public health resources to implement effective control measures. Political instability and conflict can further compromise disease surveillance and response capabilities, while also creating population displacement that facilitates the spread of disease. Table 5.2 shows key drivers of emerging infectious diseases.

5.4. Predictive Modelling and Risk Assessment

The development of sophisticated predictive modelling and risk assessment frameworks represents a critical advancement in the global capacity to anticipate, prepare for, and respond to emerging infectious disease threats. These quantitative approaches integrate diverse data sources, including epidemiological surveillance, environmental monitoring, social and economic indicators, and pathogen genomic information, to generate actionable intelligence about current and future disease risks. The evolution from reactive surveillance systems to proactive prediction and early warning capabilities represents a fundamental shift in public health strategy, with the potential to prevent or substantially mitigate future pandemic threats.

Mathematical modelling of infectious disease transmission has emerged as a crucial tool for understanding disease dynamics, evaluating intervention strategies, and informing public health decision-making during outbreaks. Dynamic transmission models simulate the spread of pathogens within populations by incorporating parameters such as transmission rates, incubation periods, infectious periods, and population contact patterns (Ogden et al., 2024). These models can generate predictions about epidemic trajectories, estimate the potential impact of various interventions, and identify optimal strategies for disease control under different scenarios.

The application of mathematical modelling to emerging infectious diseases presents unique challenges compared to modelling well-characterised endemic diseases. For emerging pathogens, key epidemiological parameters may be unknown or highly uncertain during the early stages of an outbreak, requiring models that can accommodate substantial uncertainty and update predictions as new information becomes available. Adaptive modelling approaches that incorporate real-time data updates and uncertainty quantification have become essential tools for supporting decision-making during emerging infectious disease events.

Risk assessment frameworks offer systematic approaches for evaluating the likelihood and potential impact of emerging infectious disease events across various geographic areas, populations, and time horizons. These frameworks typically integrate multiple types of information, including pathogen characteristics, environmental conditions, host population factors, and public health system capabilities, to generate comprehensive risk estimates. The development of standardised risk assessment methodologies enables consistent evaluation of diverse threats and supports resource allocation decisions at local, national, and international levels.

Environmental scanning and horizon scanning approaches complement traditional surveillance systems by monitoring trends and events that may influence future disease emergence risks. Environmental scanning involves the systematic collection and analysis of information about environmental, social, economic, and technological trends that may affect the emergence of infectious diseases. Horizon scanning focuses specifically on identifying potential future threats that may not yet be apparent through conventional surveillance systems but could emerge over medium to long-term time horizons.

The integration of artificial intelligence and machine learning technologies is transforming the capabilities of predictive modelling and risk assessment systems. Machine learning algorithms can identify complex patterns in large datasets that may not be apparent through traditional analytical approaches, enabling the detection of early warning signals for emerging infectious disease events. Natural language processing techniques can analyse vast quantities of unstructured text data from sources such as news reports, social media, and scientific literature to identify potential disease emergence signals before they appear in formal surveillance systems.

Early warning systems represent the operational culmination of predictive modelling and risk assessment activities, providing automated or semi-automated alerts when predefined risk thresholds are exceeded, or unusual patterns are detected in surveillance data. Effective early warning systems must balance sensitivity and specificity to provide timely alerts for genuine threats while minimising false alarms that could overwhelm response systems or reduce confidence in the system. The development of multi-tiered alert systems that offer different levels of warning for various types of threats enables more nuanced and appropriate responses to emerging risks.

Climate-based early warning systems have shown promise for vector-borne diseases, where environmental conditions play a direct role in determining transmission potential. These systems integrate meteorological data, satellite imagery, and epidemiological models to predict seasonal disease risk and identify areas where enhanced surveillance or preventive interventions may be warranted. For example, the Epidemic Prognosis Incorporating Disease and Environmental Monitoring for Integrated Assessment system uses environmental data to predict malaria epidemic risk in various regions of Africa.

The COVID-19 pandemic has provided an unprecedented natural experiment in the application of predictive modelling and risk assessment to an emerging infectious disease of global importance. Models developed during the pandemic have been used to predict epidemic trajectories, evaluate the potential impact of non-pharmaceutical interventions, guide vaccine allocation strategies, and support decisions about social distancing measures. The experience has highlighted both the tremendous potential of modelling approaches and their limitations, particularly when applied to novel pathogens with uncertain characteristics and in rapidly evolving social and policy environments.

Risk-based surveillance approaches represent an evolution from traditional surveillance systems that monitor all populations equally toward targeted approaches that focus surveillance efforts on areas, populations, or time periods with elevated risk. These approaches use predictive models and risk assessment frameworks to identify high-risk settings and deploy surveillance resources more efficiently. Risk-based surveillance can enable earlier detection of emerging threats while making more efficient use of limited surveillance resources.

5.5. Examples: SARS, MERS, COVID-19, Mpox

The examination of specific emerging infectious disease events provides critical insights into the diverse patterns of disease emergence, the factors that influence pandemic potential, and the effectiveness of different response strategies. The cases of SARS, MERS, COVID-19, and mpox represent a spectrum of emergence patterns, from successfully contained outbreaks to global pandemics, illustrating both the potential for effective response and the challenges of predicting and controlling emerging infectious diseases.

5.5.1. Severe Acute Respiratory Syndrome (SARS)

The emergence of SARS in 2003 marked the first major emerging infectious disease event of the 21st Century. It demonstrated both the pandemic potential of novel coronaviruses and the effectiveness of traditional public health measures when applied systematically. SARS-CoV was first recognised in Guangdong Province, China, in November 2002. Still, the virus spread rapidly to other regions within China and to Hong Kong, Vietnam, Singapore, Taiwan, and Toronto, Canada, in the early half of 2003 (Bell, 2004).

The epidemiological characteristics of SARS-CoV distinguished it from other respiratory viruses in several essential ways, ultimately contributing to the success of control efforts. Unlike influenza viruses, SARS-CoV demonstrated relatively low transmissibility during the early stages of illness, with most transmission occurring after symptom onset and particularly among severely ill patients. This characteristic enabled public health authorities to identify and isolate cases before peak infectiousness, breaking chains of transmission more effectively than would be possible with more readily transmissible pathogens.

The global response to SARS demonstrated the potential for international cooperation and coordination in controlling emerging infectious diseases. The World Health Organisation played a central coordinating role, issuing global alerts, providing technical guidance, and facilitating the sharing of information between affected countries. The rapid identification of the causative agent through international laboratory networks enabled the development of diagnostic tests and the implementation of case-based surveillance systems. Travel advisories and screening measures at international borders helped limit the geographic spread of the outbreak. The containment of SARS was achieved through the aggressive application of traditional public health measures, including case finding and isolation, contact tracing and quarantine, infection control measures in healthcare settings, and community-level interventions such as school closures and restrictions on mass gatherings. The success of these measures demonstrated that even novel emerging infectious diseases could be controlled through well-coordinated public health responses, provided that the epidemiological characteristics of the pathogen were favourable for control.

The economic and social impacts of the SARS outbreak, although significant, were relatively limited compared to those of subsequent pandemic events. The outbreak cost the global economy billions of dollars through impacts on travel, tourism, and trade. Still, these effects were primarily concentrated in directly affected regions and resolved relatively quickly after the outbreak was contained. The SARS experience provided valuable lessons about the potential for emerging infectious diseases to cause substantial economic disruption even when successfully contained from a public health perspective.

5.5.2. Middle East Respiratory Syndrome (MERS)

The emergence of MERS-CoV in 2012 highlighted a distinct pattern of emerging infectious disease persistence, characterised by sporadic spillover events from animal reservoirs that resulted in limited chains of human-to-human transmission, ultimately failing to achieve sustained pandemic spread. MERS was first identified in Saudi Arabia in 2012 and has continued to cause sporadic outbreaks for over a decade, primarily in the Middle East region, with occasional exportation to other countries through international travel.

The epidemiological characteristics of MERS-CoV demonstrate significant differences from those of SARS-CoV, which have influenced its transmission patterns and control challenges. MERS-CoV exhibits higher case fatality rates than SARS-CoV, with approximately 35% of reported cases resulting in death, but demonstrates lower efficiency of human-to-human transmission. Most human infections result from direct or indirect contact with infected dromedary camels, which serve as the primary intermediate host for the virus. Human-to-human transmission typically requires close contact and has been most commonly observed in healthcare settings.

The persistence of MERS as a recurring threat reflects the continued circulation of the virus in camel populations throughout the Middle East and the ongoing exposure of human populations to infected animals. Unlike SARS-CoV, which appears to have been successfully eliminated from both human and animal populations, MERS-CoV maintains a stable reservoir in dromedary camels, creating the potential for continued spillover events. This pattern illustrates the challenges of controlling emerging infectious diseases when animal reservoirs remain infected and human-animal contact continues.

The healthcare-associated transmission of MERS-CoV has been a particular concern, with several large outbreaks occurring in hospital settings due to inadequate infection control measures. The 2015 outbreak in South Korea, which resulted from a single imported case, demonstrated how MERS-CoV could spread rapidly within healthcare facilities and highlighted the critical importance of early recognition and the implementation of appropriate infection control measures for preventing nosocomial transmission.

The limited international spread of MERS, despite its circulation for more than a decade, reflects both the epidemiological characteristics of the virus and the implementation of enhanced surveillance and response measures based on lessons learned from SARS. Improved global surveillance systems enabled rapid detection and reporting of MERS cases, while enhanced infection control measures in healthcare settings helped prevent large-scale nosocomial outbreaks in most affected countries.

Table 5.3. Comparative analysis of major 21st century emerging infectious diseases

Disease	Pathogen	Year	Geographic Origin	Transmission Efficiency	Case Fatality Rate	Global Spread	Control Status
SARS	SARS-CoV	2003	China	Low ($R_0 \approx 2$-3)	~10%	Limited (30 countries)	Successfully contained
MERS	MERS-CoV	2012	Saudi Arabia	Very Low ($R_0 < 1$)	~35%	Limited (27 countries)	Ongoing sporadic cases
COVID-19	SARS-CoV-2	2019	China	High ($R_0 \approx 2$-6)	~1-3%	Global pandemic	Endemic circulation
Mpox (Clade II)	MPXV	2022	Nigeria	Moderate ($R_0 \approx 1$-2)	<1%	Global (100+ countries)	Controlled but ongoing
Mpox (Clade I)	MPXV	2023	DRC	Moderate	~3%	Regional spread	Active response

5.5.3. COVID-19

The COVID-19 pandemic represents the most significant emerging infectious disease event of the modern era, demonstrating the devastating potential of novel pathogens when they acquire characteristics that enable efficient human-to-human transmission and global spread. SARS-CoV-2 was first identified in Wuhan, China, in December 2019 and spread rapidly across the globe, prompting the World Health Organisation to declare a pandemic in March 2020.

The epidemiological characteristics of SARS-CoV-2 that enabled its pandemic spread differed fundamentally from those of previous emerging coronaviruses. Unlike SARS-CoV, SARS-CoV-2 demonstrated high transmissibility during the presymptomatic and asymptomatic phases of infection, enabling infected individuals to spread the virus before they were aware of their infection. This characteristic made traditional public health measures such as case isolation and contact tracing much more challenging and contributed to the virus's rapid global spread.

The pandemic demonstrated the vulnerability of modern societies to emerging infectious diseases, despite substantial advances in medical knowledge, public health infrastructure, and global coordination mechanisms. Healthcare systems in many countries became overwhelmed during successive waves of infection, leading to excess mortality both from COVID-19 and from other conditions that could not be adequately treated due to healthcare system strain. The social and economic impacts of the pandemic were unprecedented in modern times, with lockdowns, travel restrictions, and other control measures causing massive economic disruption and social upheaval.

The development and deployment of COVID-19 vaccines represented an unprecedented scientific achievement, with multiple effective vaccines developed and authorised for use within one year of the pandemic declaration. The rapid development was enabled by prior research on coronavirus vaccines, particularly work conducted after the SARS and MERS outbreaks, as well as technological advances in vaccine platforms such as mRNA vaccines. However, vaccine distribution was highly unequal, with high-income countries obtaining access to vaccines months or years before they became available in many low-income countries.

The evolution of SARS-CoV-2 during the pandemic has illustrated the dynamic nature of emerging infectious diseases and the challenges of maintaining control measures against rapidly evolving pathogens. The emergence of variants such as Alpha, Delta, and Omicron, each with distinct characteristics regarding transmissibility, virulence, and immune evasion, necessitated the constant adaptation of public health strategies and vaccine formulations. This ongoing evolution demonstrates the need for surveillance systems that can rapidly detect and characterise new variants, as well as response systems that can adapt quickly to changing pathogen characteristics.

5.5.4. Mpox

The mpox outbreaks of 2022-2024 illustrate yet another pattern of emerging infectious disease, involving a pathogen that had circulated for decades in limited geographic areas before acquiring characteristics that enabled broader spread to new populations and geographic regions. Mpox, caused by the monkeypox virus, was first identified in humans in 1970 in the

Democratic Republic of the Congo, where it remained largely confined to Central and West Africa for several decades.

The global mpox outbreak that began in 2022 was caused by a variant of the clade IIb monkeypox virus that demonstrated enhanced transmission capability, particularly through sexual contact networks. This outbreak spread rapidly through multiple countries, primarily affecting men who have sex with men, before expanding to other populations. By the time the World Health Organisation declared the outbreak a public health emergency of international concern in January 2020, the virus had spread to more than 75 countries and caused thousands of infections (WHO, 2024).

The 2023-2024 emergence of clade I mpox in Central Africa represents a separate but related emerging infectious disease event, characterised by distinct epidemiological characteristics and higher case fatality rates compared to the global clade II outbreak. Clade I mpox has caused more than 29,000 cases with over 800 fatalities in the Democratic Republic of the Congo and neighbouring countries, prompting the World Health Organisation to declare another public health emergency of international concern in August 2024 (ECDC, 2024).

The mpox outbreaks illustrate several key principles about the dynamics of emerging infectious diseases. First, pathogens that have circulated in limited areas for extended periods can acquire new characteristics, enabling them to expand into new populations and geographic regions. Second, different clades or variants of the same pathogen can have substantially different epidemiological characteristics, requiring tailored response strategies. Third, stigma and discrimination can significantly complicate outbreak response efforts, particularly when diseases disproportionately affect marginalised populations.

The response to mpox outbreaks has benefited from existing smallpox vaccines, which provide cross-protection against the monkeypox virus, allowing for vaccination strategies targeting high-risk populations. However, vaccine availability has been limited, particularly in African countries where the highest case burdens occur, illustrating ongoing challenges in ensuring equitable access to medical countermeasures during emerging infectious disease events. Table 5.3 presents a comparative analysis of the significant emerging contagious diseases of the 21st Century.

5.6. Preparedness Frameworks and Response Strategies

The development of comprehensive preparedness frameworks and response strategies represents a critical evolution in global health security, moving from reactive crisis management toward proactive risk reduction and rapid response capabilities. These frameworks integrate lessons learned from previous emerging infectious disease events with advances in scientific understanding, technological capabilities, and international cooperation mechanisms to create more effective and equitable approaches to pandemic prevention and control.

The International Health Regulations (2005) provide the foundational legal framework for global infectious disease preparedness and response, establishing core capacities that countries must develop and maintain for detecting, reporting, and responding to public health risks and emergencies. These core capacities encompass surveillance systems, laboratory networks, response capabilities, risk communication systems, and coordination mechanisms that enable effective national and international response to emerging infectious disease threats. Regular assessment of IHR implementation through mechanisms such as the State Party Self-Assessment Annual Reporting and Joint External Evaluations helps identify gaps and track progress in preparedness capacities.

Assessment of global preparedness capacities reveals significant disparities between countries and regions, with many low- and middle-income countries lacking the necessary infrastructure, resources, and technical capacity for effective detection and response to emerging infectious diseases (Oppenheim et al., 2019). Analysis of IHR capacity data from 186 countries between 2018 and 2022 indicates that most countries demonstrate intermediate levels of preparedness across key capacity areas, with substantial room for improvement in areas such as laboratory systems, emergency response, and operational readiness.

The One Health approach has become central to modern preparedness frameworks, recognising that effective emerging infectious disease prevention and control requires integration across human health, animal health, and environmental health sectors. This approach acknowledges that most emerging infectious diseases originate from animal sources and that sustainable prevention strategies must address the ecological and social factors that facilitate pathogen spillover. Implementation of One Health approaches requires coordination mechanisms that enable collaboration between sectors with different mandates, cultures, and operational procedures.

Risk-based preparedness strategies have evolved to focus resources and attention on the most likely and consequential emerging infectious disease threats. These approaches use risk assessment frameworks to identify priority pathogens, geographic areas, and populations for enhanced surveillance and preparedness activities. The WHO R&D Blueprint exemplifies this approach by maintaining a priority list of pathogens requiring urgent research and development attention, enabling focused investment in medical countermeasures for the most concerning threats.

The concept of medical countermeasures has expanded beyond traditional vaccines and therapeutics to encompass a broader range of tools and strategies for preventing and controlling emerging infectious diseases. Modern preparedness frameworks emphasise the importance of platform technologies that can be rapidly adapted to new pathogens, such as mRNA vaccine platforms and monoclonal antibody technologies. The development of prototype vaccines for entire pathogen families, rather than specific pathogens, represents an evolution toward more comprehensive preparedness strategies.

Emergency Use Authorisation mechanisms have been refined based on experience during the COVID-19 pandemic to enable more rapid deployment of medical countermeasures during public health emergencies while maintaining appropriate safety and efficacy standards. These mechanisms balance the need for speed during emergencies with the requirement for adequate evidence of safety and effectiveness, enabling earlier access to potentially life-saving interventions when standard approval timelines would be inadequate.

Global supply chain resilience has emerged as a crucial component of pandemic preparedness, following the disruptions experienced during the COVID-19 pandemic. Preparedness frameworks now emphasise the importance of distributed manufacturing capabilities, strategic stockpiles, and international cooperation mechanisms to ensure equitable access to essential medical countermeasures during emergencies. The establishment of regional manufacturing networks and technology transfer agreements aims to reduce dependence on single sources of supply and improve access in resource-limited settings.

Surveillance system integration represents a fundamental shift toward more comprehensive and sensitive detection capabilities for emerging infectious disease threats. Modern surveillance frameworks integrate traditional indicator-based surveillance with event-based surveillance systems that monitor informal information sources, such as media reports and social media, for early warning signals. The integration of genomic surveillance capabilities enables rapid characterisation of emerging pathogens and real-time monitoring of pathogen evolution during outbreaks.

Risk communication and community engagement have been recognised as essential components of adequate preparedness and response frameworks. The COVID-19 pandemic underscored the crucial importance of clear, consistent, and culturally sensitive communication strategies for maintaining public trust and promoting adherence to public health measures. Preparedness frameworks now emphasise the need for pre-planned communication strategies, community partnership development, and counter-misinformation capabilities.

International cooperation mechanisms have been strengthened through initiatives such as the Pandemic Prevention, Preparedness and Response Accord, being developed under WHO auspices, which aims to establish more robust and equitable frameworks for global pandemic preparedness and response. These mechanisms address challenges identified during previous outbreaks, including information sharing, resource allocation, technology transfer, and coordination of international response activities.

The integration of artificial intelligence and digital technologies is transforming preparedness and response capabilities through applications such as predictive modelling, automated surveillance, digital contact tracing, and telemedicine platforms. These technologies enable more sophisticated risk assessment, faster detection of emerging threats, and more efficient deployment of response resources. However, their implementation requires careful attention to privacy, equity, and digital divide considerations to ensure that technological solutions enhance rather than exacerbate existing health disparities.

Financing mechanisms for pandemic preparedness and response have evolved to address the chronic underinvestment that has limited global preparedness capabilities. Innovative financing approaches, including pandemic bonds, advance market commitments, and international financing facilities, aim to provide sustainable funding for preparedness activities and ensure rapid resource mobilisation during emergencies. The economic analysis of preparedness investments demonstrates that prevention and preparedness activities offer substantial returns on investment compared to the costs of responding to major pandemic events.

Conclusion

Emerging infectious diseases in the 21st century reveal a complex and evolving landscape of health threats that demand sophisticated global responses. The accelerating frequency and severity of disease emergence events, from SARS in 2003 to the ongoing COVID-19 and mpox outbreaks, demonstrate the growing risks associated with anthropogenic environmental changes and the critical importance of robust preparedness systems.

Disease emergence patterns reflect the convergence of multiple drivers, including climate change, globalisation, urbanisation, land-use modifications, and agricultural intensification.

These have increased spillover frequency from animal reservoirs and enhanced potential for rapid global dissemination through international travel and trade networks.

Advances in predictive modelling, artificial intelligence, and risk assessment frameworks enable more sophisticated analysis of emergence risk. Evolution toward One Health approaches represents a fundamental advancement in global health security strategy, integrating surveillance across human, animal, and environmental sectors.

COVID-19 provided unprecedented insights into both the devastating potential and remarkable scientific achievements, including the rapid development of vaccines. Ongoing environmental changes, demographic shifts, and technological advancements will shape future challenges. Investment in preparedness represents both a moral imperative and an economic necessity, with preparedness costs minimal compared to the impacts of a pandemic. Sustained political commitment, adequate resources, and effective international coordination remain essential for protecting global health security.

Acknowledgments

The authors would like to extend our appreciation to those who offered helpful commentary during the drafting process of this manuscript. We also acknowledge the role Nova Science Publishers played in enabling the work described herein.

References

Baker, R. E., Mahmud, A. S., Miller, I. F., Rajeev, M., Rasambainarivo, F., Rice, B. L., Takahashi, S., Tatem, A. J., Wagner, C. E., Wang, L. F., Wesolowski, A., & Metcalf, C. J. E. (2022). Infectious disease in an era of global change. *Nature Reviews Microbiology*, 20(4), 193-205. https://doi.org/10.1038/s41579-021-00639-z.

Bell, D. M. (2004). Public health interventions and SARS spread, 2003. *Emerging Infectious Diseases*, 10(11), 1900-1906. https://doi.org/10.3201/eid1011.040729.

European Centre for Disease Prevention and Control. (2024). Epidemiological update – Week 36/2024: Mpox due to monkeypox virus clade I. https://www.ecdc.europa.eu/en/news-events/mpox-epidemiological-update-week-36-2024-clade-i.

Ogden, N. H., Acheson, E. S., Brown, K., Champredon, D., Colijn, C., Diener, A., Dushoff, J., Earn, D. J. D., Gabriele-Rivet, V., Gangbè, M., Guillouzic, S., Hennessy, D., Hongoh, V., Hurford, A., Kanary, L., Li, M., Ng, V., Otto, S. P., Papst, I., Rees, E. E., Tuite, A., MacLeod, M. R., Murall, C. L., Waddell, L., Wasfi, R., & Wolfson, M. (2024). Mathematical modelling for pandemic preparedness in Canada. *Canada Communicable Disease Report*, 50(10), 329-339. https://doi.org/10.14745/ccdr.v50i10a01.

Oppenheim, B., Gallivan, M., Madhav, N. K., Brown, N., Serhiyenko, V., Wolfe, N. D., & Ayscue, P. (2019). Assessing global preparedness for the next pandemic: development and application of an Epidemic Preparedness Index. *BMJ Global Health*, 4(1), e001157. https://doi.org/10.1136/bmjgh-2018-001157.

Ryu, S., Kim, B. I., Lim, J. S., Tan, C. S., & Chun, B. C. (2017). One Health perspectives on emerging public health threats. *Journal of Preventive Medicine and Public Health*, 50(6), 411-414. https://doi.org/10.3961/jpmph.17.097.

Today's Clinical Lab. (2024). Emerging pathogens: A look toward 2024. https://www.clinicallab.com/emerging-pathogens-a-look-toward-2024-27676.

Wang, L. F., & Crameri, G. (2014). Emerging zoonotic viral diseases. *Revue Scientifique et Technique*, 33(2), 569-581. https://doi.org/10.20506/rst.33.2.2311.

World Health Organization. (2024). Prioritising diseases for research and development in emergency contexts. https://www.who.int/activities/prioritizing-diseases-for-research-and-development-in-emergency-contexts.

World Health Organization. (2024). WHO Director-General declares mpox outbreak a public health emergency of international concern. https://www.who.int/news/item/14-08-2024-who-director-general-declares-mpox-outbreak-a-public-health-emergency-of-international-concern.

Woolhouse, M. E. J., & Brierley, L. (2018). Epidemiological characteristics of human-infective RNA viruses. *PLoS ONE*, 13(9), e0204644. https://doi.org/10.1371/journal.pone.0204644.

Zhou, P., Yang, X. L., Wang, X. G., Hu, B., Zhang, L., Zhang, W., Si, H. R., Zhu, Y., Li, B., Huang, C. L., Chen, H. D., Chen, J., Luo, Y., Guo, H., Jiang, R. D., Liu, M. Q., Chen, Y., Shen, X. R., Wang, X., Zheng, X. S., Zhao, K., Chen, Q. J., Deng, F., Liu, L. L., Yan, B., Zhan, F. X., Wang, Y. Y., Xiao, G. F., & Shi, Z. L. (2020). A pneumonia outbreak associated with a new coronavirus of probable bat origin. *Nature*, 579(7798), 270-273. https://doi.org/10.1038/s41586-020-2012-7.

Chapter 6

Disease Risk Assessment and Emergency Response Planning

Chhaya Mahesh Suryawanshi[1] and Maajid Mohi Ud Din Malik[2,*], PhD

[1]Department of Anesthesiology, Dr. D. Y. Patil Medical College, Hospital and Research Centre, Dr. D. Y. Patil Vidyapeeth, Pune (Deemed to be University)- Sant Tukaram Nagar, Pimpri, Pune, India
[2]Department of Radiology and Imaging Technology, Dr. D. Y. Patil School of Allied Health Sciences, Dr. D. Y. Patil Vidyapeeth· Pune (Deemed to be University), Sant Tukaram Nagar, Pimpri, Pune, India

Abstract

Disease risk assessment and emergency response planning represent critical components of global health security, requiring systematic evaluation of threats, vulnerabilities, and response capacities. This chapter examines contemporary methodologies for assessing disease risks, including quantitative and qualitative approaches that integrate epidemiological, environmental, and social determinants. The analysis encompasses vulnerability mapping techniques that identify geographic and demographic hotspots, enabling targeted interventions and resource allocation. Emergency response protocols are explored through multi-sector coordination frameworks that bridge public health, healthcare systems, and community engagement mechanisms. Communication strategies during health emergencies are examined, emphasising risk communication, community engagement, and information management systems. The chapter synthesises lessons learned from recent outbreaks, including COVID-19, Ebola, and Zika virus epidemics, highlighting strengths and gaps in preparedness systems. The integration of One Health approaches, digital surveillance technologies, and equity considerations in emergency planning is emphasised as an essential element for sustainable health security. These findings contribute to achieving Sustainable Development Goal 3 (Good Health and Well-being) by strengthening the resilience and emergency preparedness capabilities of health systems.

Keywords: disease surveillance, risk assessment, emergency preparedness, vulnerability mapping, outbreak response, health security, One Health, Sustainable Development Goal 3

---

* Corresponding Author's Email: maajid.malik@dpu.edu.in

In: Advances in the One Health Approach
Editors: Maajid Mohi Ud Din Malik, Abhay Saraf, Harshal Tukaram Pandve et al.
ISBN: 979-8-90134-202-2

Introduction

Disease risk assessment and emergency response planning have emerged as critical components of contemporary public health practice, particularly in an era characterised by increasing frequency and complexity of health emergencies. The global interconnectedness of modern society, coupled with environmental changes and emerging infectious disease threats, necessitates sophisticated approaches to anticipating, preparing for, and responding to health crises. The conceptual framework for emergency preparedness has evolved significantly from reactive disaster response models toward proactive risk management systems that emphasise prevention, early detection, and rapid response capabilities (Nelson et al., 2007).

The integration of One Health approaches, which recognise the interconnections among human, animal, and environmental health, has fundamentally transformed risk assessment methodologies and response planning frameworks (Kahn, 2006). Contemporary emergency preparedness systems must address complex, multi-sectoral challenges that require coordination across diverse organisational boundaries and jurisdictional levels. The lessons learned from recent major outbreaks, including the 2014-2016 West Africa Ebola epidemic and the COVID-19 pandemic, have highlighted both the critical importance of robust preparedness systems and the substantial gaps that persist in global health security capabilities (Kruk et al., 2015). This chapter examines the current state of disease risk assessment and emergency response planning, analysing methodological approaches, operational frameworks, and lessons learned that inform contemporary practice and future directions for strengthening health security systems.

6.1. Risk Assessment Methodologies

Risk assessment methodologies in disease surveillance and emergency preparedness have undergone significant evolution, incorporating sophisticated analytical frameworks integrating multiple data sources and modelling approaches (Brownstein et al., 2009). Contemporary approaches encompass both quantitative and qualitative methods, each offering distinct advantages for evaluating complex epidemiological landscapes.

Quantitative methodologies rely on mathematical modelling and statistical analysis, utilising compartmental models such as the susceptible-infected-recovered (SIR) model to estimate outbreak probability and potential impact. Advanced approaches integrate machine learning algorithms and artificial intelligence techniques, processing vast heterogeneous data, including social media trends, climate data, mobility patterns, and genomic information, to identify early warning signals.

Qualitative methodologies complement quantitative approaches by incorporating expert knowledge and contextual factors through structured frameworks, such as failure mode and effects analysis (FMEA) and hazard analysis and critical control points (HACCP). Expert elicitation techniques, including Delphi surveys, capture professional judgment where historical data is limited.

The integration of social determinants—such as socioeconomic status, housing conditions, and healthcare access—has gained recognition as essential for comprehensive threat evaluation. Environmental risk factors, particularly climate change and ecological degradation, have become central considerations.

Geographic information systems and spatial analysis techniques have revolutionised risk assessment capabilities, enabling the visualisation of spatial patterns and risk clusters. Temporal aspects incorporate seasonal patterns and long-term trends through the analysis of time series. Multi-hazard approaches address complex interactions between different health threats, while uncertainty quantification acknowledges inherent limitations. Participatory methodologies are increasingly engaging communities, incorporating local knowledge and fostering ownership of preparedness initiatives. Table 6.1 presents a comparison of risk assessment methodologies.

Table 6.1. Risk assessment methodology comparison

Methodology	Data Requirements	Time Frame	Strengths	Limitations
Quantitative Modeling	Historical data, population parameters, transmission parameters	Days to weeks	Precise estimates, scenario testing	Data dependency, assumption sensitivity
Qualitative Assessment	Expert knowledge, stakeholder input	Hours to days	Rapid implementation incorporates judgment	Subjective, limited precision
Hybrid Approaches	Mixed quantitative and qualitative data	Days	Balances precision and practicality	Complexity in integration
Machine Learning	Large datasets, computational resources	Variable	Pattern recognition, adaptive	A black box requires training data

6.2. Vulnerability Mapping and Hotspot Identification

Vulnerability mapping and hotspot identification are critical components of disease risk assessment, enabling targeted interventions and efficient resource allocation during public health emergencies. These approaches combine geographic analysis with epidemiological intelligence to identify areas and populations at highest risk (Paquet et al., 2006).

The conceptual framework integrates three fundamental components: exposure (degree of population exposure to disease agents, including population density and proximity to vectors), sensitivity (intrinsic characteristics influencing susceptibility, including age distribution, underlying health conditions, and immunisation coverage), and adaptive capacity (ability to respond effectively, including healthcare infrastructure, human resources, and institutional mechanisms).

Geographic information systems serve as the primary technological platform, enabling integration and analysis of diverse spatial datasets. Multi-criteria decision analysis techniques create composite vulnerability indices by assigning weights to different risk factors. Hotspot identification methodologies employ statistical methods, including spatial clustering algorithms and spatial scan statistics, to detect areas with significantly elevated risk levels.

Social vulnerability mapping has gained prominence, with the CDC's Social Vulnerability Index incorporating factors such as poverty, minority status, language barriers, and housing characteristics. Environmental vulnerability mapping integrates climate data and ecosystem characteristics to assess ecological factors that influence disease risk.

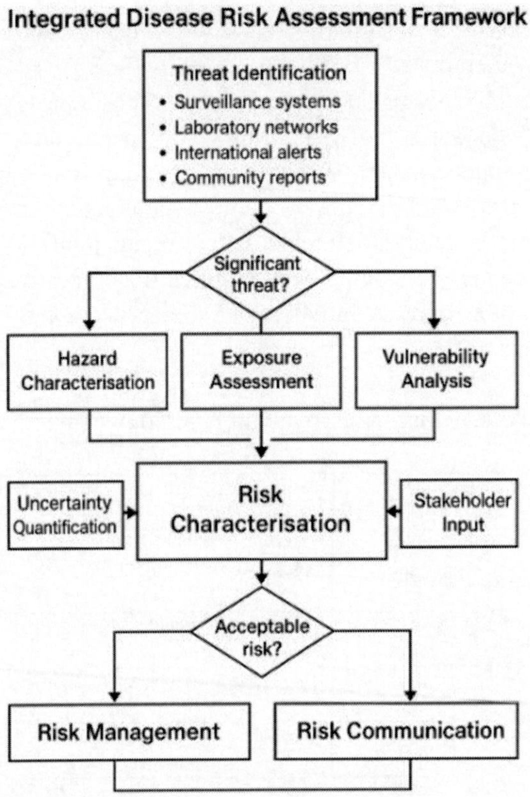

Figure 9. Integrated disease risk assessment framework.

Digital data sources, including mobile phone location data and social media trends, provide dynamic vulnerability mapping capabilities. Community engagement ensures the incorporation of local knowledge, while machine learning approaches enable the analysis of complex, high-dimensional datasets, identifying non-linear relationships between risk factors.

Figure 9 shows A comprehensive flowchart depicting the integrated disease risk assessment process, beginning with threat identification from multiple sources (surveillance systems, laboratory networks, international alerts, community reports). The framework shows parallel assessment pathways for hazard characterisation, exposure assessment, and vulnerability analysis, which feed into a risk characterisation module. The process incorporates feedback loops for uncertainty quantification and stakeholder input, culminating in informed risk management decisions and practical communication outputs. Decision points are indicated at each significant stage, along with the criteria for proceeding to the next level of assessment.

6.3. Emergency Response Protocols

Emergency response protocols form the operational backbone of public health emergency management, providing systematic frameworks for coordinating rapid and effective responses to disease outbreaks and other health emergencies (Centres for Disease Control and Prevention, 2018). These protocols establish transparent chains of command, define roles and responsibilities, and specify standardised procedures for key response functions including detection, verification, investigation, and control of health threats. The development and implementation of robust emergency response protocols require careful consideration of local contexts, resource constraints, and institutional capabilities while adhering to international guidelines and best practices.

The Incident Command System (ICS) has been widely adopted as the organisational framework for emergency response operations, providing a standardised approach to command, control, and coordination of response activities. The ICS structure establishes clear hierarchical relationships and functional divisions that can be scaled up or down based on the magnitude and complexity of the emergency. Key functional areas include operations, planning, logistics, finance and administration, and information management, each with clearly defined responsibilities and reporting relationships.

Activation protocols specify the criteria and procedures for initiating emergency response operations, including trigger mechanisms that determine when routine surveillance activities should escalate to emergency response mode. These triggers may be based on quantitative thresholds, such as case numbers, attack rates, or geographic spread, as well as qualitative factors, including disease severity, public concern, or potential for international spread. Early activation protocols emphasise the importance of rapid response to prevent or minimise the spread of infectious diseases and reduce adverse health outcomes. Table 6.2 shows the activation response.

Detection and verification protocols establish systematic procedures for identifying potential health threats through surveillance systems, laboratory networks, and community reporting mechanisms. These protocols outline the necessary information to verify the occurrence of a public health emergency, including case definitions, laboratory confirmation requirements, and epidemiological criteria for diagnosis. Rapid verification procedures are essential for distinguishing true emergencies from routine disease occurrences and preventing unnecessary activation of resource-intensive response operations.

Investigation protocols provide detailed guidance for conducting field investigations to characterise disease outbreaks and inform control measures. These protocols specify the formation and deployment of investigation teams, data collection procedures, laboratory sample collection and testing, and analytical methods for identifying the source, mode of transmission, and risk factors associated with disease occurrence. Standardised investigation protocols ensure consistency in data collection and analysis across different outbreaks, facilitating the comparison of findings.

Table 6.2. Emergency response activation criteria

Threat Level	Epidemiological Criteria	Impact Assessment	Response Level	Coordination Requirements
Low	Sporadic cases, no clusters	Limited geographic spread	Local response	Department coordination
Medium	Small clusters, limited transmission	Multiple jurisdictions	Regional response	State/provincial coordination
High	Sustained transmission, rapid spread	Multi-state/provincial impact	National response	Federal coordination
Critical	Pandemic potential, severe outcomes	International spread	International response	Global coordination

Case management protocols establish clinical guidelines for diagnosing, treating, and caring for patients affected by a health emergency. These protocols specify case definitions, diagnostic criteria, treatment algorithms, and infection prevention and control measures for healthcare facilities. Protocols for severe or novel diseases may include guidance for experimental treatments, clinical trials, and compassionate use of investigational therapies. Case management protocols must be regularly updated based on emerging scientific evidence and clinical experience.

Contact tracing protocols define systematic procedures for identifying, monitoring, and managing individuals who have been exposed to infectious disease cases. These protocols specify criteria for identifying contacts, methods for contact investigation and follow-up, quarantine and isolation procedures, and provision of preventive interventions such as prophylactic treatment or vaccination. Digital contact tracing technologies have been increasingly incorporated into protocols, particularly following experiences during the COVID-19 pandemic.

Communication protocols establish procedures for sharing information among response partners and communicating with the public, media, and other stakeholders. Internal communication protocols specify reporting requirements, information sharing agreements, and coordination mechanisms among different levels of government and response organisations. External communication protocols address public information management, media relations, and community engagement strategies that support response operations and maintain public trust.

Resource mobilisation protocols define procedures for requesting, deploying, and managing human resources, supplies, equipment, and financial support during emergency response operations. These protocols outline mutual aid agreements, resource-sharing mechanisms, and procedures for accessing national and international assistance. Emergency procurement protocols enable rapid acquisition of necessary supplies and services while maintaining accountability and fiscal responsibility.

Laboratory protocols establish procedures for specimen collection, transportation, testing, and reporting of laboratory results during public health emergencies. These protocols specify biosafety requirements, quality assurance procedures, and result reporting timelines that support rapid diagnostic confirmation and epidemiological investigation. Laboratory protocols must address capacity limitations and surge procedures for managing increased testing demands during emergencies.

Border health protocols address the management of disease threats that may cross international boundaries, including screening procedures at ports of entry, travel restrictions, and coordination with global partners. These protocols must strike a balance between public health protection and trade and travel considerations, adhering to international guidelines such as the World Health Organisation's International Health Regulations.

Recovery and transition protocols guide the scaling down of emergency response operations and the transition to routine public health activities as the immediate threat subsides. These protocols address the continuation of essential public health functions, evaluation of response performance, and documentation of lessons learned. Long-term recovery protocols may address ongoing health monitoring, rehabilitation services, and mental health support for affected populations.

Quality assurance and performance monitoring protocols establish mechanisms for evaluating the effectiveness and efficiency of response operations. These protocols outline performance indicators, data collection procedures, and evaluation methodologies that facilitate the continuous improvement of response capabilities. After-action reviews and improvement planning processes are essential components of quality assurance protocols.

Training and exercise protocols ensure that response personnel are prepared to implement emergency procedures effectively. These protocols outline the training requirements for various response roles, exercise scenarios and objectives, and evaluation criteria for assessing preparedness levels. Regular training and exercises are essential for maintaining response readiness and identifying areas for improvement in emergency protocols.

6.4. Multi-Sector Coordination Mechanisms

Multi-sector coordination mechanisms represent fundamental elements of effective emergency response systems, recognising that public health emergencies require coordinated action across diverse organisations, institutions, and sectors (Kapucu, 2008). These mechanisms establish formal and informal networks that facilitate information sharing, resource coordination, and joint decision-making among government agencies, healthcare organisations, non-governmental organisations, private sector entities, and community groups. The complexity of modern health emergencies necessitates sophisticated coordination frameworks that can operate across multiple jurisdictional levels and organisational boundaries.

Government coordination mechanisms typically operate through emergency management agencies that serve as focal points for multi-sector coordination during public health emergencies. These agencies maintain relationships with diverse stakeholders during non-emergency periods and activate coordination structures when emergencies occur. The emergency operations centre serves as the physical and virtual hub for coordination activities, providing communications infrastructure, information management systems, and meeting spaces that support collaborative decision-making processes.

Inter-agency coordination committees bring together representatives from different government departments and agencies to ensure alignment of policies, procedures, and resource allocation decisions. These committees typically include representatives from health departments, emergency management agencies, law enforcement, military organisations, transportation authorities, and social services agencies. Regular meetings during non-emergency periods help build relationships and establish a shared understanding of roles and responsibilities, which facilitates effective coordination during emergencies.

Healthcare system coordination mechanisms address the unique challenges of coordinating response activities across diverse healthcare organisations, including hospitals, clinics, emergency medical services, and public health agencies. Healthcare coalitions have emerged as essential coordination entities that bring together healthcare stakeholders within defined geographic regions to plan for and respond to emergencies collectively. These coalitions facilitate resource sharing, coordinate patient movement and medical surge responses, and provide forums for joint planning and training activities.

Information sharing mechanisms are essential components of multi-sector coordination systems, enabling the timely exchange of situational awareness information, operational updates, and resource status reports among response partners. Health information exchanges and surveillance networks provide platforms for sharing epidemiological data and laboratory results among public health agencies and healthcare organisations. Emergency communication networks, including dedicated radio systems and secure internet platforms, ensure reliable communications capabilities during emergencies when routine communication systems may be compromised.

Mutual aid agreements formalise resource-sharing arrangements among different organisations and jurisdictions, enabling the rapid mobilisation of personnel, equipment, and supplies during emergencies when local resources are insufficient. These agreements outline procedures for requesting assistance, deployment protocols, cost-sharing arrangements, and the legal frameworks governing mutual aid operations. The Emergency Management Assistance Compact (EMAC) in the United States exemplifies a comprehensive framework for mutual aid that enables interstate assistance during major emergencies.

Private sector coordination mechanisms recognise the critical roles that private companies play in emergency response, particularly in areas such as healthcare delivery, supply chain management, telecommunications, and transportation. Public-private partnerships establish formal relationships between government agencies and private sector entities, facilitating coordination during emergencies. Business continuity planning and critical infrastructure protection initiatives help ensure that essential private sector services remain operational during emergencies.

Community engagement mechanisms involve local communities, voluntary organisations, and faith-based groups in emergency planning and response activities. Community emergency response teams (CERT) and medical reserve corps (MRC) provide frameworks for training and organising community volunteers to support emergency response operations. Community health workers and promotoras serve as essential links between formal response organisations and affected communities, particularly in underserved or marginalised populations.

International coordination mechanisms address the management of health emergencies that cross national boundaries or require international assistance. The World Health Organisation's Health Emergencies Programme provides a framework for international coordination during public health emergencies of global concern. Regional coordination mechanisms, such as the European Centre for Disease Prevention and Control, facilitate coordination among neighbouring countries that may be affected by the same health threats.

Non-governmental organisation coordination mechanisms integrate the capabilities of humanitarian organisations, professional associations, academic institutions, and advocacy groups into emergency response operations. These organisations often possess specialised expertise, community relationships, and operational capabilities that complement government and healthcare system responses. Coordination mechanisms must address the diverse mandates, operating procedures, and accountability frameworks of different types of non-governmental organisations.

Logistics and supply chain coordination mechanisms address the complex challenges of managing resource flows during emergencies when demand for medical supplies, equipment, and personnel typically exceeds normal capacity. Strategic national stockpiles and regional cache systems provide reserve supplies that can be rapidly deployed during emergencies. Vendor-managed inventory systems and just-in-time delivery arrangements with private sector suppliers help ensure adequate supply availability while minimising storage costs during non-emergency periods.

Technology platforms increasingly support multi-sector coordination by providing common operating pictures, resource tracking systems, and communication platforms that enable real-time information sharing among diverse response partners. Geographic information systems integrate spatial data from multiple sources to support situational awareness and resource allocation decisions. Social media monitoring and analysis tools help response organisations track public sentiment and identify emerging issues that require attention.

Legal and regulatory coordination mechanisms address the complex legal frameworks that govern emergency response operations, particularly when responses involve multiple jurisdictions or require deviation from routine regulatory requirements. Emergency declarations activate special legal authorities that enable rapid response actions while maintaining appropriate oversight and accountability. Mutual aid agreements and memoranda of understanding establish legal frameworks for inter-organisational cooperation during emergencies.

Evaluation and improvement mechanisms ensure that coordination systems are regularly assessed and refined based on lessons learned from exercises and actual emergency responses. After-action reviews involving all participating organisations help identify strengths and weaknesses in coordination mechanisms and develop improvement plans. Performance metrics and indicators help track the effectiveness of coordination systems and identify areas requiring additional attention or resources.

6.5. Communication Strategies During Emergencies

Communication strategies during health emergencies serve multiple critical functions, including informing the public about health risks and protective measures, maintaining stakeholder coordination, and preserving public trust in response institutions (Savoia et al., 2013). Effective emergency communication requires a careful balance between providing sufficient information to enable informed decision-making while avoiding panic or misinformation that could undermine response efforts. The modern information environment, characterised by diverse communication channels and rapid information flow, presents both opportunities and challenges for emergency communication that require sophisticated strategic approaches.

Risk communication principles form the foundation of effective emergency communication strategies, emphasising the importance of providing accurate, timely, and actionable information that enables individuals and communities to make informed decisions about protective behaviours. Risk communication acknowledges that the public's perception of risk may differ from technical risk assessments and seeks to address both the objective and subjective dimensions of risk. Effective risk communication builds trust through transparency, consistency, and empathy while acknowledging uncertainty and limitations in knowledge during rapidly evolving emergencies.

Message development processes require careful consideration of audience characteristics, communication objectives, and available communication channels. Primary messages typically address the nature of the health threat, recommended protective actions, and available resources for assistance. Messages must be tailored to different audience segments, considering factors such as age, education level, language preferences, cultural background, and risk perception. Clear, simple language and concrete action steps are essential for ensuring message comprehension and uptake across diverse populations.

Multi-channel communication strategies recognise that different population segments prefer different sources and methods of receiving information during emergencies (Sanderson et al., 2004). Traditional media channels, including television, radio, and newspapers, continue to be essential sources of information for many populations, particularly older adults and those with limited internet access. Digital platforms, including websites, social media, and mobile applications, provide opportunities for rapid information dissemination and two-way communication with affected populations. Direct communication methods such as emergency alert systems, door-to-door outreach, and community meetings may be necessary to reach specific populations or geographic areas. Table 6.3 illustrates the effectiveness of communication channels by audience.

Spokesperson designation and training ensure that official communications are delivered by credible, knowledgeable individuals who can effectively represent response organisations and maintain public confidence. Lead spokespersons should possess subject matter expertise, communication skills, and institutional authority to speak on behalf of response organisations. Backup spokespersons and specialised technical experts should be identified and trained to ensure communication continuity and provide specialised expertise when needed. Media training helps spokespersons develop skills for effective interaction with journalists and manage challenging interview situations.

Social media strategies have become increasingly important components of emergency communication, offering opportunities for rapid information dissemination, community engagement, and real-time monitoring of public sentiment and concerns. Social media platforms enable response organisations to share updates, correct misinformation, and engage directly with affected communities. However, social media also presents challenges, including information overload, the spread of misinformation, and difficulty in controlling message framing. Social media monitoring tools help response organisations track online conversations, identify emerging concerns, and respond rapidly to misinformation.

Cultural competency and linguistic accessibility are essential considerations for ensuring that emergency communications reach and resonate with diverse population groups. Translation services and multilingual communication materials help ensure that language barriers do not prevent access to critical health information. Cultural mediators and community liaisons can help adapt messages to align with the cultural values and communication preferences of different population groups. Visual communication aids, including pictographs and infographics, can help overcome literacy and language barriers.

Table 6.3. Communication channel effectiveness by audience

Audience Segment	Primary Channels	Trust Level	Message Preferences	Special Considerations
General Public	Television, social media	Moderate	Simple, actionable	Multiple languages needed
Healthcare Workers	Professional networks, e-mail	High	Technical, detailed	Clinical guidance emphasis
Community Leaders	Direct meetings, phone calls	High	Community-specific	Cultural sensitivity
Media	Press releases, briefings	Variable	Newsworthy, accurate	Fact verification important

Misinformation management has emerged as a critical component of emergency communication strategies, particularly in the digital age, where false or misleading information can spread rapidly and undermine public health responses. Misinformation monitoring systems help identify false claims or conspiracy theories that may be circulating in traditional or social media. Fact-checking initiatives and partnerships with credible information sources help provide accurate information to counter false claims. Prebunking strategies involve anticipating potential misinformation themes and proactively providing precise information to reduce susceptibility to false claims.

Community engagement strategies recognise that effective emergency communication requires two-way dialogue between response organisations and affected communities rather than one-way information dissemination. Community listening sessions, surveys, and focus groups help response organisations understand community concerns, preferences, and information needs. Community advisory groups and stakeholder coalitions provide ongoing forums for dialogue and input from diverse community representatives. Community health workers and peer educators can serve as trusted messengers, helping to relay information and gather feedback from their communities.

Crisis communication protocols establish procedures for managing communication during high-stress, rapidly evolving situations when information may be incomplete or uncertain. These protocols specify decision-making authorities for communication activities, approval processes for key messages, and coordination mechanisms among different response organisations. Protocols should address procedures for correcting inaccurate information, managing conflicting messages from various sources, and communicating uncertainty while maintaining credibility.

Health literacy considerations recognise that communication effectiveness depends on the audience's ability to understand and act on health information. Health literacy-informed communication uses plain language, avoids medical jargon, and provides clear explanations of technical concepts. Numeracy considerations address the challenges of communicating statistical information and probability estimates to lay audiences. Visual aids, analogies, and storytelling techniques can help make complex health information more accessible and easier to remember.

Media relations strategies establish frameworks for productive working relationships with journalists and news organisations that serve as critical intermediaries between response organisations and the public. Regular press briefings and media advisories help ensure that journalists have access to accurate, up-to-date information from authoritative sources. Background briefings and technical briefings provide opportunities for more detailed discussions with specialised reporters. Media kits and resource libraries provide journalists with access to key information, images, and expert contacts necessary for accurate reporting.

Internal communication strategies ensure adequate information flow among response organisations and their personnel. Internal communication needs may differ from external communication in terms of content, timing, and channels. Staff briefings, situation reports, and internal newsletters help ensure that response personnel have the information needed to perform their roles effectively and represent their organisations accurately when interacting with external audiences. Rumour control mechanisms help address misinformation or confusion that may arise within response organisations.

Communication evaluation mechanisms assess the effectiveness of communication strategies and provide feedback for continuous improvement. Communication monitoring tracks reach, engagement, and sentiment associated with different communication channels and messages. Audience research, including surveys, focus groups, and social media analysis, helps assess message comprehension, credibility, and behavioural impact. Communication after-action reviews identify lessons learned and areas for improvement in communication strategies and implementation.

6.6. Lessons Learned from Recent Outbreaks

The analysis of lessons learned from recent outbreaks provides invaluable insights for improving future emergency preparedness and response capabilities (Gostin et al., 2016). Major disease outbreaks of the past two decades, including the 2003 SARS outbreak, the 2009 H1N1 influenza pandemic, the 2014-2016 West Africa Ebola epidemic, the 2015-2016 Zika virus outbreak, and the ongoing COVID-19 pandemic, have revealed both strengths and significant gaps in global health security systems. These experiences have fundamentally transformed the understanding of pandemic preparedness requirements and highlighted the need for more robust, equitable, and adaptive response systems.

The COVID-19 pandemic has provided the most comprehensive stress test of global health systems in modern history, revealing critical vulnerabilities while also demonstrating remarkable innovations and adaptations. Early pandemic response challenges included delayed recognition of human-to-human transmission, inadequate surveillance systems for detecting novel pathogens, and insufficient surge capacity in healthcare systems worldwide (Bell et al., 2009). The initial global response was hampered by competition for scarce medical supplies, inconsistent public health messaging, and limited coordination mechanisms among countries and international organisations.

Healthcare system resilience emerged as a critical vulnerability during the COVID-19 pandemic, with many countries experiencing overwhelming demand that exceeded their capacity for intensive care beds, ventilators, and specialised healthcare personnel. The pandemic revealed significant disparities in healthcare access and quality that influenced disease outcomes across different population groups. Long-term care facilities proved particularly vulnerable to COVID-19 transmission, highlighting the need for enhanced infection prevention and control measures in these settings. Healthcare worker safety has become a paramount concern, with shortages of personal protective equipment and occupational transmission risks posing a threat to the sustainability of healthcare responses.

Supply chain vulnerabilities were dramatically exposed during the COVID-19 pandemic, with global shortages of personal protective equipment, diagnostic tests, and subsequently, vaccines and therapeutics. The concentration of manufacturing capacity in limited geographic regions created single points of failure, affecting global supply availability. Just-in-time inventory systems that minimise storage costs during normal times proved inadequate for managing surge demand during emergencies. The pandemic highlighted the importance of strategic reserves, diversified supply chains, and domestic manufacturing capacity for critical medical supplies.

Digital health innovations accelerated significantly during the COVID-19 pandemic, demonstrating both the potential and limitations of technology-enabled responses to the pandemic. Telemedicine adoption expanded rapidly, enabling continued healthcare delivery while minimising transmission risks. Digital contact tracing applications were deployed in many countries with varying degrees of success, highlighting technical, privacy, and uptake challenges. Vaccine passport systems and digital health certificates emerged as tools for managing movement and access during the pandemic, raising important questions about equity and privacy.

The 2014-2016 West Africa Ebola epidemic revealed critical gaps in infectious disease preparedness in resource-limited settings and highlighted the importance of community engagement in outbreak response. Initial response efforts were hampered by weak health systems, limited surveillance capacity, and cultural barriers to case detection and isolation. The epidemic demonstrated the importance of community health workers and traditional healers as partners in outbreak response rather than obstacles to overcome. Safe burial practices required culturally sensitive approaches that respected traditional customs while preventing the transmission of disease.

International coordination challenges were evident throughout the Ebola response, with delayed activation of international assistance and coordination mechanisms that struggled to scale up rapidly enough to match the epidemic's growth. The epidemic highlighted gaps in the International Health Regulations framework and led to significant reforms in the WHO's emergency response capabilities. Travel restrictions and border closures implemented by many countries demonstrated the tension between public health protection and international trade and travel considerations.

The 2015-2016 Zika virus outbreak illustrated the challenges of responding to emerging threats with limited scientific knowledge and uncertain health impacts. The initially mild clinical presentation of Zika virus infection led to delayed recognition of its association with severe congenital disabilities and neurological complications. The outbreak highlighted gaps in reproductive health services and vector control capabilities in affected regions. Communication challenges arose regarding recommendations for pregnancy and travel, necessitating a balance between uncertain risks and potential social and economic consequences.

Mental health and psychosocial impacts have been increasingly recognised as essential dimensions of outbreak responses, with COVID-19 highlighting the substantial mental health toll of pandemic control measures. Social isolation, economic disruption, and fear of infection contributed to increased rates of depression, anxiety, and substance abuse. The pandemic revealed significant gaps in mental health services and the need for psychological support systems that can be rapidly scaled during emergencies. The evaluation of non-pharmaceutical interventions has shown both their effectiveness and the importance of considering their broader social and economic impacts (Aledort et al., 2007).

Equity considerations have emerged as central themes in lessons learned from recent outbreaks, with COVID-19 revealing and exacerbating existing health disparities. Marginalised populations, including racial and ethnic minorities, low-income communities, and undocumented immigrants, experienced disproportionate infection rates and severe outcomes. Vaccine distribution highlighted global inequities in access to medical countermeasures, with wealthy countries securing the majority shares of initial vaccine supplies. The pandemic emphasised the importance of addressing social determinants of health as essential components of emergency preparedness.

Economic impacts of outbreak responses have proven far more severe than initially anticipated, with COVID-19 control measures contributing to the worst global recession since the Great Depression. The pandemic highlighted the complex tradeoffs between public health protection and economic sustainability that characterise significant outbreak responses. Economic support systems, including unemployment insurance, business assistance programs, and social safety nets, proved essential for maintaining public support for public health measures.

The governance and political dimensions of outbreak responses have emerged as critical factors influencing the effectiveness of responses. Political polarisation around public health measures during COVID-19 demonstrated the importance of maintaining public trust and political support for evidence-based responses. Federal systems faced particular challenges in coordinating responses across multiple levels of government with different authorities and priorities. The pandemic highlighted the importance of science communication and the risks associated with the politicisation of public health decision-making.

Research and development capabilities demonstrated both remarkable achievements and significant limitations during recent outbreaks. COVID-19 vaccine development achieved unprecedented speed through advanced platform technologies and parallel development processes, while therapeutic development faced greater challenges. The pandemic underscored the importance of research infrastructure, regulatory flexibility, and international collaboration in accelerating the development of medical countermeasures. Equitable access to research benefits emerged as an important consideration for future research planning.

Conclusion

Disease risk assessment and emergency response planning represent fundamental pillars of global health security requiring continuous evolution based on emerging threats and technological advances (World Health Organisation, 2019). Effective preparedness systems must integrate sophisticated risk assessment methodologies with robust emergency response protocols, multi-sector coordination mechanisms, and strategic communication approaches.

The evolution toward integrated, dynamic, and participatory approaches, incorporating big data analytics, machine learning, and artificial intelligence, offers unprecedented opportunities for early detection. However, technological advances must strike a balance with equity considerations, ensuring that benefits reach all populations. Vulnerability mapping and hotspot identification have emerged as critical tools for targeting preparedness investments toward the highest-risk areas and populations.

Emergency response protocols must balance standardised approaches with flexibility to adapt to specific threats and local contexts. Multi-sector coordination mechanisms have proven essential for managing complex health emergencies. Communication strategies have become increasingly complex, necessitating sophisticated approaches to combat misinformation while preserving public trust.

Recent outbreaks, particularly COVID-19, highlight the catastrophic consequences of inadequate preparedness while demonstrating remarkable innovation capacity. Key themes guiding future preparedness include equity as a central consideration, community engagement and participatory approaches, One Health approaches that address interconnections, and global cooperation for addressing transboundary threats.

Climate change integration into risk assessment represents an emerging priority, altering the geographic distribution and seasonal patterns of diseases. The International Health Regulations framework provides essential guidance for strengthening national surveillance and response capacities (World Health Organisation, 2016). Investment in health system strengthening represents a critical foundation for improved preparedness capabilities.

Future research priorities should address knowledge gaps in disease emergence and transmission dynamics, particularly for novel pathogens. Implementation research is necessary for translating scientific knowledge into actionable policies, particularly in resource-constrained settings (Garza et al., 2016). Global health security development represents a shared responsibility requiring sustained commitment from governments, international organisations, the private sector, and civil society.

Acknowledgments

The authors would like to extend our appreciation to those who offered helpful commentary during the drafting process of this manuscript. We also acknowledge the role Nova Science Publishers played in enabling the work described herein.

References

Aledort, J. E., Lurie, N., Wasserman, J., & Bozzette, S. A. (2007). Non-pharmaceutical public health interventions for pandemic influenza: An evaluation of the evidence base. *BMC Public Health*, 7(1), 208-221. https://doi.org/10.1186/1471-2458-7-208.

Bell, D. M., Weisfuse, I. B., Hernandez-Avila, M., Del Rio, C., Bustamante, X., & Rodier, G. (2009). Pandemic influenza as 21st century urban public health crisis. *Emerging Infectious Diseases*, 15(12), 1963-1969. https://doi.org/10.3201/eid1512.091232.

Brownstein, J. S., Freifeld, C. C., & Madoff, L. C. (2009). Digital disease detection—harnessing the Web for public health surveillance. *New England Journal of Medicine*, 360(21), 2153-2157. https://doi.org/10.1056/NEJMp0900702.

Centers for Disease Control and Prevention. (2018). *Public health emergency preparedness and response capabilities: National standards for state, local, tribal, and territorial public health departments*. U.S. Department of Health and Human Services.

Garza, K. B., Owensby, J. K., Braxton Lloyd, K., Wood, S. M., Hansen, R. A., Reed, B. M., Brown, J. D., Robinson, E. T., & Renfro, C. P. (2016). Pilot study to test the effectiveness of different knowledge translation strategies in emergency departments. *International Journal of Emergency Medicine*, 9(1), 1-8. https://doi.org/10.1186/s12245-016-0101-3.

Gostin, L. O., Tomori, O., Wibulpolprasert, S., Jha, A. K., Frenk, J., Moon, S., Piot, P., Stocking, B., Dziuban, E. J., & Leung, G. M. (2016). Toward a common secure future: Four global commissions in the wake of Ebola. *PLoS Medicine*, 13(5), e1002042. https://doi.org/10.1371/journal.pmed.1002042.

Kahn, L. H. (2006). Confronting zoonoses, linking human and veterinary medicine. *Emerging Infectious Diseases*, 12(4), 556-561. https://doi.org/10.3201/eid1204.051539.

Kapucu, N. (2008). Collaborative emergency management: Better community organising, better public preparedness and response. *Disasters*, 32(2), 239-262. https://doi.org/10.1111/j.1467-7717.2008.01037.x.

Kruk, M. E., Myers, M., Varpilah, S. T., & Dahn, B. T. (2015). What is a resilient health system? Lessons from Ebola. *The Lancet*, 385(9980), 1910-1912. https://doi.org/10.1016/S0140-6736(15)60755-3.

Nelson, C., Lurie, N., Wasserman, J., & Zakowski, S. (2007). Conceptualising and defining public health emergency preparedness. *American Journal of Public Health*, 97(S1), S9-S11. https://doi.org/10.2105/AJPH.2007.114496.

Paquet, C., Coulombier, D., Kaiser, R., & Ciotti, M. (2006). Epidemic intelligence: A new framework for strengthening disease surveillance in Europe. *Eurosurveillance*, 11(12), 212-214. https://doi.org/10.2807/esm.11.12.00665-en.

Sanderson, T. M., Caldera, S., Gracely, E., Kirschke, D., Marano, N., Buehler, J., & Whitney, E. (2004). Public health emergency preparedness and response communications with 911 dispatch. *Prehospital Emergency Care*, 8(4), 388-394. https://doi.org/10.1016/j.prehos.2004.06.001.

Savoia, E., Lin, L., & Viswanath, K. (2013). Communications in public health emergency preparedness: A systematic review of the literature. *Biosecurity and Bioterrorism*, 11(3), 170-184. https://doi.org/10.1089/bsp.2013.0038.

World Health Organization. (2016). *International health regulations (2005): Areas of work for implementation*. WHO Press.

World Health Organization. (2019). *Health emergency and disaster risk management framework*. WHO Press.

Chapter 7

Cross-Species Transmission: When Pathogens Jump Boundaries

Bhavini Bushan Shah[1]
and Maajid Mohi Ud Din Malik[2,*]**, PhD**

[1]Department of Anesthesiology, Dr. D. Y. Patil Medical College, Hospital and Research Centre, Dr. D. Y. Patil Vidyapeeth, Pune (Deemed to be University), Sant Tukaram Nagar, Pimpri, Pune, India
[2]Department of Radiology and Imaging Technology, Dr. D. Y. Patil School of Allied Health Sciences, Dr. D. Y. Patil Vidyapeeth, Pune (Deemed to be University), Sant Tukaram Nagar, Pimpri, Pune, India

Abstract

Cross-species transmission, also known as spillover, represents one of the most significant threats to global health security, accounting for approximately 75% of emerging infectious diseases and 60% of known human pathogens. This chapter examines the complex mechanisms underlying zoonotic transmission, including the molecular, ecological, and evolutionary factors that enable pathogens to overcome species barriers and establish infection in novel hosts. The analysis encompasses host range expansion processes, the role of amplification hosts in spillover events, and the molecular mechanisms facilitating host switching through genetic recombination, reassortment, and adaptive mutations. Detailed case studies of influenza viruses, coronaviruses, and rabies virus illustrate the diverse pathways of cross-species transmission and the factors that influence pandemic potential. The chapter explores contemporary prevention and control strategies, emphasising One Health approaches that integrate human, animal, and environmental health perspectives. Spillover events are increasingly driven by anthropogenic factors, including habitat encroachment, agricultural intensification, climate change, and wildlife trade, which alter human-animal interfaces and create new opportunities for transmission. The integration of advanced surveillance technologies, molecular epidemiology, and predictive modelling represents promising directions for anticipating and preventing future spillover events. These findings contribute directly to achieving Sustainable Development Goal 3 (Good Health and Well-being) by addressing the animal-human-environment interface that serves as the source of most emerging infectious disease threats.

---

* Corresponding Author's Email: maajid.malik@dpu.edu.in

In: Advances in the One Health Approach
Editors: Maajid Mohi Ud Din Malik, Abhay Saraf, Harshal Tukaram Pandve et al.
ISBN: 979-8-90134-202-2

Keywords: zoonotic transmission, spillover events, host switching, pathogen evolution, One Health, emerging infectious diseases, cross-species barriers, Sustainable Development Goal 3

Introduction

Cross-species transmission events represent fundamental processes in the emergence of new infectious diseases, serving as the primary mechanism through which novel pathogens enter human populations and potentially cause epidemics or pandemics. The phenomenon of pathogen spillover from animal reservoirs to human hosts has shaped the evolutionary history of infectious diseases. It continues to pose significant challenges to global health security in the contemporary era. Approximately 60% of known human infectious diseases have zoonotic origins. In comparison, 75% of emerging infectious diseases have animal sources, highlighting the critical importance of understanding cross-species transmission dynamics (Centres for Disease Control and Prevention, 2025).

The increasing frequency of spillover events in recent decades reflects the complex interplay between ecological disruption, climate change, globalisation, and intensified human-animal interactions that characterise the Anthropocene epoch (Petrovan et al., 2021). Major pandemic threats of the 21st century, including severe acute respiratory syndrome (SARS), Middle East respiratory syndrome (MERS), influenza H1N1, and COVID-19, all originated through cross-species transmission events that enabled animal pathogens to adapt to human hosts (Ellwanger et al., 2021). The economic and social costs of these events, exemplified by the COVID-19 pandemic's devastating global impact, underscore the urgent need for a comprehensive understanding of spillover mechanisms and the development of effective prevention strategies.

The One Health approach has emerged as the conceptual framework for addressing cross-species transmission through integrated consideration of human, animal, and environmental health dimensions. This paradigm recognises that effective prevention and control of zoonotic diseases requires collaborative efforts across multiple sectors and disciplines, moving beyond traditional boundaries between human and veterinary medicine to embrace ecosystem-level perspectives on Health (Roche et al., 2022). Understanding the mechanisms of cross-species transmission is essential for developing evidence-based strategies to prevent future pandemic threats and protect global health security.

7.1. Mechanisms of Zoonotic Transmission

Zoonotic transmission mechanisms encompass a complex array of biological, ecological, and environmental processes that enable pathogens to cross species barriers and establish infection in novel hosts (Plowright et al., 2017). These mechanisms operate at multiple scales, from molecular interactions between pathogens and host cells to landscape-level ecological dynamics that influence pathogen circulation and human-animal contact patterns. Understanding these diverse mechanisms is essential for developing comprehensive strategies to prevent and control zoonotic diseases.

Direct transmission represents the most straightforward mechanism of zoonotic disease transfer, involving immediate contact between infected animals and susceptible human hosts (Centres for Disease Control and Prevention, 2025). This pathway requires transmission through animal bites, scratches, or contact with infected bodily fluids, including saliva, blood, urine, or faeces. Rabies virus exemplifies direct transmission through animal bites, as infected animals shed the virus in their saliva and transmit the infection through bite wounds that provide direct access to the nervous tissue. The efficiency of direct transmission depends on factors including viral load in infected animal secretions, duration and intensity of contact, and the susceptibility of exposed human individuals.

Indirect transmission pathways involve environmental intermediates that facilitate pathogen transfer from animal reservoirs to human hosts without direct contact with the animals. Environmental persistence is a crucial factor in indirect transmission, as pathogens exhibit significant variations in their ability to survive outside host organisms. Some pathogens, such as Bacillus anthracis spores, can persist in soil for decades, whereas others, like influenza viruses, have limited environmental survival. Contaminated water sources serve as important indirect transmission routes for pathogens such as Leptospira species, which are shed in animal urine and can survive in aquatic environments for extended periods.

Vector-borne transmission involves arthropod intermediates that acquire pathogens from infected animal hosts and subsequently transmit them to humans through blood feeding. This mechanism is exemplified by arboviruses such as West Nile virus, which circulates between bird reservoirs and mosquito vectors before occasionally infecting humans as incidental hosts. Vector competence, the ability of arthropod species to acquire, maintain, and transmit specific pathogens, varies significantly among vector species and is influenced by genetic, physiological, and environmental factors. Climate change and ecological modification can alter the distribution and abundance of vectors, affecting the geographic range and intensity of vector-borne zoonotic transmission.

Foodborne transmission represents another critical pathway for zoonotic disease transfer, involving the consumption of contaminated animal products, including meat, milk, eggs, or other foods of animal origin. Foodborne zoonoses can result from the consumption of products from infected animals, cross-contamination during food processing, or inadequate food safety practices. Salmonella species exemplify foodborne zoonotic transmission, with numerous animal species serving as reservoirs and transmission occurring through consumption of contaminated eggs, meat, or dairy products. The globalisation of food systems has increased the potential for widespread foodborne zoonotic disease outbreaks.

Airborne transmission, while less common for zoonotic pathogens, can occur through inhalation of aerosols containing infectious agents generated by infected animals. This mechanism is exemplified by certain influenza viruses and coronaviruses that can be transmitted through respiratory droplets or aerosols produced by infected animals. Enclosed spaces with high animal densities, such as intensive livestock operations or live animal markets, can facilitate the transmission of airborne diseases through aerosol generation and inadequate ventilation.

The role of intermediate hosts adds complexity to zoonotic transmission pathways, with some pathogens requiring amplification or adaptation in intermediate species before acquiring the ability to infect humans efficiently. Intermediate hosts may serve as "mixing vessels" where genetic reassortment or recombination events occur, generating novel pathogen variants with enhanced potential for human transmission. Swine populations serve as critical intermediate hosts for influenza viruses, harbouring both avian and human virus strains and facilitating genetic reassortment that can produce pandemic strains.

Molecular factors influencing zoonotic transmission include pathogen characteristics such as receptor binding specificity, host range determinants, and genetic variability. Many zoonotic pathogens must overcome species-specific barriers, including differences in cellular receptors, immune recognition patterns, and physiological conditions between animal reservoirs and human hosts. RNA viruses, characterised by high mutation rates and genetic plasticity, are particularly adept at adapting to new hosts through rapid evolutionary processes.

Host factors that affect susceptibility to zoonotic transmission include immune status, age, genetic background, and concurrent infections or underlying health conditions. Immunocompromised individuals may be at increased risk for zoonotic diseases, while certain genetic polymorphisms can influence susceptibility to specific pathogens. The concept of "pathogen pollution" describes how environmental contamination with infectious agents can increase exposure risks for human populations, particularly in areas with poor sanitation infrastructure.

Ecological factors influencing zoonotic transmission include biodiversity patterns, habitat fragmentation, and ecosystem disruption, which can alter the dynamics of pathogen circulation and human-animal contact patterns. The "dilution effect" hypothesis suggests that biodiversity loss can increase the risk of zoonotic transmission by reducing the diversity of host species that can regulate pathogen prevalence in reservoir populations. Conversely, intact ecosystems with high biodiversity may provide natural regulation of pathogen circulation, thereby reducing the risk of spillover.

Anthropogenic drivers of zoonotic transmission include deforestation, agricultural expansion, urbanisation, and climate change, which alter ecological systems and create new pathways for human-animal interactions. Land use change can bring human populations into closer contact with wildlife reservoirs while simultaneously disrupting natural environmental processes that regulate pathogen circulation. Intensive animal agriculture creates concentrated populations of genetically similar animals, which can facilitate the amplification and evolution of pathogens.

Surveillance and detection systems play a crucial role in identifying zoonotic transmission events and enabling a rapid response to prevent further spread of the disease. Traditional surveillance approaches focus on clinical case detection and laboratory confirmation, while emerging approaches incorporate environmental sampling, molecular epidemiology, and predictive modelling to identify transmission events earlier in their development. The integration of human, animal, and environmental surveillance data through One Health platforms can provide a comprehensive picture of zoonotic transmission dynamics.

7.2. Host Range Expansion and Adaptation

Host range expansion represents a fundamental evolutionary process through which pathogens acquire the ability to infect new host species, often leading to novel infectious diseases with pandemic potential (Gibson & Bruckner, 2024). This process involves complex interactions between pathogen genetics, host biology, and environmental factors determining whether cross-species transmission results in transient infections or sustained circulation.

Pathogen adaptation to new hosts requires overcoming multiple biological barriers. Receptor compatibility necessitates that pathogens bind to and enter the cells of new host species. For example, influenza viruses demonstrate a preference for different sialic acid linkages, with avian viruses binding to α2,3-linked variants and human viruses preferring α2,6-linked variants. Cellular and tissue tropism represents another barrier, requiring adaptations to diverse cellular environments and metabolic conditions. Immune system compatibility poses significant challenges, as different host species have evolved distinct immune recognition patterns and defence mechanisms.

Genetic factors underlying host range expansion include specific mutations, gene duplications, or recombination events. RNA viruses, characterised by high mutation rates and genetic plasticity, are particularly prone to host range expansion through adaptive evolution. However, many mutations that facilitate adaptation to new hosts may be deleterious in the original reservoir hosts, creating evolutionary trade-offs that influence the likelihood of sustained expansion (Ellwanger & Chies, 2021).

The phylogenetic distance between the donor and recipient host species significantly influences the likelihood of expansion. Closely related species share similar cellular receptors and physiological characteristics, facilitating pathogen adaptation. Intermediate hosts may serve as evolutionary stepping stones, allowing gradual adaptation through sequential host switches. Domestic animals often serve this role due to close contact with both wildlife reservoirs and human populations.

Experimental evolution studies using bacteriophages and RNA viruses demonstrate that host range expansion can occur rapidly under appropriate selective pressures. Population genetics factors—including adequate population size, genetic diversity, and demographic history—influence expansion success. Environmental factors, such as temperature, humidity, and pH, affect pathogen survival and transmission efficiency, with climate change potentially altering conditions that facilitate host range expansion.

Quantitative approaches predicting expansion potential include phylogenetic analysis, machine learning models, and experimental studies assessing cross-species transmission risk. Pre-adaptation refers to situations where pathogens possess characteristics that facilitate host range expansion before exposure to new hosts. Evolutionary constraints, including trade-offs between adapting to different host environments and pleiotropic effects, explain why many transmission events result in dead-end infections rather than sustained circulation.

7.3. Spillover Events and Amplification Hosts

Spillover events represent critical transitions where pathogens cross species barriers and establish infections in novel host populations, serving as the initial step in the emergence of infectious diseases (Nyamai et al., 2022). These events require a careful distinction between different transmission outcomes. Primary spillover involves the initial transmission from natural reservoir hosts to a new species. Secondary spillover occurs when pathogens subsequently transmit between individuals within the same species. Spillback describes the reverse transmission from spillover hosts back to the original reservoir species.

Ecological factors influencing spillover frequency include habitat modification, climate change, and biodiversity loss, which alter the contact probability between reservoir hosts and potential spillover species. Deforestation and agricultural expansion increase human-wildlife contact while displacing wildlife populations. Urbanisation creates ecological niches where synanthropic species may serve as bridge hosts between wildlife reservoirs and human populations.

Host density and distribution patterns significantly affect spillover risk, with higher reservoir host densities generally associated with increased pathogen prevalence and transmission potential. Amplification hosts play crucial roles by providing intermediate steps in transmission chains and opportunities for pathogen adaptation, sometimes serving as "mixing vessels" where genetic recombination generates novel variants with enhanced human transmission potential.

Competent reservoirs maintain pathogen circulation indefinitely through intraspecific transmission, thereby serving as permanent sources of spillover risk. Bridge species facilitate spillover by serving as intermediate hosts with ecological characteristics that increase contact between both reservoir hosts and human populations. Environmental contamination serves as a crucial pathway for pathogens to survive outside hosts for extended periods.

Anthropogenic drivers include the wildlife trade and markets, which bring together diverse animal species under conditions that facilitate pathogen transmission and amplification. Intensive animal agriculture creates high-density populations of genetically similar animals, particularly susceptible to pathogen emergence.

Prevention strategies focus on reducing contact between reservoir hosts and potential spillover species, managing amplification host populations, and monitoring high-risk interfaces to prevent disease transmission. One Health approaches, integrating human, animal, and environmental health perspectives, are crucial for developing comprehensive spillover prevention strategies.

Case studies of specific spillover events provide valuable insights into the factors that contribute to successful cross-species transmission and the dynamics of pathogen emergence. Analysis of events such as the emergence of SARS-CoV-2, MERS-CoV, and pandemic influenza strains has revealed common patterns and risk factors that can inform future prevention efforts. Table 7.1 shows characteristics of major spillover events in recent decades.

Table 7.1. Characteristics of major spillover events in recent decades

Pathogen	Reservoir Host	Intermediate Host	Spillover Year	Transmission Route	Pandemic Potential
SARS-CoV	Bats	Palm civets	2002	Respiratory/Contact	Limited
MERS-CoV	Bats	Dromedary camels	2012	Respiratory/Contact	Limited
SARS-CoV-2	Bats	Unknown	2019	Respiratory/Aerosol	High
H1N1 Influenza	Swine	None	2009	Respiratory	High
Ebola virus	Bats	None	2014	Contact/Bodily fluids	Limited

7.4. Molecular Mechanisms of Host Switching

Molecular mechanisms of host switching encompass genetic and biochemical processes that enable pathogens to overcome species barriers and establish infections in new host organisms. These mechanisms operate at multiple levels, from initial pathogen-host cell interactions to complex adaptations affecting immune evasion, replication efficiency, and transmission characteristics.

Receptor binding represents the initial and most critical step, determining whether pathogens can successfully enter cells of new host species. Many pathogens exhibit strict specificity for cellular receptors, with cross-species transmission requiring pre-existing compatibility or adaptive mutations enabling binding to orthologous receptors. Influenza viruses exemplify the importance of receptor specificity, with human-adapted strains preferentially binding to α2,6-linked sialic acids, while avian-adapted strains bind to α2,3-linked variants (Barclay et al., 2018). Single-nucleotide changes can sometimes confer the ability to utilise receptors from new host species.

Entry pathway modifications represent another critical aspect, as pathogens may need to adapt to different cellular entry mechanisms. Replication machinery adaptation enables pathogens to function effectively within the cellular environments of new host species, often involving trade-offs between efficiency in new and original hosts. Host range determinants represent specific genetic elements controlling a pathogen's ability to infect host species.

Immune evasion mechanisms must often be modified, as different host species have evolved distinct immune recognition patterns and defence strategies. Genetic recombination and reassortment provide mechanisms for generating novel pathogen variants with altered host range characteristics, potentially creating chimeric organisms with new host specificity patterns. Influenza viruses demonstrate pandemic potential of genetic reassortment.

Pathogen genetic diversity plays a crucial role in host switching success—larger, more diverse pathogen populations are more likely to contain variants capable of adapting to new hosts. Experimental approaches include reverse genetics systems, cell culture models, and structural biology methods that elucidate molecular interactions between pathogens and host factors.

Evolutionary constraints include genetic linkage between adaptive and deleterious mutations, pleiotropic effects, and epistatic interactions between genetic elements. These constraints explain why host-switching events are relatively rare, despite apparent genetic plasticity. Computational approaches predicting molecular host switching potential include phylogenetic analysis, machine learning models, and molecular dynamics simulations.

Molecular pre-adaptation refers to situations where pathogens possess characteristics that, coincidentally, facilitate host switching before exposure to a new host species. Therapeutic implications include developing broad-spectrum antivirals that target conserved pathogen functions, vaccines protecting against multiple related pathogens, and surveillance strategies that monitor molecular signatures associated with host adaptation.

Figure 10 shows A detailed molecular pathway diagram depicting the key steps and barriers in cross-species pathogen transmission. The diagram illustrates changes in receptor binding specificity, cellular entry adaptations, modifications to the replication machinery, and immune evasion mechanisms. Specific examples are shown for influenza virus (hemagglutinin receptor switching), coronavirus (spike protein adaptations), and general mechanisms including genetic recombination and reassortment. Success and failure pathways are illustrated with barriers and facilitating factors clearly marked. The diagram illustrates the effects of phylogenetic distance and the role of intermediate hosts in facilitating adaptation.

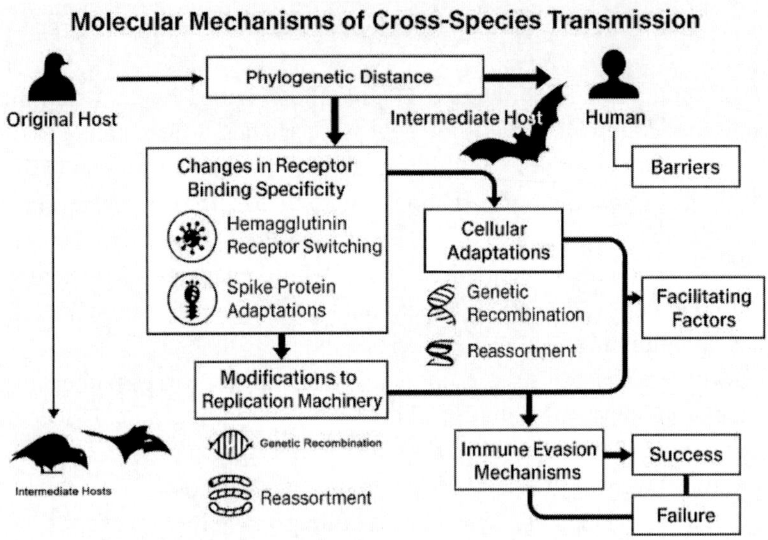

Figure 10. Molecular mechanisms of cross-species transmission.

7.5. Examples: Influenza, Coronavirus, Rabies

The examination of specific pathogen examples provides crucial insights into the diverse mechanisms and evolutionary pathways underlying cross-species transmission events. Influenza viruses, coronaviruses, and rabies virus represent three distinct viral families that have demonstrated remarkable success in crossing species barriers and establishing infection in human populations, each employing different molecular strategies and transmission pathways that illustrate the complexity of zoonotic emergence.

Influenza viruses exemplify the pandemic potential of segmented RNA viruses, which are capable of genetic reassortment and have resulted in multiple spillover events that have led to major human pandemics throughout history. The 2009 H1N1 pandemic strain emerged through a complex reassortment event involving gene segments from human, avian, and swine influenza viruses, demonstrating the role of intermediate hosts in generating novel pandemic strains. Swine populations serve as critical "mixing vessels" for influenza evolution because they possess receptors compatible with both human and avian virus strains, enabling co-infection and genetic reassortment events (Schultz-Cherry et al., 2021).

The molecular basis of influenza host switching centres on hemagglutinin receptor specificity, with avian viruses typically binding to α2,3-linked sialic acids present in avian respiratory and intestinal tissues, while human-adapted viruses preferentially bind to α2,6-linked sialic acids found in the human upper respiratory tract. The transition from avian to human receptor specificity typically requires specific amino acid substitutions in the hemagglutinin receptor binding site, though the exact mutations required vary among different influenza subtypes. Additional adaptations affecting viral polymerase function, such as the PB2 E627K mutation, which enhances replication at mammalian body temperatures, are often necessary for efficient human infection.

The ongoing threat posed by H5N1 highly pathogenic avian influenza demonstrates the continued spillover potential of avian influenza viruses. While H5N1 has caused sporadic human infections with extremely high case fatality rates exceeding 50%, the virus has not acquired the ability for efficient human-to-human transmission. However, experimental studies have identified specific mutations that could confer airborne transmission capability, highlighting the potential for future pandemic emergence through continued viral evolution.

Coronaviruses represent another major group of zoonotic pathogens that have caused multiple spillover events leading to significant human disease outbreaks. The emergence of SARS-CoV in 2002, MERS-CoV in 2012, and SARS-CoV-2 in 2019 demonstrates the repeated spillover potential of bat-origin coronaviruses. Each of these viruses likely originated in bat reservoirs before potentially adapting in intermediate hosts and subsequently spreading to human populations (Harvey & Holmes, 2024).

SARS-CoV-2 represents the most significant coronavirus spillover event to date, resulting in the COVID-19 pandemic that has caused millions of deaths worldwide and massive social and economic disruption. The virus demonstrates remarkable adaptability in human hosts, with the spike protein exhibiting a high affinity for the human ACE2 receptor and facilitating efficient human-to-human transmission through respiratory droplets and aerosols. The furin cleavage site in the SARS-CoV-2 spike protein, absent in closely related bat coronaviruses, may contribute to enhanced transmission efficiency and pathogenicity in humans.

The continued evolution of SARS-CoV-2 through variants of concern illustrates the ongoing adaptation of spillover pathogens to human hosts. Variants such as Alpha, Delta, and Omicron have acquired mutations affecting transmissibility, immune evasion, and pathogenicity, demonstrating the capacity for continued viral evolution following initial spillover events. The emergence of these variants has been facilitated by extensive global circulation and selective pressures imposed by immunity from infection and vaccination.

Coronaviruses demonstrate the importance of receptor compatibility in determining host range and spillover potential. The ability of SARS-CoV-2 to utilise ACE2 receptors, which are widely conserved among mammalian species, has enabled infection of numerous animal species, including domestic cats, dogs, ferrets, and mink, as well as wildlife species such as white-tailed deer (Wardeh et al., 2021). This broad host range has raised concerns about potential spillback transmission to animal populations and the establishment of animal reservoirs.

Rabies virus represents a distinct example of cross-species transmission involving a neurotropic virus with nearly universal mammalian host range but limited pandemic potential due to its transmission characteristics and pathogenesis. The rabies virus can infect virtually all mammalian species and demonstrates remarkable stability in its basic biological properties across diverse host species, suggesting an ancient evolutionary adaptation to mammalian hosts rather than recent spillover events.

The transmission characteristics of the rabies virus, which require direct contact with infected saliva, typically through animal bites, limit its potential for causing large-scale human outbreaks despite its lethality and broad host range. However, rabies remains a significant public health threat in many regions, causing an estimated 59,000 human deaths annually worldwide, primarily in Asia and Africa, where dog-mediated transmission predominates (World Health Organisation, 2024).

The rabies virus exhibits distinct epidemiological patterns in different host species and geographic regions, with various mammalian species serving as primary reservoirs, including dogs, bats, foxes, raccoons, and skunks. Each reservoir species maintains distinct viral variants adapted to specific host characteristics, though cross-species transmission between reservoir species and spillover to humans occurs regularly. The maintenance of rabies in multiple reservoir species complicates control efforts and provides various sources of human exposure risk.

The molecular mechanisms of rabies virus neurotropism involve specific interactions with neuronal receptors, including acetylcholine receptors and neural cell adhesion molecules, which enable the virus to enter peripheral nerves and travel to the central nervous system. Once in the nervous system, the rabies virus can manipulate host behaviour to enhance transmission, causing the characteristic aggressive behaviour in rabid animals that facilitates virus transmission through biting.

Prevention and control strategies for these three viral examples illustrate different approaches appropriate for pathogens with varying transmission characteristics and spillover potential. Influenza prevention relies heavily on annual vaccination programs that must be updated regularly to match circulating strains, combined with surveillance systems that monitor for novel variants with pandemic potential (Webster & Govorkova, 2014). Pandemic preparedness encompasses stockpiling antiviral drugs and developing rapid-response vaccination strategies.

Coronavirus prevention strategies have evolved rapidly in response to the COVID-19 pandemic, emphasising the importance of non-pharmaceutical interventions including masking, social distancing, and ventilation improvements, combined with vaccine development and deployment. The rapid growth of COVID-19 vaccines utilising novel platforms, including mRNA technology, underscores the potential for accelerated vaccine development in response to emerging threats.

Rabies prevention strategies focus on mass vaccination of domestic animal populations, particularly dogs, which serve as the primary source of human exposure in most endemic regions. The "Zero by 30" global initiative aims to eliminate human deaths from dog-mediated rabies by 2030 through coordinated vaccination campaigns and improved access to post-exposure prophylaxis (Shafaati et al., 2023). Wildlife rabies control often involves oral vaccination programs using vaccine-laden baits distributed in natural habitats.

7.6. Prevention and Control Strategies

Prevention and control strategies for cross-species transmission encompass a comprehensive array of interventions designed to reduce spillover risk, detect emergence events early, and respond effectively to limit the spread of novel zoonotic pathogens. These strategies operate across multiple scales and sectors, requiring coordination between human Health, animal health, environmental management, and policy domains to address the complex factors underlying zoonotic disease emergence.

One Health approaches represent the foundational framework for zoonotic disease prevention, emphasising the interconnected nature of human, animal, and environmental Health, and the need for collaborative action across traditional sectoral boundaries. The implementation of One Health strategies requires the establishment of multisectoral coordination mechanisms that bring together diverse stakeholders, including public health agencies, veterinary services, wildlife management authorities, environmental protection agencies, and academic institutions (Roche et al., 2022).

Surveillance systems designed to detect spillover events represent critical components of prevention strategies, requiring integrated monitoring of pathogen circulation in reservoir hosts, environmental contamination, and early human cases. Traditional passive surveillance approaches, which rely on clinical case reporting, may miss early spillover events, necessitating active surveillance programs that systematically monitor high-risk interfaces between humans and animals. Syndromic surveillance systems that monitor patterns of illness in humans and animals can provide early warning of unusual disease activity.

Pathogen discovery and characterisation efforts aim to identify novel zoonotic threats before spillover events occur, using techniques including viral metagenomics, serological surveys, and environmental sampling to detect unknown pathogens in reservoir species. The Global Virome Project represents an ambitious effort to characterise viral diversity in wildlife populations and identify pathogens with high spillover potential before emergence occurs. Predictive modelling approaches integrate information about pathogen genetics, host ecology, and environmental factors to prioritise surveillance efforts.

Risk assessment frameworks provide systematic approaches for evaluating the potential for spillover and informing preventive investments. These frameworks typically consider factors including pathogen characteristics, reservoir host abundance and distribution, human-animal contact patterns, and environmental conditions that influence transmission risk. Quantitative risk assessment models can estimate the probability of spillover events and evaluate the potential effectiveness of different intervention strategies.

Habitat conservation and ecosystem management strategies address the environmental drivers of spillover events by maintaining intact ecosystems that support natural pathogen regulation mechanisms. Protected areas and wildlife corridors can reduce human-wildlife contact while preserving biodiversity that may buffer against pathogen emergence. Sustainable land use practices that minimise ecosystem disruption can reduce spillover risk while supporting human development needs.

Animal trade and market regulation represent another essential component of spillover prevention, as these activities can bring together diverse animal species under conditions that facilitate the transmission and amplification of pathogens. Enhanced biosecurity measures, stringent health screening requirements, and limitations on high-risk species can minimise transmission opportunities in trade and market settings. The closure of live animal markets during the COVID-19 pandemic highlighted both the potential importance of these settings for spillover events and the challenges of implementing effective regulations.

Vaccination strategies for spillover prevention include both animal vaccination programs that reduce pathogen circulation in reservoir and amplification host populations, as well as human vaccination programs that protect against known zoonotic threats. Mass vaccination of domestic animals, particularly dogs, for rabies control, is one of the most successful strategies for preventing zoonotic diseases. Wildlife vaccination programs using oral baits have proven effective for rabies control in specific settings, but they remain technically challenging and expensive.

Education and behaviour change interventions aim to reduce high-risk human behaviours that increase spillover exposure, while promoting practices that support prevention efforts. These interventions may target specific occupational groups with high animal exposure, such as farmers, veterinarians, and wildlife workers, as well as general populations in high-risk areas. Cultural and social factors that influence human-animal interactions must be carefully considered in designing effective behaviour change programs.

Rapid response systems enable quick action when spillover events are detected, potentially preventing limited spillover events from developing into larger outbreaks or pandemics. These systems require pre-positioned resources, trained personnel, and clear protocols for investigation and control measures. International coordination mechanisms, such as the World Health Organisation's health emergency programs, facilitate the rapid sharing of information and the deployment of resources across national boundaries.

Antimicrobial and antiviral development efforts focus on creating medical countermeasures that can prevent or treat infections caused by novel zoonotic pathogens. Broad-spectrum antivirals that target conserved viral functions may protect against multiple related pathogens. At the same time, platform technologies for vaccine development can accelerate the creation of specific vaccines for newly emerged threats. Stockpiling of medical countermeasures requires careful consideration of shelf life, storage requirements, and equitable distribution strategies.

Technology applications for spillover prevention include remote sensing for environmental monitoring, molecular diagnostics for rapid pathogen detection, and artificial intelligence for predictive modelling and analysis of surveillance data. Mobile health technologies can facilitate reporting from remote areas and support contact tracing efforts. Blockchain and other distributed technologies may improve supply chain transparency and traceability for animal products.

Policy and governance frameworks provide the regulatory foundation for spillover prevention efforts, establishing authorities, responsibilities, and resources for controlling zoonotic diseases. International agreements, such as the Convention on Biological Diversity and the World Trade Organisation's Sanitary and Phytosanitary Agreement, influence national policies that affect spillover risk. Pandemic preparedness treaties and agreements are being developed to strengthen global coordination for prevention and response efforts.

Economic incentives and financing mechanisms can support spillover prevention by aligning economic interests with public health goals. Payment for ecosystem services programs can compensate landowners for conservation practices that reduce spillover risk. Insurance and risk transfer mechanisms may encourage private sector actors to adopt biosecurity measures. Development financing can support capacity building in low-income countries where spillover risk may be highest.

Community engagement and participatory approaches recognise that effective spillover prevention requires the support and participation of local communities, who are often the first to encounter spillover events. Community-based surveillance programs can extend monitoring coverage while building local capacity and expertise. Traditional ecological knowledge can offer valuable insights into wildlife behaviour and environmental changes that may influence spillover risk.

Figure 11 shows A comprehensive diagram illustrating the multiple factors contributing to zoonotic spillover risk and potential intervention points. The diagram illustrates interconnected pathways from wildlife reservoirs to potential intermediate hosts and ultimately to human populations. Risk factors are shown, including habitat encroachment, agricultural intensification, climate change, and wildlife trade. Intervention points are highlighted, including habitat protection, surveillance systems, animal vaccination, market regulation, and behaviour change programs. The diagram emphasises the One Health approach with interconnected circles representing human Health, animal health, and environmental health sectors.

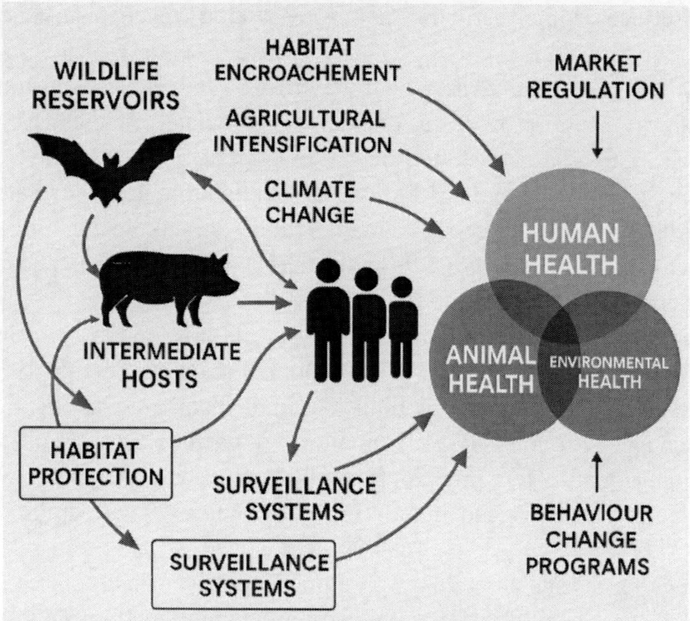

Figure 11. Zoonotic spillover risk factors and intervention points.

Table 7.2 shows prevention strategies for major zoonotic pathogens.

Table 7.2. Prevention strategies for major zoonotic pathogen groups

Pathogen Group	Primary Prevention	Secondary Prevention	Tertiary Prevention	Key Challenges
Respiratory Viruses	Animal vaccination, market regulation	Early detection, isolation	Antiviral treatment, ventilation	Airborne transmission
Vector-borne Diseases	Vector control, habitat management	Surveillance, personal protection	Clinical treatment	Climate change impacts
Contact-transmitted	Animal vaccination, behaviour change	Wound care, prophylaxis	Clinical treatment	Animal reservoir persistence
Foodborne Pathogens	Food safety measures, animal health	Testing, recall systems	Clinical treatment	Complex food chains

Conclusion

Cross-species transmission represents one of the most significant threats to global health security, accounting for the majority of emerging infectious diseases and all major pandemic events in recorded history. The comprehensive analysis reveals that spillover events arise from intricate interactions among pathogen evolution, host ecology, environmental change, and human activities, thereby creating opportunities for pathogens to cross species barriers.

Molecular mechanisms reveal remarkable pathogen adaptability, particularly in RNA viruses with segmented genomes, which are capable of genetic reassortment. However, most cross-species transmission events result in dead-end infections. Ecological factors—habitat destruction, climate change, agricultural intensification, and urbanisation—are creating new human-animal interfaces while disrupting natural regulatory mechanisms limiting pathogen circulation.

Case studies of influenza viruses, coronaviruses, and rabies illustrate the diverse transmission pathways and prevention challenges associated with these diseases. The emergence of SARS-CoV-2 demonstrates the continued relevance of spillover threats and the potential for unprecedented global disruption. Prevention requires integrated One Health approaches coordinating action across human health, animal health, and environmental management sectors. Rabies control through mass dog vaccination demonstrates the effectiveness of source-focused prevention.

Recognition of spillover prevention as a global public good has renewed interest in strengthening international cooperation. The economic costs of COVID-19 far exceed the investments in prevention programs, providing substantial economic justification. Technology applications—such as environmental DNA monitoring, machine learning risk prediction, and rapid vaccine platforms—offer promising tools that require significant infrastructure investment, particularly in low- and middle-income countries where spillover risk may be highest.

Climate change represents an increasingly important driver that requires urgent attention in prevention planning. Changing temperature and precipitation patterns alter the geographic distribution of reservoir hosts and vectors, while affecting pathogen survival and transmission dynamics.

Preventing cross-species transmission requires sustained, coordinated efforts across multiple sectors and scales, from local community engagement to global policy coordination. The stakes are enormous, as demonstrated by the ongoing impacts of COVID-19, but tools and knowledge for effective prevention are increasingly available. The critical question is whether the global community will invest adequately in prevention efforts to reduce future pandemic threats.

Acknowledgments

The authors would like to extend our appreciation to those who offered helpful commentary during the drafting process of this manuscript. We also acknowledge the role Nova Science Publishers played in enabling the work described herein.

References

Barclay, W. S., Cauldwell, A. V., & Long, J. S. (2018). Host and viral determinants of influenza A virus species specificity. *Nature Reviews Microbiology*, 16(12), 738-750. https://doi.org/10.1038/s41579-018-0115-z.

Centers for Disease Control and Prevention. (2025). About zoonotic diseases. *One Health*. Retrieved from https://www.cdc.gov/one-health/about/about-zoonotic-diseases.html.

Ellwanger, J. H., & Chies, J. A. B. (2021). Zoonotic spillover: Understanding basic aspects for better prevention. *Genetics and Molecular Biology*, 44(1), e20200355. https://doi.org/10.1590/1678-4685-GMB-2020-0355.

Ellwanger, J. H., Kulmann-Leal, B., Kaminski, V. L., Valverde-Villegas, J. M., Veiga, A. B. G., Spilki, F. R., Fearnside, P. M., Caesar, L., Giatti, L. L., Wallau, G. L., Almeida, S. E. M., Santos, B. R., & Chies, J. A. B. (2021). Beyond diversity loss and climate change: Impacts of Amazon deforestation on infectious diseases and public Health. *Anais da Academia Brasileira de Ciências*, 93(1), e20191375. https://doi.org/10.1590/0001-3765202120191375.

Gibson, L., & Bruckner, T. (2024). Spillover: Mechanisms, genetic barriers, and the role of reservoirs in emerging pathogens. *Pathogens*, 13(11), 967. https://doi.org/10.3390/pathogens13110967.

Harvey, E., & Holmes, E. C. (2024). Diversity and evolution of the animal virome. *Nature Reviews Microbiology*, 22(6), 321-334. https://doi.org/10.1038/s41579-021-00665-x.

Nyamai, M., Njenga, S. M., Bett, B., & Schelling, E. (2022). A generalisable One Health framework for the control of zoonotic diseases. *Scientific Reports*, 12(1), 8588. https://doi.org/10.1038/s41598-022-12619-1.

Petrovan, S. O., Aldridge, D. C., Bartlett, H., Bladon, A. J., Booth, H., Broad, S., Broom, D. M., Burgess, N. D., Cleaveland, S., Ferri, M., Hinsley, A., Hua, F., Hughes, A. C., Jones, K. E., Kelly, M., King, T., Kirkland, T., MaCDonald, D. W., Newman, C., ... & Smith, R. K. (2021). Post COVID-19: A solution scan of options for preventing future zoonotic epidemics. *Biological Reviews*, 96(6), 2694-2715. https://doi.org/10.1111/brv.12774.

Plowright, R. K., Parrish, C. R., McCallum, H., Hudson, P. J., Ko, A. I., Graham, A. L., & Lloyd-Smith, J. O. (2017). Pathways to zoonotic spillover. *Nature Reviews Microbiology*, 15(8), 502-510. https://doi.org/10.1038/nrmicro.2017.45.

Roche, X., Rozstalnyy, A., TagliaCarne, A., Pittiglio, C., Kamata, A., Belot, G., Pinto, J., & Traore, T. (2022). One Health approach to address zoonotic diseases. *Zoonoses*, 2(1), 1-23. https://doi.org/10.15212/ZOONOSES-2022-0037.

Schultz-Cherry, S., Webby, R. J., Webster, R. G., Kelso, A., Barr, I. G., McCauley, J. W., Daniels, R. S., Wang, D., Shu, Y., Nobusawa, E., Itamura, S., Tashiro, M., & Xu, X. (2021). Influenza virus and SARS-CoV-2: Pathogenesis and host responses in the respiratory tract. *Nature Reviews Microbiology*, 19(7), 425-441. https://doi.org/10.1038/s41579-021-00542-7.

Shafaati, M., Akbarpour, S., Priyanka, Saied, A. A., & Choudhary, O. P. (2023). Tackling rabies by One Health approach: Pitfalls on the road to global eradication. *Frontiers in Public Health*, 11, 1137861. https://doi.org/10.3389/fpubh.2023.1137861.

Wardeh, M., Baylis, M., & Blagrove, M. S. C. (2021). Predicting mammalian hosts in which novel coronaviruses can be generated. *Nature Communications*, 12(1), 780. https://doi.org/10.1038/s41467-021-21034-5.

Webster, R. G., & Govorkova, E. A. (2014). Continuing challenges in influenza. *Annals of the New York Academy of Sciences*, 1323(1), 115-139. https://doi.org/10.1111/nyas.12462.

World Health Organization. (2024). Rabies fact sheet. Retrieved from https://www.who.int/news-room/fact-sheets/detail/rabies.

Chapter 8

Disease Detection, Identification, and Monitoring Systems

Sushil Ghanshyam Kachewar[1]
and Maajid Mohi Ud Din Malik[2,*], PhD
[1]Department of Radio-Diagnosis, Dr. D. Y. Patil Medical College, Hospital and Research Centre, Dr. D. Y. Patil Vidyapeeth, Pune (Deemed to be University)- Sant Tukaram Nagar, Pimpri, Pune, India
[2]Department of Radiology and Imaging Technology, Dr. D. Y. Patil School of Allied Health Sciences, Dr. D. Y. Patil Vidyapeeth· Pune (Deemed to be University), Sant Tukaram Nagar, Pimpri, Pune, India

Abstract

Disease detection, identification, and monitoring systems represent the foundational infrastructure for effective One Health surveillance and response, integrating advanced laboratory diagnostics, rapid testing technologies, and comprehensive monitoring approaches across human, animal, and environmental health domains. This chapter examines the evolution of diagnostic capabilities from traditional laboratory-based methods to innovative point-of-care testing, genomic sequencing platforms, and environmental monitoring systems that enable real-time detection and characterization of pathogens. Syndromic surveillance approaches are analysed as complementary systems that detect disease patterns before laboratory confirmation, while ecological monitoring through wastewater and ecosystem surveillance provides population-level insights into pathogen circulation. The integration of molecular diagnostics, including next-generation sequencing and metagenomic analysis, has revolutionised pathogen identification capabilities and enabled rapid characterization of emerging threats. Quality assurance and standardisation frameworks are essential for ensuring reliability, comparability, and interoperability of surveillance data across different sectors and geographic regions. Challenges in implementing integrated One Health surveillance systems include technical barriers, resource constraints, regulatory frameworks, and the need for multisectoral coordination. The chapter emphasises the critical role of these systems in achieving early detection of disease threats, enabling rapid response interventions, and supporting evidence-based public health decision-making. These comprehensive detection and monitoring capabilities are fundamental to achieving Sustainable Development Goal 3 (Good Health and Well-being) by strengthening health system resilience and pandemic preparedness capacity.

---

* Corresponding Author's Email: maajid.malik@dpu.edu.in

In: Advances in the One Health Approach
Editors: Maajid Mohi Ud Din Malik, Abhay Saraf, Harshal Tukaram Pandve et al.
ISBN: 979-8-90134-202-2

Keywords: disease surveillance, laboratory diagnostics, point-of-care testing, genomic sequencing, syndromic surveillance, environmental monitoring, wastewater surveillance, One Health, quality assurance, Sustainable Development Goal 3

Introduction

Disease detection, identification, and monitoring systems serve as the cornerstone of global health security, providing the essential infrastructure for early warning, rapid response, and evidence-based decision-making in public health emergencies. The evolution of these systems has been dramatically accelerated by technological advances in molecular diagnostics, digital health platforms, and integrated surveillance approaches that transcend traditional boundaries between human, animal, and environmental health sectors. Contemporary surveillance systems must address increasingly complex challenges, including emerging infectious diseases, antimicrobial resistance, climate-related health threats, and the interconnected nature of health risks in our globalised world.

The One Health approach has fundamentally transformed surveillance system design and implementation, recognising that effective disease detection requires coordinated monitoring across the entire spectrum of factors that influence health outcomes. This paradigm shift has led to the development of integrated surveillance platforms that combine traditional clinical and laboratory surveillance with innovative approaches, including environmental monitoring, digital syndromic surveillance, and real-time genomic analysis. The COVID-19 pandemic highlighted both the critical importance of robust surveillance systems and the significant gaps that exist in current detection and monitoring capabilities, particularly in resource-limited settings and at the human-animal-environment interface.

Technological innovations have revolutionised diagnostic capabilities, enabling rapid pathogen identification, real-time monitoring of disease trends, and predictive analytics that can anticipate emerging threats before they manifest as clinical outbreaks. Point-of-care testing technologies have democratised diagnostic capabilities, bringing sophisticated testing closer to patients and communities while reducing dependence on centralised laboratory infrastructure. Genomic sequencing platforms now provide unprecedented insights into pathogen evolution, transmission dynamics, and antimicrobial resistance patterns, informing both clinical care and public health interventions (Hayman et al., 2023).

The integration of environmental monitoring approaches, particularly wastewater surveillance, has emerged as a powerful tool for population-level health monitoring that complements traditional clinical surveillance systems. These approaches provide unbiased, anonymised insights into community health status and can detect pathogen circulation before clinical cases are recognised. Quality assurance and standardisation frameworks ensure that surveillance data are reliable, comparable, and actionable across different settings and jurisdictions, supporting coordinated response efforts and evidence-based policy development.

8.1. Laboratory Diagnostics in One Health

Laboratory diagnostics in One Health represent the analytical foundation enabling integrated surveillance and response across human, animal, and environmental health domains. These systems must overcome traditional sectoral boundaries to provide comprehensive pathogen detection, characterisation, and monitoring capabilities, supporting evidence-based decision-making for complex health challenges that transcend species and environmental limits.

The conceptual framework emphasises interconnected health risks, recognising that many pathogens circulate freely among humans, animals, and ecological matrices, requiring surveillance strategies that monitor all relevant compartments for comprehensive threat assessment. Traditional laboratory systems organised around specific sectors must evolve to support multisectoral collaboration while maintaining specialised expertise and regulatory compliance.

Multisectoral laboratory networks have emerged as essential infrastructure, bringing together public health laboratories, veterinary diagnostic facilities, environmental testing laboratories, and research institutions under coordinated frameworks that enable rapid information sharing and collaborative responses (Nyamai et al., 2022). These networks face significant challenges in harmonising different analytical methods, quality standards, and data management systems that have evolved independently within each sector.

The Electronic Integrated Disease Surveillance System exemplifies successful One Health laboratory integration, providing platforms for collecting and analysing epidemiological, clinical, and laboratory information across medical, veterinary, and environmental sectors. Implementation experiences in Kazakhstan demonstrate that integrated surveillance systems can enhance disease detection and response capabilities, while reducing duplication and improving cost-effectiveness, thereby enforcing One Health concepts by improving surveillance for hazardous pathogens, such as Crimean-Congo hemorrhagic fever (Burdakov & Ukharov, 2013).

Standardisation of analytical methods represents a critical component that requires harmonised protocols applied consistently across different sample types and laboratory settings. Molecular diagnostic approaches—particularly polymerase chain reaction and next-generation sequencing technologies—offer harmonisation opportunities because they can be applied to diverse sample types using similar analytical procedures.

Quality assurance programs must address complex challenges, ensuring analytical quality across different sectors with varying regulatory requirements, accreditation standards, and quality control procedures. Information management systems must support rapid data sharing and integrated analysis while respecting sectoral requirements for data security, privacy, and regulatory compliance.

Capacity building requires coordinated training programs that build expertise in cross-sectoral collaboration while maintaining specialised technical competencies. Resource-sharing mechanisms enhance efficiency by enabling laboratories to pool their specialised equipment, expertise, and materials. Emergency response capabilities must address complex logistical and coordination challenges that arise during public health emergencies, requiring rapid diagnostic support across multiple sectors simultaneously.

Regulatory frameworks must address the complex legal and policy issues that arise when laboratory services span multiple sectors with different regulatory authorities. Innovation and technology transfer mechanisms can accelerate the development and deployment of new diagnostic technologies that support One Health objectives. Performance monitoring and evaluation systems must assess both technical performance, regarding analytical quality, and operational performance, regarding cross-sectoral collaboration and integration.

8.2. Rapid Diagnostic Tools and Point-of-Care Testing

Rapid diagnostic tools and point-of-care testing represent transformative technologies that revolutionise disease detection capabilities by bringing sophisticated analytical methods closer to patients, communities, and field settings, where immediate diagnostic information is most valuable. These technologies address critical gaps in traditional laboratory-based diagnostic systems, particularly in resource-limited settings where access to centralised laboratories is limited and rapid decision-making is crucial.

Point-of-care testing encompasses a diverse range of diagnostic platforms designed to provide rapid, accurate results in non-laboratory settings with minimal training requirements. Performance characteristics have improved dramatically, with many tests achieving sensitivity and specificity levels comparable to those of traditional laboratory-based methods, while providing results in minutes rather than hours or days (Centres for Disease Control and Prevention, 2024).

Application to zoonotic and infectious disease diagnosis is crucial in One Health contexts, where rapid diagnostic information is vital for controlling the transmission of diseases. Veterinary applications have demonstrated significant potential for enhancing animal health surveillance, particularly in low- and middle-income countries; however, implementation faces unique technical, regulatory, and socioeconomic challenges (Hobbs et al., 2021).

Lateral flow assays represent the most widely deployed category, utilising simple immunochromatographic principles to detect pathogen antigens or host antibodies. Molecular point-of-care platforms, including loop-mediated isothermal amplification, recombinase polymerase amplification, and portable PCR systems, represent cutting-edge technology that enables nucleic acid detection in portable formats.

Smartphone-based diagnostic systems leverage mobile phone technology for optical detection, data analysis, and result reporting. Nanopore sequencing technology has emerged as a promising point-of-care molecular diagnostic, enabling real-time DNA and RNA sequencing in portable formats for pathogen identification and characterisation (McLean & Graham, 2022).

Multiplex testing capabilities enable the simultaneous detection of multiple pathogens in a single test procedure, particularly valuable for syndromic approaches. Quality assurance and regulatory considerations present unique challenges requiring a balance between analytical quality and practical deployment requirements.

Cost-effectiveness analysis must consider both direct costs and indirect benefits, including reduced transmission and improved treatment outcomes. Implementation barriers include technical challenges, regulatory barriers, and socioeconomic restrictions limiting access in resource-limited settings (Sikkema et al., 2023).

Innovation pathways continue evolving rapidly, with emerging technologies including artificial intelligence-enhanced interpretation and improved sample preparation systems (Zhu et al., 2025). Integration into One Health surveillance systems requires careful consideration of data management, quality assurance, and coordination mechanisms enabling distributed diagnostic capabilities to contribute effectively to broader surveillance objectives (Tegegne et al., 2024). Table 8.1 presents a comparison of point-of-care testing technologies within a one-health approach.

Table 8.1. Comparison of Point-of-Care testing technologies

Technology Platform	Typical Turnaround Time	Sample Types	Multiplexing Capability	Training Requirements	Cost Level
Lateral Flow Assays	10-30 minutes	Multiple	Limited (2-5 targets)	Minimal	Low
Molecular LAMP/ RPA	30-60 minutes	Multiple	Moderate (5-10 targets)	Basic	Moderate
Portable PCR	1-3 hours	Multiple	High (10+ targets)	Intermediate	High
Nanopore Sequencing	1-6 hours	DNA/RNA	Unlimited	Advanced	High
Smartphone-based	Variable	Multiple	Moderate	Basic	Low-Moderate

8.3. Genomic Sequencing and Phylogenetic Analysis

Genomic sequencing and phylogenetic analysis have emerged as transformative technologies providing unprecedented insights into pathogen biology, evolution, transmission dynamics, and antimicrobial resistance patterns. These molecular approaches have revolutionised surveillance capabilities by enabling rapid pathogen identification, real-time monitoring of genetic changes, and detailed investigation of outbreak sources and transmission pathways.

Next-generation sequencing technologies have significantly reduced the cost and time required for whole-genome sequencing while improving data quality and throughput capabilities. Platforms can now generate complete pathogen genomes within hours, rather than weeks, enabling real-time genomic surveillance that informs immediate public health response decisions. The democratisation of sequencing technology has made genomic analysis accessible worldwide, although significant disparities remain in technical capacity, limiting its implementation in resource-limited settings.

Metagenomic sequencing approaches represent compelling applications that enable the simultaneous detection and characterisation of all microorganisms present in clinical, environmental, or ecological samples. This unbiased approach can identify unknown or unexpected pathogens, characterise complex microbial communities, and provide comprehensive information about antimicrobial resistance genes and virulence factors, proving particularly valuable for investigating outbreaks of unknown aetiology (Miller et al., 2021).

Phylogenetic analysis techniques utilise genomic sequence data to reconstruct evolutionary relationships among pathogens and infer transmission pathways during outbreaks, identifying outbreak sources, tracking transmission chains, and distinguishing between related and unrelated cases. Real-time genomic surveillance systems integrate sequencing technologies with bioinformatics pipelines that analyse sequence data and generate epidemiologically relevant information within hours of sample collection.

Antimicrobial resistance detection through genomic analysis has become essential, enabling the rapid identification of resistance genes and mechanisms that inform treatment decisions. Portable sequencing technologies, particularly nanopore platforms, have enabled genomic analysis in field settings and resource-limited environments where traditional sequencing infrastructure is unavailable.

Bioinformatics infrastructure represents critical components requiring sophisticated computational resources and expertise for sequence analysis, quality control, and epidemiological interpretation. Data management and sharing frameworks must address complex technical and policy challenges related to data volume, storage, analysis, and international sharing while balancing concerns about data sovereignty, privacy, and potential misuse.

Quality assurance requires specialised approaches that address the unique characteristics of sequencing technology and bioinformatics pipelines. Integration with traditional epidemiological investigations requires new approaches that combine molecular and epidemiological information to generate actionable insights. Ethical considerations encompass questions about consent, privacy, and data ownership, which differ from traditional surveillance approaches.

Cost-effectiveness analysis must consider both direct sequencing and analysis costs, as well as indirect benefits, including improved clinical outcomes, reduced transmission, and enhanced public health response capabilities. Future developments are likely to focus on increasing automation, reducing costs, and improving integration with routine surveillance systems, with artificial intelligence and machine learning approaches potentially enhancing speed and accuracy.

8.4. Syndromic Surveillance Approaches

Syndromic surveillance approaches represent innovative monitoring systems that detect disease patterns through the systematic collection and analysis of health-related data, preceding traditional diagnostic confirmation. These systems provide early warning capabilities by monitoring indicators, including clinical symptoms, healthcare utilisation patterns, pharmaceutical sales, school or workplace absenteeism, and other proxy measures that signal outbreak onset before laboratory-confirmed cases are identified.

The conceptual foundation rests on the principle that disease outbreaks produce detectable signals in various data streams before clinical diagnosis and laboratory confirmation occur. Early indicators may include increased emergency department visits for respiratory symptoms, elevated sales of over-the-counter medications, increased absenteeism, or unusual reports of animal mortality. By systematically monitoring these syndromic indicators, public health agencies can detect potential outbreaks days or weeks before they are identified through traditional surveillance methods.

Electronic syndromic surveillance systems have revolutionised the field by enabling automated data collection, analysis, and alerting from diverse sources, including hospital emergency departments, urgent care centres, pharmacies, schools, and workplaces. Systems can process thousands of daily data points and apply statistical algorithms to detect unusual patterns warranting public health investigation.

One Health applications recognise that disease patterns in human populations may be preceded or accompanied by similar patterns in animal populations or environmental indicators. Integrated syndromic surveillance systems monitor human health indicators alongside animal health reports, ecological monitoring data, and agricultural production metrics, providing comprehensive early warning capabilities particularly valuable for detecting zoonotic disease outbreaks.

Artificial intelligence and machine learning techniques have enhanced syndromic surveillance capabilities by enabling more sophisticated pattern recognition and predictive analytics (Zhou et al., 2023). These approaches identify complex patterns in multidimensional data that are not apparent through traditional statistical methods, adapting to local patterns and seasonal variations while maintaining sensitivity to unusual events that represent emerging public health threats.

Mobile health technologies and social media monitoring have emerged as new sources of syndromic surveillance data, providing real-time insights into community health. Emergency department syndromic surveillance represents one of the most mature applications, utilising chief complaint data, diagnostic codes, and clinical notes to detect unusual emergency department visit patterns. Pharmaceutical surveillance systems monitor the sales of over-the-counter medications, prescription patterns, and pharmacy inquiries, detecting early indicators of outbreaks.

School-based systems monitor student and staff absenteeism patterns, detecting disease outbreaks in educational settings. Workplace surveillance monitors employee absenteeism and occupational health indicators. Veterinary syndromic surveillance monitors animal health indicators, including clinical signs, mortality patterns, and production metrics, to detect animal disease outbreaks with zoonotic potential.

Statistical methods must address the unique characteristics of syndromic data, including high volume, real-time processing requirements, and seasonal patterns. Data quality and validation pose ongoing challenges, as factors beyond disease occurrence may influence indicators. Privacy and ethical considerations require a careful balance between public health benefits and individual privacy rights.

8.5. Environmental Monitoring and Detection

Environmental monitoring and detection systems have emerged as critical components of One Health surveillance, providing unique insights into pathogen circulation, exposure pathways, and population health status through systematic monitoring of air, water, soil, and other environmental matrices. These approaches complement traditional clinical and animal surveillance by detecting pathogens in environmental reservoirs before causing recognisable disease outbreaks, enabling early intervention and prevention strategies.

Wastewater surveillance represents the most developed and widely implemented form of environmental pathogen monitoring, leveraging the fact that many human and animal pathogens are shed in faeces and urine and can be detected in sewage systems serving defined populations (Zhang et al., 2021). This approach provides unbiased population-level monitoring, detecting pathogen circulation regardless of individual healthcare access, symptom severity, or testing behaviour. Wastewater surveillance has been successfully applied to numerous pathogens, including poliovirus, SARS-CoV-2, influenza viruses, norovirus, and antimicrobial-resistant bacteria, demonstrating its versatility and reliability (Gibas et al., 2021).

Table 8.2. Environmental monitoring applications in One Health surveillance

Environmental Matrix	Primary Applications	Detection Methods	Spatial Coverage	Temporal Resolution	One Health Integration
Wastewater	Population health monitoring	qPCR, sequencing	Community/institutional	Daily/weekly	Human-animal interface
Surface water	Recreational/drinking water safety	Culture, qPCR	Local/regional	Variable	Environmental-human
Air	Airborne pathogen detection	PCR, culture	Building/local	Real-time/hourly	Indoor environments
Soil/sediments	Environmental persistence	Culture, qPCR	Local/regional	Monthly/seasonal	Animal-environmental
Food/feed	Food safety monitoring	Multiple methods	Supply chain	Batch/continuous	Human-animal-food

Technical implementation requires careful consideration of sampling strategies, laboratory methods, and data analysis approaches, taking into account the unique characteristics of wastewater. Laboratory methods have evolved rapidly, incorporating advanced concentration techniques, molecular detection methods, and quality control procedures optimised for wastewater samples. Polymerase chain reaction (PCR) and quantitative PCR (qPCR) methods are most commonly used for pathogen detection, although metagenomic sequencing approaches are increasingly applied for broader surveillance capabilities.

Air monitoring represents an emerging area for detecting respiratory pathogens in healthcare facilities, schools, and transportation systems. Soil and surface environmental monitoring detects pathogens persisting in environmental matrices outside host organisms, particularly relevant for monitoring spore-forming bacteria and agricultural pathogens. Water quality monitoring beyond wastewater includes surveillance of drinking water, recreational water, and environmental water sources for pathogenic organisms.

One Health environmental monitoring approaches integrate surveillance of human, animal, and ecological pathogen reservoirs, providing a comprehensive understanding of pathogen ecology and transmission dynamics. Sensor technologies and automated monitoring systems enable continuous, real-time monitoring of environmental conditions and pathogen levels through biosensor technologies and Internet of Things approaches.

Quality assurance presents unique challenges because environmental samples are typically more complex and variable than clinical samples. Data integration requires sophisticated analytical approaches combining ecological monitoring data with clinical and epidemiological information, generating actionable public health insights.

Regulatory frameworks are still evolving as surveillance approaches mature and demonstrate public health value (World Health Organisation, 2024). Cost-effectiveness analysis must consider both direct sampling and laboratory analysis costs, as well as broader public health benefits, including early warning capabilities and reduced disease burden. Table 8.2 shows ecological monitoring applications in one health surveillance.

8.6. Quality Assurance and Standardisation

Quality assurance and standardisation represent fundamental requirements for reliable disease detection, identification, and monitoring systems that can support evidence-based public health decision-making and coordinated response efforts. These frameworks ensure that surveillance data are accurate, reliable, comparable across different settings and jurisdictions, and suitable for supporting critical decisions about public health interventions. The complexity of modern surveillance systems, which incorporate diverse technologies, data sources, and analytical approaches, requires sophisticated quality assurance programs that address both the technical and operational aspects of system performance.

Laboratory quality assurance programs form the foundation of reliable surveillance systems, establishing standardised procedures, performance requirements, and quality control measures that ensure analytical accuracy and precision. These programs must address all aspects of laboratory operations, including sample collection and handling, analytical procedures, equipment calibration and maintenance, personnel training and competency assessment, as well as data management and reporting. International standards such as ISO

15189 for medical laboratories and ISO/IEC 17025 for testing and calibration laboratories provide frameworks for comprehensive quality management systems.

Standardisation of analytical methods is essential for ensuring comparability of surveillance data across different laboratories, regions, and time periods. Standardised protocols must specify all aspects of analytical procedures, including sample collection, storage, and transportation requirements; pre-analytical processing steps; analytical methods and equipment; quality control procedures; and criteria for result interpretation. The development of standardised methods requires extensive validation studies that demonstrate analytical performance across diverse sample types and laboratory settings.

Proficiency testing programs provide external quality assessment by requiring laboratories to analyse standardised samples and compare their results with reference values or peer laboratory performance. These programs help identify analytical problems, assess method performance, and verify laboratory competency across different testing scenarios. Proficiency testing for surveillance applications may require specialised programs that address the unique characteristics of surveillance samples and testing requirements that differ from those of routine clinical testing.

Reference materials and standards are essential components of quality assurance systems, providing traceable benchmarks for method validation, equipment calibration, and quality control procedures. The availability of appropriate reference materials is often a limiting factor in developing quality assurance programs for emerging pathogens or novel surveillance applications. International coordination of reference material development and distribution can help ensure that quality assurance standards are achievable across different resource settings.

Data quality assurance encompasses procedures for ensuring the accuracy, completeness, consistency, and timeliness of surveillance data throughout the entire data lifecycle from collection through analysis and reporting. Data validation procedures must address potential sources of error, including data entry mistakes, missing values, coding errors, and logical inconsistencies. Automated data quality checks can identify possible problems in real-time and alert users to data quality issues that may affect analysis and interpretation.

Quality indicators and performance metrics provide objective measures of surveillance system performance that can guide quality improvement efforts and demonstrate system reliability to stakeholders. These metrics may include analytical performance measures, such as sensitivity, specificity, and detection limits, as well as operational performance measures, including turnaround time, data completeness, and system availability. Regular monitoring of quality indicators can identify trends in system performance and trigger corrective actions when performance falls below acceptable standards.

Training and competency programs ensure that personnel involved in surveillance systems possess the necessary knowledge and skills to perform their roles effectively and maintain high-quality standards. Training programs must address technical aspects of laboratory testing, data collection and management, and quality assurance procedures, as well as broader aspects of surveillance system operation, including communication, coordination, and emergency response procedures. Competency assessment and continuing education requirements help ensure that personnel maintain current knowledge and skills as surveillance systems evolve.

Quality management systems provide organisational frameworks for implementing and maintaining quality assurance programs across complex surveillance systems that may involve multiple organisations, sectors, and jurisdictions. These systems must establish clear roles and responsibilities, effective communication channels, and robust accountability mechanisms to ensure that quality standards are consistently maintained throughout the surveillance system. Document control procedures ensure that policies, procedures, and protocols remain current and are consistently applied across all system components.

External quality assessment through accreditation, certification, or recognition programs provides independent verification that surveillance systems meet established quality standards. Accreditation programs evaluate both technical competency and quality management systems to ensure comprehensive quality assurance. International recognition programs can facilitate the mutual recognition of surveillance data, supporting cross-border collaboration and information sharing.

Continuous improvement processes are essential for maintaining and enhancing quality assurance programs as surveillance systems evolve and new challenges emerge. These processes must include regular reviews and evaluations of quality assurance procedures, the incorporation of lessons learned from quality incidents or system failures, and proactive adaptation to new technologies, methods, and requirements. Feedback mechanisms from system users and stakeholders can provide valuable insights for quality improvement initiatives.

Information technology systems play increasingly essential roles in supporting quality assurance programs through automated data validation, quality control monitoring, and performance reporting capabilities. Laboratory information management systems can enforce quality procedures, track quality control results, and automatically generate quality reports. Cloud-based platforms can facilitate centralised quality monitoring across distributed surveillance networks while maintaining appropriate data security and access controls.

Regulatory compliance represents a crucial dimension of quality assurance, ensuring that surveillance systems meet applicable legal and regulatory requirements. These requirements may include laboratory licensing and certification, data privacy and security regulations, and public health reporting requirements. Compliance monitoring systems must track regulatory requirements across different jurisdictions and ensure that surveillance systems maintain appropriate compliance as regulations evolve.

International harmonisation of quality standards can facilitate global surveillance coordination and mutual recognition of surveillance data across national boundaries. International organisations, including the World Health Organisation, the World Organisation for Animal Health, and the International Organisation for Standardisation, play essential roles in developing harmonised quality standards and promoting their adoption worldwide. Regional harmonisation initiatives can address specific geographic or disease-specific requirements while contributing to broader global standardisation efforts.

Cost considerations in quality assurance program design must balance quality requirements with available resources and operational constraints. Quality assurance programs should be designed to achieve necessary quality objectives efficiently while avoiding unnecessary complexity or cost. Risk-based approaches can help prioritise quality assurance efforts on the most critical aspects of surveillance systems where quality problems would have the most significant impact on system performance and public health outcomes.

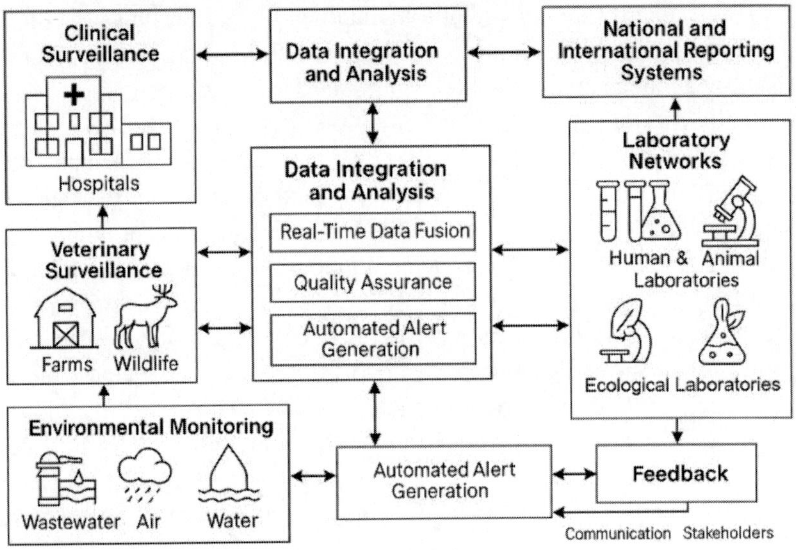

Figure 12. Integrated one health surveillance system architecture.

Figure 12 shows A comprehensive system diagram illustrating the integration of various surveillance components within a One Health framework. The diagram displays interconnected modules including clinical surveillance (hospitals, clinics), veterinary surveillance (farms, wildlife), environmental monitoring (wastewater, air, water), and laboratory networks (human, animal, ecological labs). The central data integration hub shows real-time data fusion, quality assurance systems, and automated alert generation. Information flows are depicted between sectors with bidirectional arrows showing data sharing and coordinated response pathways. The system is connected to national and international reporting systems, featuring feedback loops for continuous improvement and stakeholder communication channels.

Conclusion

Disease detection, identification, and monitoring systems represent foundational infrastructure upon which effective public health surveillance and response capabilities depend. Modern surveillance systems must integrate diverse technological approaches and operational strategies that address complex, interconnected health challenges, transcending traditional boundaries between human, animal, and environmental health domains.

The evolution of laboratory diagnostics toward One Health integration represents a fundamental paradigm shift, recognising interconnected health risks. Point-of-care testing technologies have democratised diagnostic capabilities by bringing sophisticated testing closer to patients and field settings. Genomic sequencing and phylogenetic analysis have revolutionised the understanding of pathogen biology and transmission dynamics, enabling real-time monitoring of pathogen evolution.

Syndromic surveillance approaches demonstrate significant value as early warning systems, detecting outbreaks before traditional methods. Environmental monitoring systems, particularly wastewater surveillance, have emerged as powerful tools for population-level health monitoring, providing unbiased insights into the circulation of community pathogens. Quality assurance frameworks are essential for ensuring that surveillance systems produce reliable, comparable data that supports confident decision-making.

The integration of artificial intelligence and machine learning represents an emerging frontier, promising enhanced analytical capabilities and improved early detection performance. The COVID-19 pandemic dramatically demonstrated the economic value of surveillance systems, highlighting both the catastrophic costs of inadequate preparedness and the potential benefits of early detection.

Future directions must address the integration of diverse data sources, the development of predictive analytics, the enhancement of real-time response coordination, and the improvement of equity across populations. Climate change and environmental degradation represent emerging challenges that require adaptation of surveillance systems. Globalisation requires enhanced international coordination, as pathogens transcend national boundaries.

Disease detection systems represent critical public health investments that protect population health and ensure sustainable development. Continued investment, supported by sustained political commitment and international cooperation, is essential for achieving global health security and advancing Sustainable Development Goals.

Figure 13 shows A timeline diagram depicting the evolution of surveillance technologies from traditional methods to future innovations. The timeline illustrates the progression from basic clinical reporting and laboratory culture (1900s-1970s) to molecular diagnostics and electronic surveillance (1980s-2000s), and finally to current integrated systems incorporating genomic sequencing, AI analytics, and environmental monitoring (2000s-present). Future directions (2025-2040) show predictive analytics, autonomous surveillance systems, and personalised population health monitoring. Each era shows key technologies, capabilities achieved, and remaining challenges. The diagram emphasises increasing integration, automation, and predictive capabilities over time.

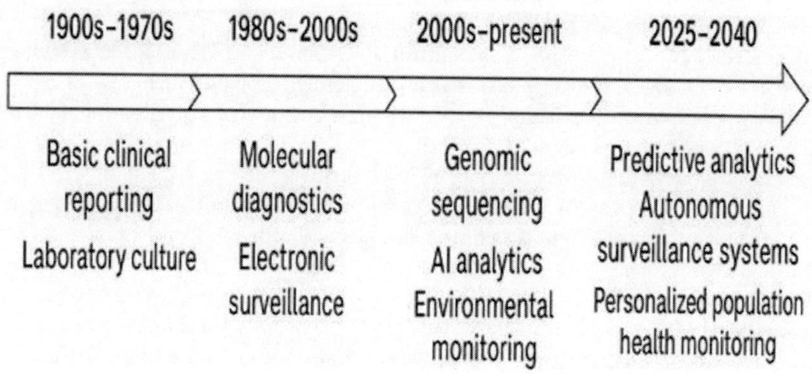

Figure 13. Surveillance technology evolution and future directions.

Acknowledgments

The authors would like to extend our appreciation to those who offered helpful commentary during the drafting process of this manuscript. We also acknowledge the role Nova Science Publishers played in enabling the work described herein.

References

Burdakov, A., & Ukharov, A. (2013). One Health surveillance with Electronic Integrated Disease Surveillance System. *BMC Proceedings*, 7(Suppl 2), P12. https://doi.org/10.1186/1753-6561-7-S2-P12.

Centers for Disease Control and Prevention. (2024). Rapid diagnostic tests for infectious diseases. In *CDC Yellow Book 2024: Health Information for International Travel*. Oxford University Press.

Gibas, C., Lambirth, K., Mittal, N., Juel, M. A. I., Barua, V. B., Brazell, L. R., Hinton, K., Lontai, J., Stark, N., Young, I., Quach, C., Russ, M., Kauer, J., Nicolosi, B., Chen, D., Akella, S., Tang, W., Schlueter, J., Munir, M., & Sikka, M. K. (2021). Implementing building-level SARS-CoV-2 wastewater surveillance on a university campus. *Science of the Total Environment*, 782, 146749. https://doi.org/10.1016/j.scitotenv.2021.146749.

Hayman, D. T. S., Adisasmito, W. B., Almuhairi, S., Barton Behravesh, C., Bilivogui, P., Bukachi, S. A., Casas, N., Cediel Becerra, N., Charron, D. F., Chaudhary, A., Ciacci Zanella, J. R., Cunningham, A. A., Dar, O., Debnath, N., Dungu, B., Farag, E., Gao, G. F., Khaitsa, M., Koopmans, M., ... & Lahariya, C. (2023). Developing One Health surveillance systems. *One Health*, 17, 100617. https://doi.org/10.1016/j.onehlt.2023.100617.

Hobbs, E. C., Colling, A., Gurung, R. B., & Allen, J. (2021). The potential of diagnostic point-of-care tests (POCTs) for infectious and zoonotic animal diseases in developing countries: Technical, regulatory and sociocultural considerations. *Transboundary and Emerging Diseases*, 68(4), 1835-1849. https://doi.org/10.1111/tbed.13880.

McLean, R. K., & Graham, S. P. (2022). The pig as an amplifying host for new and emerging zoonotic viruses. *One Health*, 14, 100384. https://doi.org/10.1016/j.onehlt.2022.100384.

Miller, S., Naccache, S. N., Samayoa, E., Messacar, K., Arevalo, S., Federman, S., Stryke, D., Pham, E., Fung, B., Bolosky, W. J., Ingebrigtsen, D., Lorizio, W., Paff, S. M., Leake, J. A., Pesano, R., Martinot, A., Yagi, S., Miller, M., Firth, C., ... & Chiu, C. Y. (2021). Laboratory validation of a clinical metagenomic sequencing assay for pathogen detection in cerebrospinal fluid. *Genome Research*, 29(6), 831-842. https://doi.org/10.1101/gr.238170.118.

Nyamai, M., Njenga, S. M., Bett, B., & Schelling, E. (2022). A generalisable One Health framework for the control of zoonotic diseases. *Scientific Reports*, 12, 8588. https://doi.org/10.1038/s41598-022-12619-1.

Sikkema, R. S., Koopmans, M. P. G., & Diederen, B. M. W. (2023). Rapid response screening for emerging zoonotic pathogens, barriers and opportunities: A study for enhanced preparedness of the Netherlands. *One Health*, 16, 100477. https://doi.org/10.1016/j.onehlt.2023.100477.

Tegegne, H. A., Freeth, F. T. A., Bogaardt, C., Reinhardt, J., Collineau, L., Prada, J. M., & Hasler, B. (2024). Implementation of One Health surveillance systems: Opportunities and challenges - lessons learned from the OH-EpiCap application. *One Health*, 18, 100704. https://doi.org/10.1016/j.onehlt.2024.100704.

U.S. Environmental Protection Agency. (2024). Quality assurance, quality control, and quality assessment measures. Retrieved from https://archive.epa.gov/water/archive/web/html/132.html.

World Health Organization. (2024). Wastewater and environmental surveillance guidance. Retrieved from https://www.who.int/teams/environment-climate-change-and-health/water-sanitation-and-health/sanitation-safety/wastewater.

Zhang, Y., Ma, Z. F., Kim, E. B., Zhao, P., Shim, S., Doherty, M., Wang, Y., & Grandjean, P. (2021). A narrative review of wastewater surveillance: Pathogens of concern, applications, detection methods, and challenges. *Journal of Environmental Management*, 294, 113011. https://doi.org/10.1016/j.jenvman.2021.113011.

Zhou, L., Wang, K., Li, C., & Zhao, F. (2023). Modern technologies and solutions to enhance surveillance and response systems for emerging zoonotic diseases. *Frontiers in Public Health*, 11, 1190824. https://doi.org/10.3389/fpubh.2023.1190824.

Zhu, L., Liu, J., Dao, T. L., Lu, D., Lu, H., Cheng, X., & Zhang, Y. (2025). Swine zoonotic viruses: Transmission and novel diagnostic technology. *One Health Advances*, 3, 3. https://doi.org/10.1186/s44280-024-00068-6.

Chapter 9

Vector-Borne Diseases and Medical Entomology

Maajid Mohi Ud Din Malik[1,*], PhD
and Rohini Adepwar[2]
[1]Department of Radiology and Imaging Technology, Dr. D. Y. Patil School of Allied Health Sciences, Dr. D. Y. Patil Vidyapeeth, Pune (Deemed to be University), Sant Tukaram Nagar, Pimpri, Pune, India
[2]Dr. D. Y. Patil School of Allied Health Sciences, Dr. D. Y. Patil Vidyapeeth, Pune (Deemed to be University), Sant Tukaram Nagar, Pimpri, Pune, India

Abstract

Vector-borne diseases represent a critical global health challenge, affecting over one billion people annually and imposing substantial health, social, and economic burdens worldwide. This chapter provides a comprehensive examination of medical entomology and the major vector-borne diseases that impact human populations, including malaria, dengue, Zika virus, and Lyme disease. The chapter explores the complex interactions among pathogens, arthropod vectors, vertebrate hosts, and environmental factors that collectively shape disease emergence, transmission dynamics, and public health impact. Topics covered include the biology and ecology of disease vectors, particularly mosquitoes and ticks, their behavioral patterns, breeding habitats, and feeding preferences. The chapter examines how climate change is fundamentally altering the geographic and temporal boundaries of vector-borne disease transmission through its effects on vector development, survival, distribution patterns, and pathogen replication rates. Integrated vector management strategies are discussed, including chemical control methods, biological control agents, environmental management approaches, and innovative technologies such as genetically modified mosquitoes and sterile insect techniques. The One Health approach is presented as an essential framework for addressing the complex ecological and social determinants of vector-borne diseases through coordinated action across human health, animal health, and environmental management sectors. Special emphasis is placed on community engagement strategies and participatory approaches as fundamental components of sustainable vector control programs. The chapter synthesizes current evidence on epidemiological patterns, control challenges, economic burden, and future directions for vector-borne disease prevention and management.

---

* Corresponding Author's Email: maajid.malik@dpu.edu.in

In: Advances in the One Health Approach
Editors: Maajid Mohi Ud Din Malik, Abhay Saraf, Harshal Tukaram Pandve et al.
ISBN: 979-8-90134-202-2

Keywords: posture, ergonomics, workplace assessment, repetitive strain injuries, pain prevention

Introduction

Vector-borne diseases represent a complex and expanding global health challenge that exemplifies the interconnected nature of human, animal, and environmental health systems. These diseases, transmitted by arthropod vectors such as mosquitoes, ticks, fleas, and flies, affect over one billion people annually and impose devastating health, social, and economic burdens, particularly on the world's most vulnerable populations. The World Health Organisation estimates that 80% of the global population lives in areas at risk for at least one primary vector-borne disease, with the burden concentrated in tropical and subtropical regions where poverty, inadequate infrastructure, and favourable climatic conditions create optimal environments for vector proliferation and disease transmission (World Health Organisation, 2024).

The epidemiological landscape of vector-borne diseases is rapidly evolving in response to multiple interconnected drivers, including climate change, globalisation, urbanisation, and environmental degradation, which collectively alter vector ecology, pathogen dynamics, and human exposure patterns. Climate change has emerged as a particularly critical factor, with warming temperatures, changing precipitation patterns, and extreme weather events expanding the geographic and temporal boundaries of vector habitat suitability while potentially increasing transmission intensity in endemic areas (Ryan et al., 2019). The economic implications of vector-borne diseases extend far beyond direct healthcare costs to include lost productivity, reduced agricultural output, decreased tourism, and impediments to economic development that perpetuate cycles of poverty in affected regions.

Traditional approaches to vector control, based primarily on chemical interventions, face mounting challenges from widespread insecticide resistance, environmental concerns, and sustainability constraints, prompting a renewed emphasis on integrated vector management strategies. The One Health approach provides a conceptual framework for addressing vector-borne diseases through coordinated action across human Health, animal health, and environmental management sectors, recognising that effective control requires understanding and intervention at multiple levels of the socioecological system (Bardosh et al., 2024). Community engagement and participatory approaches have emerged as essential components of sustainable vector control programs, built local capacity and ownership while addressed the social determinants that influence vulnerability to vector-borne diseases.

9.1. Major Vector-Borne Diseases (Malaria, Dengue, Zika, Lyme)

The global burden of vector-borne diseases encompasses a diverse array of pathogens transmitted through arthropod vectors, with four diseases—malaria, dengue, Zika virus, and Lyme disease—representing particularly significant public health challenges that illustrate the varied epidemiological patterns, clinical presentations, and control strategies characteristic of this disease category. These diseases collectively illustrate the complex interplay between pathogens, vectors, hosts, and environmental factors that influence transmission dynamics and disease outcomes in diverse geographic and socioecological contexts.

Malaria remains the deadliest vector-borne disease globally, causing an estimated 249 million cases and more than 608,000 deaths annually, with most fatalities occurring in children under five years of age in sub-Saharan Africa. The disease is caused by Plasmodium parasites transmitted through the bite of infected female Anopheles mosquitoes, with Plasmodium falciparum representing the most virulent species responsible for severe malaria and death. The complex life cycle of malaria parasites involves both human and mosquito hosts, with sexual reproduction occurring in the mosquito vector and asexual reproduction in human hosts, affecting red blood cells and liver cells. Malaria transmission is susceptible to environmental conditions, with temperature, humidity, and rainfall patterns influencing both vector abundance and parasite development rates within mosquitoes.

The epidemiology of malaria has undergone significant changes over the past two decades, with substantial progress in reducing the disease burden achieved through the scaled implementation of key interventions, including insecticide-treated bed nets, indoor residual spraying, rapid diagnostic tests, and artemisinin-based combination therapy. However, progress has stagnated in recent years, with some regions experiencing increases in malaria cases and deaths attributed to factors including insecticide resistance, drug resistance, weakened health systems, and climate variability. The emergence and spread of artemisinin resistance in Southeast Asia represents a critical threat to malaria control efforts. In contrast, insecticide resistance in Anopheles vectors has reduced the effectiveness of bed nets and indoor residual spraying in many areas where malaria is endemic.

Dengue has emerged as the most rapidly spreading mosquito-borne viral disease globally, with transmission now reported in over 100 countries, resulting in an estimated 390 million infections annually. The disease is caused by four closely related dengue virus serotypes transmitted primarily by Aedes aegypti mosquitoes, though Aedes albopictus can also serve as a competent vector. Dengue presents a complex clinical spectrum, ranging from asymptomatic infection to life-threatening dengue hemorrhagic fever and dengue shock syndrome. Sequential infections by different virus serotypes are associated with an increased risk of severe disease through immunopathological mechanisms.

The geographic distribution of dengue has expanded dramatically over the past five decades, driven by factors including urbanisation, increased global travel and trade, inadequate vector control, and climate change that has extended the suitable habitat range for Aedes vectors. Urban environments provide ideal conditions for Aedes aegypti proliferation, with water storage containers, poor sanitation, and high population density facilitating both vector breeding and virus transmission. The lack of specific antiviral treatments and the complexity of dengue pathogenesis have made disease management challenging; however, the recent development and deployment of dengue vaccines represent a significant advance in prevention strategies.

Zika virus emerged as a global public health emergency following explosive outbreaks in the Pacific region and the Americas between 2013 and 2016, highlighting the potential for previously obscure pathogens to achieve pandemic status rapidly. The Zika virus is transmitted primarily through Aedes aegypti mosquitoes. However, sexual transmission and mother-to-child transmission represent additional routes of infection that distinguish Zika from other mosquito-borne viruses. While Zika virus infection is typically asymptomatic or causes mild illness characterised by fever, rash, and joint pain, the virus has been causally linked to serious neurological complications, including microcephaly in newborns and Guillain-Barré syndrome in adults.

The rapid spread of the Zika virus through the Americas demonstrated the vulnerability of populations in regions with established Aedes aegypti populations to emerging arboviral threats. The association between Zika virus infection during pregnancy and severe congenital disabilities created unprecedented public health challenges, prompting emergency declarations and urgent research efforts to develop diagnostic tests, surveillance systems, and prevention strategies. The Zika epidemic also highlighted health equity issues, with the most significant impact falling on marginalised populations with limited access to healthcare, family planning services, and vector control measures.

Lyme disease represents the most common vector-borne disease in temperate regions of the Northern Hemisphere, with over 30,000 cases reported annually in the United States and an increasing incidence in Europe and other temperate areas. The disease is caused by Borrelia burgdorferi spirochetes, which are transmitted through the bite of infected Ixodes ticks. Multiple tick species serve as competent vectors in different geographic regions. Lyme disease typically presents as an expanding erythema migrans rash at the site of tick attachment, though early localised infection can progress to disseminated infection affecting the nervous system, cardiovascular system, and joints if left untreated.

The epidemiology of Lyme disease reflects complex ecological relationships between tick vectors, reservoir hosts (including rodents and birds), and environmental factors that influence tick survival and host-seeking behaviour. Climate change has been linked to the expansion of tick populations and extended activity seasons in many regions, potentially increasing the risk of human exposure to tick-borne pathogens. Forest fragmentation and suburban development in tick habitat areas have increased human-tick contact opportunities, while changes in deer populations and land use patterns have influenced tick abundance and distribution. The prevention of Lyme disease primarily relies on personal protective measures, including avoiding ticks, wearing protective clothing, using repellents, and promptly removing ticks. However, environmental management strategies and targeted acaricide applications may also provide additional protection in high-risk areas. Table 9.1 shows epidemiological characteristics of major vector-borne diseases.

Table 9.1. Epidemiological characteristics of major vector-borne diseases

Disease	Pathogen	Primary Vector	Global Cases/Year	Geographic Distribution	Case Fatality Rate	Prevention Tools
Malaria	Plasmodium spp.	Anopheles mosquitoes	249 million	Tropical/ subtropical	0.2-0.3%	ITNs, IRS, antimalarials
Dengue	Dengue virus	Aedes mosquitoes	390 million	Urban tropical/ subtropical	<1%	Vector control, vaccine
Zika	Zika virus	Aedes mosquitoes	Variable (epidemic)	Tropical/ subtropical	<0.1%	Vector control, personal protection
Lyme	Borrelia burgdorferi	Ixodes ticks	>300,000	Temperate forests	<0.1%	Personal protection, early treatment

9.2. Vector Biology and Ecology

Understanding vector biology and ecology represents a fundamental requirement for developing effective vector-borne disease prevention and control strategies. Arthropod vectors have evolved complex life cycles and behavioural adaptations that enable efficient host location and blood feeding, while maintaining pathogen populations through both horizontal and vertical transmission mechanisms. Ecological relationships between vectors, pathogens, and host populations are influenced by environmental factors, including climate, habitat characteristics, and human activities modifying natural ecosystems.

Mosquito vectors represent the most epidemiologically significant group globally, with Anopheles, Aedes, and Culex species responsible for transmitting viruses, parasites, and bacteria causing major human diseases. Mosquito life cycles involve four developmental stages—egg, larva, pupa, and adult—with aquatic immature stages requiring water for development and terrestrial adult stages engaging in host-seeking and blood-feeding behaviours that are essential for reproduction and pathogen transmission. Development duration is highly temperature-dependent, with warmer conditions accelerating development rates and potentially increasing the number of generations per year.

Anopheles mosquitoes, the exclusive vectors of human malaria, exhibit species-specific preferences for larval breeding sites, adult resting locations, and host blood meal sources, which influence their vectorial capacity and susceptibility to control interventions. Host-seeking behaviour involves complex sensory mechanisms that detect carbon dioxide, lactic acid, heat, and other chemical cues. Anthropophilic species exhibit strong human blood meal preferences, while zoophilic species may prefer cattle or domestic animals.

Aedes mosquitoes, including Aedes aegypti and Aedes albopictus, are highly efficient urban disease vectors that transmit dengue, Zika, chikungunya, and yellow fever viruses. These species have adapted to urban environments by utilising artificial water containers as breeding sites and exhibiting strong anthropophilic feeding preferences, increasing human-vector contact rates. The container-breeding habit creates unique challenges, as breeding sites are typically small, numerous, and closely associated with human habitations.

Tick vectors exhibit distinct ecological strategies, as their parasitic lifestyle necessitates successful host attachment and extended feeding periods lasting several days. Ticks exhibit a complex life cycle involving three feeding stages—larva, nymph, and adult—with each stage requiring blood meals from vertebrate hosts to support moulting and reproduction. Ixodes ticks, which are responsible for transmitting Lyme disease, exhibit seasonal activity patterns that correspond to peak human outdoor activities in temperate regions.

Climate and environmental factors profoundly influence vector biology through their effects on development rates, survival, reproductive success, and behavioural patterns, collectively determining vectorial capacity and disease transmission potential. Temperature affects multiple aspects, including developmental rates, longevity, feeding behaviour, and pathogen replication rates within vectors. Humidity and precipitation patterns have a significant influence on vector survival and the availability of breeding sites.

Figure 14 shows A comprehensive diagram illustrating the life cycles of major disease vectors and their pathogen transmission pathways. The diagram displays four panels showing: (1) Anopheles mosquito life cycle with malaria parasite development stages in both human and mosquito hosts, 2) Aedes mosquito life cycle highlighting container breeding sites and viral transmission mechanisms for dengue/Zika, (3) Ixodes tick life cycle showing three-host feeding pattern and Lyme disease transmission, and (4) Environmental factors affecting vector development including temperature, humidity, and habitat characteristics. Each panel includes detailed annotations of key developmental stages, feeding behaviours, and critical control points for intervention strategies.

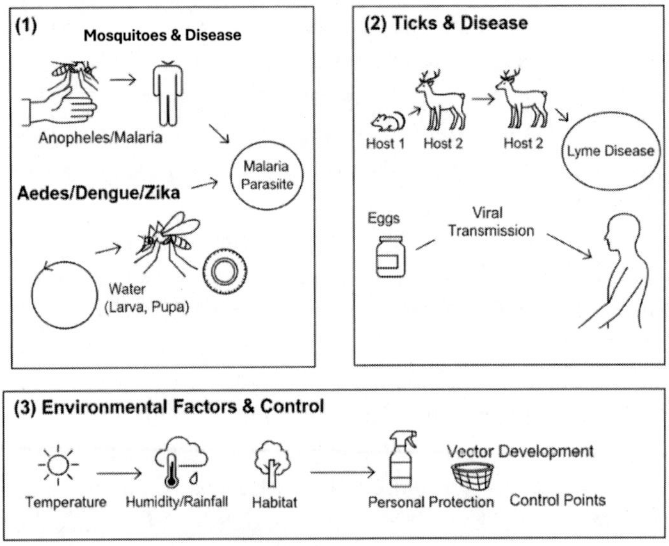

Figure 14. Vector Life Cycles and Transmission Pathways.

9.3. Climate Change Impacts on Vector Distribution

Climate change represents one of the most significant contemporary drivers of vector-borne disease emergence and re-emergence, fundamentally altering geographic and temporal boundaries of disease transmission through direct and indirect effects on vector biology, pathogen development, and host-pathogen interactions.

Temperature increases exert multiple effects on the transmission of vector-borne diseases through various biological and ecological mechanisms. Higher temperatures generally accelerate arthropod development rates within physiological tolerance limits, potentially reducing generation times and increasing reproductive cycles per transmission season. Warmer temperatures also increase adult activity levels and feeding frequencies, resulting in more frequent host contact and potentially higher pathogen transmission rates.

Temperature effects on pathogen development within arthropod vectors represent particularly critical determinants of transmission potential. Most vector-borne pathogens require specific temperature thresholds for successful replication within arthropod hosts. Higher temperatures typically accelerate pathogen development rates and reduce the extrinsic incubation period required before vectors become infectious, enhancing transmission efficiency. Mathematical models incorporating temperature-dependent parameters have projected substantial increases in the transmission potential of many vector-borne diseases under climate change scenarios. However, some regions may become too hot for efficient transmission (Couper et al., 2021).

Table 9.2. Climate change impacts on major vector-borne disease systems

Disease System	Climate Driver	Vector Response	Geographic Impact	Transmission Impact	Adaptation Needs
Malaria	Temperature increase	Faster development, extended seasons	Altitudinal expansion	Increased potential	Enhanced surveillance
Dengue/Zika	Temperature + precipitation	Urban adaptation, drought storage	Latitudinal expansion	Extended seasons	Container management
Lyme Disease	Temperature increase	Range expansion, longer seasons	Northward expansion	Earlier onset	Personal protection
West Nile	Temperature + extreme events	Heat tolerance, flood breeding	Geographic spread	Epidemic potential	Integrated surveillance

Precipitation patterns influence transmission through effects on vector breeding site availability, humidity levels, and environmental pathogen persistence. Drought conditions may intensify transmission by concentrating vectors and hosts around limited water sources, while extreme precipitation events create extensive temporary breeding sites.

Vector geographic range expansion represents one of the most visible consequences of climate change. Aedes albopictus exemplifies successful climate-driven range expansion, establishing populations across temperate regions of Europe, North America, and other previously unsuitable areas. Similarly, Ixodes ticks, responsible for Lyme disease transmission, have expanded their ranges northward and to higher elevations in response to warming temperatures, extending their activity seasons and improving overwinter survival rates.

Altitudinal shifts represent another consequence, with vectors establishing populations at higher elevations. Highland regions, historically protected by cooler temperatures, are increasingly experiencing disease transmission. Timing and duration of vector activity seasons have also been modified, with earlier spring onset and extended fall activity periods providing more opportunities for pathogen circulation.

Sea-level rise and coastal flooding create additional pathways by modifying coastal ecosystems and creating new breeding habitats for salt-tolerant mosquito species. Climate variability and extreme weather events have acute effects that differ from gradual, long-term trends. Interactions between climate change and other anthropogenic factors—such as urbanisation, land use change, and global trade—create complex synergies that potentially accelerate the emergence of vector-borne diseases beyond the effects of climate change alone. Table 9.2 illustrates the impacts of climate change on major vector-borne disease systems.

9.4. Vector Control Strategies and Resistance Management

Vector control strategies have evolved significantly from early approaches that relied primarily on environmental management and chemical interventions to contemporary integrated management programs, which combine multiple intervention types while addressing the growing challenges of insecticide resistance. The World Health Organisation's Global Vector Control Response provides a strategic framework for strengthening vector control as a fundamental disease prevention approach, emphasising increased technical capacity, improved surveillance systems, and enhanced community mobilisation for sustainable disease control outcomes.

Chemical control methods, particularly insecticides for adult mosquito and larval control, have formed the backbone of vector control programs for decades and continue to represent essential tools. Long-lasting insecticidal nets and indoor residual spraying represent two primary WHO-recommended malaria prevention interventions, demonstrating substantial impact on reducing malaria transmission and mortality when implemented at scale with high coverage levels. Mass LLIN distribution across sub-Saharan Africa contributed significantly to significant reductions in the malaria burden between 2000 and 2015, with an estimated 663 million cases averted. However, the effectiveness of LLINs has declined in many areas due to insecticide resistance in Anopheles vectors, prompting the development of next-generation bed nets incorporating additional active ingredients and novel modes of action.

Indoor residual spraying involves applying residual insecticides to interior wall surfaces where mosquitoes rest after feeding on blood, providing prolonged killing effects that persist for several months. Insecticide resistance represents one of the most significant contemporary challenges to controlling vector-borne diseases, with resistance mechanisms evolving in vector populations exposed to repeated applications of insecticides. Molecular mechanisms include target site modifications that reduce insecticide binding affinity, metabolic resistance involving enhanced detoxification enzyme activity, and behavioural resistance characterised by changes that minimise exposure to insecticidal intervention.

Insecticide resistance management strategies aim to preserve the effectiveness of available insecticides through rotation strategies, mosaic applications, and combination approaches that exploit different resistance mechanisms. The development of new insecticides with novel modes of action represents a critical component in resistance management. Chlorfenapyr, a pro-insecticide that targets mitochondrial respiration, has shown promise in controlling pyrethroid-resistant mosquito populations.

Biological control methods offer alternatives to chemical interventions, less prone to resistance development and more environmentally sustainable. Microbial control agents, including bacteria, fungi, viruses, and protozoa, can cause mortality in vector larvae or adults. Bacillus thuringiensis israelensis and Bacillus sphaericus are well-established bacterial larvicides demonstrating mosquito control effectiveness in diverse aquatic habitats.

The sterile insect technique and related genetic control methods represent innovative approaches to vector population suppression, exploiting reproductive biology for population reduction without the use of insecticides or environmental modification. Genetically modified mosquitoes represent an emerging technology that achieves population suppression through various mechanisms. Oxitec's genetically modified Aedes aegypti mosquitoes carry lethal genes causing offspring mortality before reproduction. Field trials have demonstrated proof of concept for population suppression, although regulatory approval processes and public acceptance remain essential considerations (Huang et al., 2024).

Environmental management approaches target vector breeding sites by modifying habitats, reducing sources, and implementing landscape management strategies to minimise vector production capacity. Integrated vector management represents a comprehensive approach that combines multiple intervention types within rational decision-making frameworks, considering local vector ecology, disease epidemiology, resource availability, and community preferences. The success of the IVM program depends on a strong technical capacity, adequate resource allocation, and sustained political commitment from national and local authorities (Bellinger et al., 2025).

9.5. One Health Approaches to Vector Control

One Health approaches to vector control recognise that effective vector-borne disease management requires coordinated action across human health, animal health, and environmental management sectors to address the complex ecological and social factors that determine vector population dynamics and disease transmission patterns. This integrated framework acknowledges that vector-borne disease systems operate within socioecological systems where human activities, animal populations, and environmental conditions interact, creating opportunities for pathogen emergence, amplification, and spread.

The conceptual foundation rests on the understanding that vectors, pathogens, and hosts exist within complex ecological networks that span multiple species and environments. Many vector-borne pathogens maintain enzootic transmission cycles involving wildlife reservoirs and arthropod vectors before spilling over into domestic animal or human populations. Effective prevention and control strategies must therefore consider entire transmission networks, rather than focusing solely on human infection endpoints, and require collaboration among professionals with expertise in human health, veterinary medicine, wildlife biology, entomology, and environmental science.

Surveillance systems designed according to One Health principles integrate the monitoring of pathogen circulation in humans, domestic animals, wildlife, and vectors, providing comprehensive early warning capabilities that detect emerging threats before they cause a significant human disease burden. West Nile virus surveillance exemplifies this approach, which includes monitoring of dead bird populations, mosquito pool testing, and equine case reports, alongside human surveillance.

Zoonotic arboviral diseases—such as West Nile virus, eastern equine encephalitis, and Rift Valley fever—exemplify the importance of the One Health approach, as these pathogens maintain complex transmission cycles involving multiple vertebrate host species and arthropod vectors. Birds serve as amplifying hosts, developing high viremia levels that enable efficient transmission of the virus to feeding vectors. In contrast, mammals typically serve as dead-end hosts, contributing minimally to ongoing transmission cycles.

Environmental management strategies implemented through One Health frameworks can address multiple vector-borne disease risks simultaneously while providing co-benefits for ecosystem health and biodiversity conservation. Urban planning and design represent critical applications, as urban environments concentrate human, domestic animal, and vector populations, while creating novel ecological conditions that facilitate disease transmission.

Climate adaptation strategies exemplify the needs of the One Health approach, as climate change impacts all components of the vector-borne disease system, including vector biology and distribution, pathogen development and survival, host population dynamics and susceptibility, and human exposure patterns and vulnerability. International cooperation frameworks provide essential coordination mechanisms for initiatives addressing vector-borne diseases crossing national boundaries.

Capacity building requires interdisciplinary education and training programs preparing professionals to work effectively across traditional sectoral boundaries. Community engagement strategies recognise local communities interact with vectors, pathogens, and hosts across multiple domains, including agriculture, animal husbandry, recreation, and household management. Policy frameworks necessitate coordination mechanisms facilitating collaboration among government agencies with diverse mandates. Evaluation presents methodological challenges because outcomes may be distributed across multiple sectors, with indirect effects that are difficult to measure using traditional health outcome indicators.

Figure 15 shows A comprehensive systems diagram illustrating the One Health approach to integrated vector management. The diagram displays three interconnected circles representing human Health, animal health, and environmental health sectors, with vector control activities shown at their intersections. Key components include coordinated surveillance systems that monitor humans, livestock, wildlife, and vectors; integrated control strategies addressing breeding sites, host protection, and pathogen interruption; community engagement platforms spanning all sectors; environmental management addressing habitat modification and ecosystem services; and policy coordination mechanisms that enable multisectoral collaboration. Arrows indicate the flow of information, resource sharing, and coordinated interventions across sectors. The framework emphasises prevention, early detection, and sustainable management strategies that address root causes of vector-borne disease vulnerability.

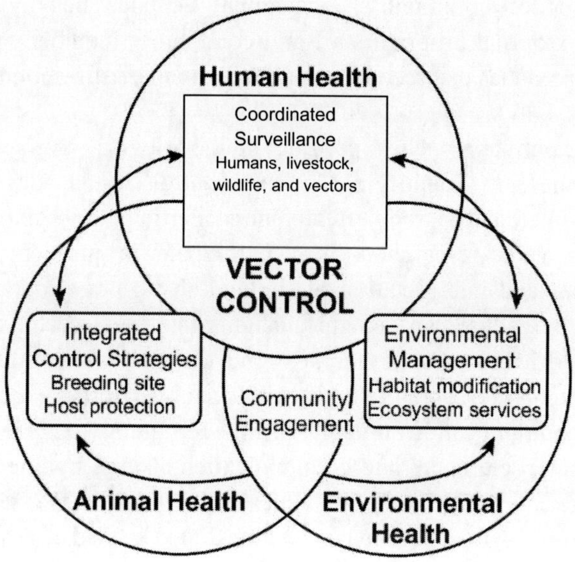

Figure 15. One Health Integrated Vector Management Framework.

9.6. Community Engagement in Vector Control

Community engagement represents a fundamental component of sustainable vector control programs, recognising that effective management of vector-borne diseases requires active participation and ownership by local populations who interact daily with vectors, breeding sites, and transmission environments. Traditional top-down approaches to vector control, which rely primarily on external interventions, have demonstrated limited sustainability and effectiveness, particularly in resource-constrained settings where ongoing program support may be intermittent. Contemporary vector control strategies increasingly emphasise participatory approaches that build local capacity, address community priorities, and integrate vector control activities with broader community development and health promotion initiatives.

The theoretical foundation for community engagement in vector control draws from multiple disciplines, including public health, social psychology, anthropology, and development studies, recognising that complex interactions between individual knowledge and attitudes, social norms and support systems, and structural factors —such as resource availability and institutional capacity — influence health behaviours and community practices. Successful community engagement requires an understanding of local cultural contexts, existing knowledge and practices related to vector control, and social and economic factors that influence community members' ability and willingness to adopt and maintain vector control behaviours.

Community-based vector control programs typically involve multiple phases, including community mobilisation and organising, participatory assessment of local vector control needs and priorities, collaborative development of intervention strategies, implementation of community-led activities, and participatory monitoring and evaluation of program outcomes. Each phase requires specific approaches and tools that are adapted to local contexts while maintaining focus on building community capacity and ownership for sustained vector control activities. The success of community engagement depends heavily on the quality of relationships between external program staff and community members, requiring respectful, culturally sensitive approaches that recognise and build upon existing community strengths and resources.

Participatory research approaches provide methodological frameworks for engaging communities as partners in identifying vector control needs, developing appropriate interventions, and evaluating program effectiveness. Participatory action research involves community members as co-researchers who participate in problem identification, data collection and analysis, and interpretation of findings that guide program development and modification. These approaches can generate insights into local vector ecology, community practices, and social determinants of vector-borne disease vulnerability that may not be apparent through traditional research methods conducted by external experts.

Educational and communication strategies within community engagement programs must address diverse learning preferences and communication channels while building on existing community knowledge and practices. Health education approaches that rely solely on didactic methods to convey technical information have demonstrated limited effectiveness in promoting sustained behaviour change. In contrast, participatory educational approaches that engage community members in dialogue, problem-solving, and skill-building activities are more likely to result in meaningful learning and application. Cultural and linguistic adaptation of educational materials and messages is essential for ensuring accessibility and relevance across diverse community populations.

Community health worker programs provide essential platforms for community engagement in vector control by training residents to serve as health educators, service providers, and advocates within their own communities. Community health workers can provide ongoing support for vector control activities, serve as liaisons between communities and formal health systems, and contribute local knowledge and perspectives to program planning and implementation. The effectiveness of community health worker programs depends on the implementation of appropriate selection, training, and ongoing supervision systems, as well as integration with broader health system structures and the establishment of adequate compensation or incentive systems.

Behavioural change interventions within community engagement programs typically focus on specific practices that reduce vector breeding sites, prevent vector-human contact, or enhance recognition and treatment of vector-borne diseases. Effective behavioural change requires understanding the multiple factors that influence health behaviours, including individual knowledge and self-efficacy, social norms and support, as well as environmental factors that enable or constrain specific behaviours. Social cognitive theory and other behavioural change frameworks offer guidance for developing interventions that target multiple levels of influence on health behaviours.

Table 9.3. Community engagement strategies for vector-borne disease control

Disease Context	Primary Vectors	Community Actions	Engagement Approach	Key Challenges	Success Indicators
Urban Aedes diseases	Aedes aegypti/ albopictus	Container elimination, water management	Household education, neighbourhood mobilisation	Water storage needs, poverty	Reduced breeding sites, knowledge
Rural malaria	Anopheles species	Net use, environmental management	Community health workers, participatory planning	Resource constraints, seasonal patterns	Net utilisation, case reduction
Peri-urban Chagas	Triatomine bugs	Housing improvement, vector control	Participatory research, technical support	Housing quality, economic barriers	Housing improvements, vector reduction
Lyme disease prevention	Ixodes ticks	Personal protection, environmental management	Education campaigns, tick surveillance	Outdoor recreation, tick awareness	Protective behaviours, tick encounters

For Aedes-borne disease control, community engagement typically focuses on eliminating container breeding sites through source reduction activities, including the removal of unnecessary containers, proper management of water storage containers, and modification of environments that collect rainwater. These activities require sustained community participation because container breeding sites are continuously created through household and community activities. Educational programs must therefore address not only the technical aspects of container management but also the social and economic factors that influence water storage practices and waste management behaviours.

Malaria prevention programs are increasingly incorporating community engagement strategies that complement the distribution of insecticide-treated nets and other vector control interventions. Community-based approaches to net distribution and maintenance can improve coverage and utilisation rates compared to clinic-based distribution systems. Meanwhile, community education programs can address misconceptions about malaria transmission and prevention, while also building support for vector control activities. Community case management programs that train local volunteers to provide rapid diagnostic tests and treatment for malaria cases can improve access to care while reducing transmission through prompt treatment.

Social marketing approaches apply commercial marketing principles to promote the adoption of vector control behaviours and products, using market research methods to understand community preferences and barriers while developing communication strategies that emphasise benefits and address concerns. Social marketing campaigns for insecticide-treated nets, for example, may emphasise multiple benefits including protection from malaria and nuisance mosquitoes while addressing concerns about safety, durability, and cost. Successful social marketing requires an understanding of local social and economic contexts that influence decision-making about health-related purchases and behaviours.

Environmental management activities offer significant opportunities for community engagement, as many vector breeding sites and control measures are situated in community spaces, necessitating collective action for effective management. Community-based environmental management may involve organising clean-up campaigns, establishing community gardens that eliminate standing water, or developing community-led mosquito control programs that address public breeding sites. These activities can build social cohesion and collective efficacy while achieving vector control objectives.

Participatory monitoring and evaluation systems engage community members in tracking the implementation and outcomes of vector control programs, building local capacity for ongoing program management, and generating information that can guide adaptive management decisions. Community members can be trained to conduct household surveys, monitor vector breeding sites, and assess behaviour change outcomes using simple data collection tools. Participatory evaluation approaches can generate insights into program strengths and weaknesses from community perspectives while building ownership for program improvement efforts.

Sustainability of community engagement programs requires attention to institutional and financial factors that can support ongoing community activities after external program support ends. Community-based organisations, religious institutions, schools, and other existing social structures can provide platforms for continuing vector control activities. In contrast, local government support can give legitimacy and resources for sustained programming. Integration of vector control activities with existing community programs and priorities can enhance sustainability by reducing the burden of additional activities while leveraging existing organisational capacity.

Challenges to effective community engagement in vector control include competing community priorities, resource constraints that limit community participation, and social and cultural factors that may create barriers to behaviour change. Power dynamics within communities may limit participation by marginalised groups, while conflicting interests among community members may impede collective action. External factors, including poverty, political instability, and weak institutional capacity, can constrain community engagement efforts despite strong local motivation and leadership.

Evaluation of community engagement programs requires assessing both process indicators, which reflect the quality and extent of community participation, and outcome indicators, which reflect changes in vector control behaviours, vector populations, and disease transmission. Process evaluation can assess the reach and engagement of target populations, the quality of participatory activities, and the development of community capacity for ongoing vector control activities. Outcome evaluation requires the use of appropriate comparison groups and longitudinal study designs that can account for temporal trends and external factors influencing vector control outcomes (Van Den Berg et al., 2023). Table 9.3 above shows community engagement strategies for vector-borne disease control.

Conclusion

Vector-borne diseases represent complex global health challenges that embody intricate relationships between pathogens, arthropod vectors, vertebrate hosts, and environmental factors, collectively determining disease emergence, transmission, and impact. Effective management requires multifaceted approaches integrating biological understanding of vector ecology with social, environmental, and technological interventions tailored to local epidemiological contexts. Disease burden disproportionately falls on vulnerable populations in tropical and subtropical regions, where poverty, inadequate infrastructure, and favourable climatic conditions create optimal environments for vector proliferation.

The four major vector-borne diseases examined—malaria, dengue, Zika virus, and Lyme disease—illustrate diversity in pathogen types, vector species, transmission patterns, and control challenges. Climate change has emerged as a critical driver, fundamentally altering geographic and temporal disease transmission boundaries through its effects on vector development, survival, and distribution patterns.

Vector control strategies face mounting challenges from widespread insecticide resistance, which reduces the effectiveness of chemical interventions. Innovative technologies, including genetically modified mosquitoes, sterile insect techniques, and biological control agents, provide promising alternatives that require careful evaluation of effectiveness, safety, and community acceptance. One Health approaches have gained recognition as essential frameworks for addressing complex ecological and social determinants, while optimising interventions across human health, animal health, and environmental management domains.

Community engagement represents a fundamental component of sustainable programs, recognising that local populations possess essential knowledge and resources for effective disease control. Economic burden extends beyond direct healthcare costs to include lost productivity and impediments to economic development. Future directions must address the development of new control tools, climate change adaptation, strengthening health system capacity, and enhanced international cooperation. Technology transfer and capacity-building efforts must prioritise equitable access while building local research, development, and implementation capacity.

Acknowledgments

The authors would like to extend our appreciation to those who offered helpful commentary during the drafting process of this manuscript. We also acknowledge the role Nova Science Publishers played in enabling the work described herein.

References

Bardosh, K., Inthavong, N., Jaques, N., Homsana, A., Pongvongsa, T., Phommasone, K., Elliott, I., Moore, C., Thanapongtharm, W., Robinson, M. T., & Brey, P. T. (2024). One Health prevention and preparedness to vector-borne diseases: How should we deal with a multisectoral, multilevel and multigroup governance? *One Health Outlook*, 2(1), 19. https://doi.org/10.1186/s42522-024-00114-8.

Bellinger, M. R., Reed, J., Wood, S., Holley, D., & Reeves, L. E. (2025). One Health, many approaches: Integrated vector management strategies support One Health goals. *Frontiers in Insect Science*, 4, 1549348. https://doi.org/10.3389/finsc.2025.1549348.

Couper, L. I., Farner, J. E., Lyberger, K. P., Lee, A. S., & Mordecai, E. A. (2021). Evolutionary adaptation under climate change: Aedes sp. demonstrates potential to adapt to warming. *Proceedings of the National Academy of Sciences*, 122(2), e2418199122. https://doi.org/10.1073/pnas.2418199122.

Huang, Y., Ling, L., Tuu, S., Huang, M. H., Liu, N., McBride, C. S., & Montell, C. (2024). Innovative strategies and challenges mosquito-borne disease control amidst climate change. *Frontiers in Microbiology*, 15, 1488106. https://doi.org/10.3389/fmicb.2024.1488106.

Ryan, S. J., Carlson, C. J., Mordecai, E. A., & Johnson, L. R. (2019). Global expansion and redistribution of Aedes-borne virus transmission risk with climate change. *PLoS Neglected Tropical diseases*, 13(3), e0007213. https://doi.org/10.1371/journal.pntd.0007213.

Van Den Berg, H. H. J., De Urioste-Stone, S. M., Bargues, M. D., Willott, E., Mas-Coma, S., & Catalá, L. (2023). Adoption of community-based strategies for sustainable vector control and prevention. *BMC Public Health*, 23, 1785. https://doi.org/10.1186/s12889-023-16516-8.

Wellcome Trust. (2025). How climate change affects vector-borne diseases. Retrieved from https://wellcome.org/news/how-climate-change-affects-vector-borne-diseases.

World Health Organization. (2024). Global Vector Control Response 2017–2030: Vector-borne diseases. Retrieved from https://www.who.int/news-room/fact-sheets/detail/vector-borne-diseases.

World Health Organization. (2024). Updated WHO guidance for controlling vector-borne diseases through indoor residual spraying. Retrieved from https://www.who.int/news/item/15-02-2024-updated-who-guidance-for-controlling-vector-borne-diseases-through-indoor-residual-spraying.

World Health Organization Special Programme for Research and Training in Tropical Diseases. (2025). One Health and vector-borne diseases in the context of climate change. Retrieved from https://tdr.who.int/activities/one-health-and-vector-borne-diseases.

Chapter 10

Environmental and Social Determinants of Disease Emergence

Maajid Mohi Ud Din Malik[1,*], PhD and Tanuja S. Deshmukh[2]

[1]Department of Radiology and Imaging Technology, Dr. D. Y. Patil School of Allied Health Sciences, Dr. D. Y. Patil Vidyapeeth· Pune (Deemed to be University), Sant Tukaram Nagar, Pimpri, Pune, India
[2]Dr. D. Y. Patil School of Allied Health Sciences, Dr. D. Y. Patil Vidyapeeth· Pune (Deemed to be University), Sant Tukaram Nagar, Pimpri, Pune, India

Abstract

The emergence and re-emergence of infectious diseases represent critical threats to global health security, driven by complex interactions between environmental and social determinants. This chapter examines how ecological changes, including urbanisation, climate change, and ecosystem disruption, create conditions conducive to disease emergence. Meanwhile, social determinants such as poverty, inequality, and human behaviour patterns influence disease transmission and vulnerability. Environmental drivers, including deforestation, agricultural intensification, and habitat fragmentation, facilitate zoonotic spillover events and the expansion of vectors. Climate change amplifies these risks through altered precipitation patterns, temperature increases, and extreme weather events that affect vector ecology and disease transmission dynamics. Social determinants, including access to healthcare, housing quality, population density, and socioeconomic status, create differential vulnerability patterns that exacerbate health inequities. The intersection of environmental and social factors produces syndemic conditions where multiple health threats converge, disproportionately affecting marginalised populations. Understanding these interconnected determinants is crucial for developing effective prevention strategies, enhancing the resilience of health systems, and achieving sustainable development goals related to health equity and environmental sustainability. This chapter synthesises current evidence on these relationships and identifies priority areas for research and intervention to mitigate future disease emergence risks.

* Corresponding Author's Email: maajid.malik@dpu.edu.in

In: Advances in the One Health Approach
Editors: Maajid Mohi Ud Din Malik, Abhay Saraf, Harshal Tukaram Pandve et al.
ISBN: 979-8-90134-202-2

Keywords: disease emergence, environmental determinants, social determinants, climate change, urbanisation, health equity, zoonotic diseases, One Health, Sustainable Development Goal 3, ecosystem health

Introduction

The emergence and re-emergence of infectious diseases represent one of the most pressing challenges facing global public Health in the 21st century, with environmental and social factors playing increasingly critical roles in determining when, where, and how new pathogen threats arise and spread through human populations. The complex interplay between human activities that modify natural environments, social structures that create differential vulnerability patterns, and ecological processes that govern pathogen transmission creates a dynamic landscape of disease emergence risk, requiring a comprehensive understanding and coordinated response efforts (McMichael, 2004). Recent decades have witnessed unprecedented rates of environmental change driven by human activities, including deforestation, urbanisation, climate change, and ecosystem disruption, creating novel ecological conditions that facilitate pathogen spillover from animal reservoirs into human populations. Simultaneously, persistent social inequities in healthcare access, housing quality, education, and economic opportunities create differential patterns of vulnerability that determine which populations bear the most significant burden when disease emergence events occur (Patz et al., 2004). The interconnected nature of these environmental and social determinants means that effective disease emergence prevention requires integrated approaches that address multiple risk factors simultaneously while recognising the complex feedback relationships between human Health, animal health, and environmental Health. Understanding these relationships is crucial for developing effective prevention strategies, building resilient health systems, and achieving the health equity goals outlined in the Sustainable Development Goals framework, particularly SDG 3, which aims to ensure healthy lives and promote well-being for all people at all ages.

10.1. Environmental Drivers of Disease Emergence

Environmental changes represent fundamental drivers of infectious disease emergence and re-emergence across global populations, creating novel ecological conditions that facilitate pathogen spillover, vector expansion, and transmission dynamics (Jones et al., 2008). The relationship between environmental modification and disease emergence operates through multiple interconnected pathways that disrupt natural ecological barriers, creating new opportunities for pathogen-host interactions. Human activities that alter natural environments, including deforestation, agricultural expansion, mining, and infrastructure development, serve as primary catalysts for zoonotic disease emergence by increasing contact between humans, domestic animals, and wildlife reservoirs carrying novel pathogens. These activities fundamentally alter the structure and function of ecosystems in ways that can eliminate natural barriers to pathogen transmission, while creating conditions favourable to disease amplification and spread.

Deforestation and habitat fragmentation create edge effects that bring humans into closer proximity with wildlife populations, facilitating the cross-species transmission of pathogens that were previously contained within intact ecosystems (Gottdenker et al., 2014). These activities not only reduce biodiversity, which can serve as a buffer against disease transmission through dilution effects, but also stress wildlife populations, potentially increasing viral shedding and susceptibility to infection. The fragmentation of natural habitats forces wildlife into smaller, more densely populated areas, creating conditions that favour rapid pathogen transmission within wildlife populations and increasing the probability of spillover into human communities. Forest edges typically experience elevated temperatures, reduced humidity, and increased light penetration compared to intact forest interiors, creating environmental conditions that may be more suitable for some disease vectors while stressing wildlife populations in ways that could increase pathogen shedding.

Agricultural intensification and livestock expansion further amplify disease emergence risks through several interconnected mechanisms that create favourable conditions for pathogen evolution and transmission. Intensive farming practices create dense populations of genetically similar animals, providing ideal conditions for pathogen amplification and evolution, particularly for respiratory and enteric pathogens that benefit from high host density and frequent contact opportunities. The expansion of agricultural lands into previously wild areas creates interfaces where domestic animals, wildlife, and humans interact regularly, providing bridges for pathogen transmission across species barriers that may have evolved over millennia. Additionally, the widespread use of antimicrobials in agricultural settings contributes to the development of antimicrobial resistance, which complicates treatment options when zoonotic pathogens successfully transmit to human populations and reduces the effectiveness of prophylactic interventions.

Water resource development projects, including dam construction, irrigation systems, and water diversions, create new aquatic habitats that can serve as breeding sites for disease vectors while disrupting natural water flow patterns that historically controlled vector populations (Keiser et al., 2005). These modifications can lead to the emergence or re-emergence of water-associated diseases by creating favourable conditions for vector reproduction and extending the geographic range of vector-borne pathogens into areas where human populations may have limited previous exposure or immunity. The construction of large water infrastructure projects also typically involves the movement of large numbers of workers from diverse geographic regions, creating opportunities for pathogen introduction and transmission in previously unexposed populations while establishing new population centres in areas that may be environmentally suitable for disease transmission.

Mining and extractive industries contribute to disease emergence through multiple pathways, including environmental degradation, population displacement, and the creation of new ecological niches favourable to disease vectors and reservoirs. Mining activities often involve extensive deforestation and soil disruption, which can release dormant pathogens from environmental reservoirs. This creates disturbed habitats that favour opportunistic species, potentially serving as disease reservoirs or vectors. The influx of workers into remote mining areas can introduce pathogens to indigenous populations with limited previous exposure and inadequate healthcare infrastructure to respond effectively to disease outbreaks. Additionally, mining operations often result in environmental contamination that can compromise immune function in both human and wildlife populations, potentially increasing susceptibility to infectious diseases when exposure to novel pathogens occurs.

Table 10.1. Major environmental drivers of disease emergence and associated health risks

Environmental Driver	Primary Mechanisms	Examples of Associated Diseases	Most Vulnerable Populations	Evidence-Based Prevention Strategies
Deforestation & Habitat Loss	Human-wildlife interface expansion, biodiversity reduction, and microclimate changes	Ebola virus, Nipah virus, Leishmaniasis, Lyme disease	Forest-dependent communities, agricultural workers, and indigenous populations	Protected area establishment, sustainable forestry practices, buffer zones
Intensive Agriculture	High animal density, genetic uniformity, and antimicrobial overuse	Avian influenza, Swine flu, MRSA infections, Salmonellosis	Farmers, food processing workers, and rural communities	One Health surveillance systems, biosecurity protocols, and antimicrobial stewardship
Urbanisation	Population density, inadequate infrastructure, and human mobility	Dengue fever, Tuberculosis, COVID-19, Cholera	Urban slum residents, migrants, and homeless populations	Integrated urban planning, infrastructure investment, and housing improvements
Water Development Projects	Vector breeding habitat creation, population mixing, ecosystem disruption	Schistosomiasis, Malaria, Rift Valley fever	Construction workers, resettled communities, and downstream populations	Environmental health impact assessments, vector control, and community health programs
Climate Change	Temperature shifts, precipitation changes, and extreme weather events	Malaria, Zika virus, West Nile virus, Heat-related illnesses	Tropical and subtropical populations, older people, and outdoor workers	Climate adaptation strategies, early warning systems, and vector surveillance

Environmental contamination resulting from industrial activities, waste disposal, and chemical pollution creates conditions that can compromise immune function in both human and animal populations, thereby increasing susceptibility to infectious diseases while potentially altering the virulence and transmission dynamics of pathogens. Heavy metal contamination, pesticide exposure, and other forms of chemical pollution can disrupt immune system function at multiple levels, making populations more vulnerable to infection when exposed to novel pathogens while potentially reducing the effectiveness of vaccination and other preventive interventions. Additionally, environmental contamination can affect the Health and behaviour of wildlife species that serve as disease reservoirs, potentially altering their role in disease transmission cycles and creating novel transmission patterns that may be difficult to predict or control (Woolhouse & Gowtage-Sequeria, 2005). Table 10.1 presents the major environmental drivers of disease emergence and their associated health risks.

10.2. Urbanisation and Land Use Changes

Rapid urbanisation represents one of the most significant demographic and environmental transitions of the modern era, creating novel disease emergence risks through the concentration of large populations in areas with often inadequate infrastructure while simultaneously modifying local ecological systems in ways that can facilitate pathogen transmission (Neiderud, 2015). Urban environments create unique epidemiological conditions that can reduce disease transmission through high population density, increased social mixing, and environmental modifications, while simultaneously providing opportunities for improved healthcare access, disease surveillance, and coordinated public health responses when properly managed. The pace and scale of contemporary urbanisation, particularly in low- and middle-income countries, often outstrip the capacity of local governments to provide adequate housing, sanitation, water supply, and healthcare services, creating conditions that are conducive to both disease emergence and rapid transmission once outbreaks occur.

Unplanned urbanisation frequently results in the formation of slums and informal settlements characterised by overcrowding, poor sanitation, inadequate water supply, and limited access to healthcare services, creating ideal environments for the transmission of multiple categories of communicable diseases. These conditions develop environments where respiratory infections can spread rapidly through airborne transmission in poorly ventilated housing, diarrheal diseases can flourish due to inadequate sanitation and water contamination, and vector-borne illnesses can emerge as inadequate waste management creates breeding sites for mosquitoes and other disease vectors. High population density in poorly constructed and maintained housing facilitates the transmission of airborne diseases. At the same time, inadequate spacing between structures can create conditions that allow vector-borne diseases to spread rapidly through entire communities. The proximity of dense human settlements to agricultural areas and natural habitats increases the likelihood of zoonotic disease spillover, while also providing favourable conditions for rapid human-to-human transmission once spillover events occur.

Urban heat island effects, created by the concentration of concrete, asphalt, and other heat-absorbing materials in urban environments, alter local climate conditions in ways that can significantly affect disease vector ecology and pathogen survival patterns. Elevated urban temperatures can extend the breeding seasons of mosquito vectors while accelerating pathogen development within vectors, potentially increasing transmission rates of vector-borne diseases and extending their seasonal transmission windows. These temperature effects can be particularly pronounced in tropical and subtropical urban areas, where temperature increases may cause vector and pathogen development rates to exceed optimal ranges. This can also extend the geographic range of temperature-sensitive vectors into previously unsuitable urban environments. Conversely, extreme heat events associated with urban heat islands can stress human populations and compromise immune function, increasing susceptibility to infectious diseases during periods of high vector activity while potentially overwhelming healthcare systems during concurrent heat and infectious disease emergencies.

Land use changes associated with urban expansion often involve the conversion of agricultural land, wetlands, and natural habitats into residential and commercial areas, disrupting existing ecological systems and creating edge effects that can facilitate the emergence of diseases through novel human-wildlife-domestic animal interfaces. Peri-urban areas, where urban development meets rural and natural environments, represent critical interfaces for disease emergence as they combine high human population density with ongoing contact with agricultural and wildlife disease reservoirs. These transition zones often lack adequate infrastructure development and regulatory oversight, creating conditions that elevate disease emergence risks. Still, surveillance and response capacity may be limited due to unclear jurisdictional responsibilities and resource constraints.

Urban transportation systems, while essential for economic development and social connectivity, can facilitate the rapid spread of disease both within metropolitan areas and between connected urban centres through high-volume passenger flows and frequent social mixing. High-capacity public transportation systems can enable rapid pathogen transmission during the early phases of disease outbreaks, particularly for respiratory pathogens that can be transmitted through close contact or airborne routes during daily commuting periods. International transportation hubs, including airports and ports, which are typically located in or near major urban areas, serve as critical nodes for the global spread of emerging diseases. They connect high-density population centres with international travel networks that can rapidly distribute pathogens across continents before their emergence is detected or control measures can be implemented.

The modification of water systems associated with urbanisation, including river channelisation, wetland drainage, surface water diversions, and groundwater extraction, can alter local hydrology in ways that significantly affect disease vector ecology, while creating new pathways for pathogen transmission. Urban drainage systems and water storage infrastructure can create new breeding sites for mosquito vectors while disrupting natural predator-prey relationships that historically controlled vector populations in pre-urban environments. Inadequate urban water treatment and distribution systems can facilitate waterborne disease outbreaks while providing pathways for antimicrobial-resistant organisms to persist and spread within urban environments through contaminated water supplies and inadequate sewage treatment systems. The concentration of industrial activities in urban areas can also lead to water contamination, compromising immune function and creating environmental conditions favourable to specific pathogens.

10.3. Climate Change and Health Impacts

Climate change represents a fundamental threat multiplier for infectious disease emergence, operating through complex mechanisms that alter pathogen survival, vector ecology, host susceptibility, and transmission dynamics across multiple spatial and temporal scales, while creating novel environmental conditions that facilitate disease emergence and geographic expansion (Altizer et al., 2013). Rising global temperatures, changing precipitation patterns, and the increasing frequency and intensity of extreme weather events create environmental conditions that expand the geographic ranges of disease vectors, extend transmission seasons, and facilitate pathogen emergence previously limited by climatic constraints. Health impacts are particularly pronounced in vulnerable populations and regions with limited adaptive capacity, exacerbating existing health inequities while creating new challenges to global health security.

Temperature increases directly affect the biology and ecology of disease vectors, particularly arthropod vectors—such as mosquitoes, ticks, and flies—that transmit significant proportions of emerging infectious diseases and are highly sensitive to temperature variations. Higher temperatures can accelerate vector development rates, increase reproductive frequency, and enhance feeding behaviour, while shortening the extrinsic incubation periods of pathogens within vectors, potentially increasing transmission rates and basic reproductive numbers. However, extreme heat can negatively impact vector survival and reproductive success, creating complex, non-linear relationships between temperature and disease transmission that vary by vector species, pathogen characteristics, and local environmental conditions.

Changing precipitation patterns create complex, often contradictory effects on disease emergence through their influences on vector breeding sites, water quality and availability, and broader ecosystem dynamics that affect vector and pathogen survival. Increased precipitation and flooding create new breeding habitats for mosquito vectors, while flooding events contaminate water supplies and overwhelm sanitation infrastructure, facilitating waterborne disease outbreaks. Conversely, drought conditions concentrate vectors and human populations around limited water sources, intensifying transmission opportunities while potentially compromising immune function through malnutrition and physiological stress.

Extreme weather events—hurricanes, floods, droughts, heatwaves, and severe storms—create acute conditions triggering disease outbreaks through multiple interconnected pathways, overwhelming regular prevention and control systems. Natural disasters disrupt healthcare systems, sanitation infrastructure, and disease surveillance capacity, while creating environmental and social conditions highly favourable to disease transmission through population displacement, crowding in emergency shelters, environmental contamination, and the breakdown of regular hygiene practices.

Sea level rise and coastal flooding pose particular challenges, including saltwater intrusion into freshwater systems, population displacement into crowded urban areas, and disruption of coastal ecosystems that have historically provided natural barriers against disease vectors and pathogens. Natural ecosystem disruption alters disease emergence risks through its effects on biodiversity, ecosystem services, and wildlife behaviour patterns, which in turn influence pathogen transmission dynamics and spillover risk. Climate-induced shifts in species distributions create novel species assemblages and interaction patterns, which can potentially facilitate pathogen spillover events. Biodiversity loss can reduce dilution effects provided by diverse ecological communities, potentially increasing disease transmission rates (Semenza & Menne, 2009).

10.4. Social Determinants and Health Equity

Social determinants of health encompass the conditions in which people are born, grow, live, work, and age, fundamentally shaping their vulnerability to disease emergence and determining their capacity for effective prevention and response when disease outbreaks occur (Bambra et al., 2010). These determinants operate through multiple intersecting pathways, influencing exposure risk, susceptibility to infection, access to healthcare services, and health outcomes following infection, thereby creating systematic health inequality patterns that become particularly pronounced during disease emergence events, when novel health threats amplify existing vulnerabilities.

Socioeconomic status represents a fundamental determinant influencing disease emergence risk through multiple interconnected mechanisms, including occupational exposures, housing conditions, healthcare access, and nutritional status, creating complex pathways through which poverty and inequality translate into differential health outcomes. Individuals in lower socioeconomic positions are more likely to work in occupations involving direct contact with disease reservoirs or vectors, such as agricultural work, food processing, waste management, and healthcare services, often lacking adequate personal protective equipment or workplace safety protections. Economic constraints usually force vulnerable populations to live in housing conditions that facilitate disease transmission, including overcrowded dwellings with poor ventilation, inadequate sanitation facilities, and proximity to environmental hazards, while simultaneously limiting their ability to engage in protective behaviours that require financial resources.

Educational attainment influences disease emergence vulnerability through its effects on health literacy, risk perception, and the adoption of protective behaviours, creating differential capacities for understanding and responding to disease threats across populations. Higher education levels are associated with improved knowledge of disease transmission mechanisms, greater awareness of prevention strategies, and more effective navigation of the healthcare system.

Housing quality and living conditions represent critical determinants of disease emergence risk, particularly for infectious diseases transmitted through airborne, vector-borne, or person-to-person contact pathways. Overcrowding facilitates the transmission of respiratory diseases by increasing the frequency and intensity of interpersonal contact, while reducing the effectiveness of social distancing measures. Inadequate ventilation systems increase exposure intensity and duration to airborne pathogens, while poor housing construction creates entry points for disease vectors and pest species that serve as disease reservoirs.

Healthcare service access has a significant influence on individual and population-level outcomes during disease emergence events, affecting early detection, timely treatment initiation, and effective prevention service delivery. Healthcare access barriers—financial constraints, geographic isolation, provider shortages, language barriers, and discrimination based on race, ethnicity, or immigration status—delay diagnosis and treatment while limiting disease prevention and health promotion intervention opportunities.

Social cohesion and community trust influence disease emergence vulnerability through their effects on collective efficacy, information sharing, and cooperation with public health interventions, thereby creating a differential capacity for coordinated community responses. Strong social networks provide both material and emotional support during health crises, facilitating the rapid dissemination of accurate health information and enabling coordinated response efforts that protect vulnerable community members. Mistrust in government institutions and healthcare systems, often rooted in historical experiences of discrimination, neglect, or exploitation, can undermine public health response efforts.

Cultural factors—beliefs about health and illness, traditional healing practices, and religious observances—shape disease emergence patterns, vulnerability, and response by influencing healthcare-seeking behaviour, the acceptance of prevention interventions, and the interpretation of public health recommendations. Effective disease emergence prevention and response strategies must be culturally sensitive and developed in partnership with affected communities, ensuring appropriateness and acceptability while respecting cultural values and practices.

10.5. Human Behaviour and Disease Risk

Human behaviour patterns represent critical determinants of disease emergence risk, influencing exposure opportunities, transmission dynamics, and the effectiveness of prevention and control interventions across individual, community, and population levels through complex interactions with biological, environmental, and social factors (Funk et al., 2010). Behavioural factors operate through multiple interconnected pathways that determine who is exposed to potential pathogens, under what circumstances exposure occurs, and how individuals and communities respond once exposure or infection has taken place, creating differential patterns of disease vulnerability while shaping the trajectory of outbreaks once they begin. Understanding the behavioural influences on disease emergence is essential for developing targeted interventions that can effectively reduce transmission while being acceptable and sustainable within diverse cultural and social contexts. This requires careful attention to the social, economic, and cultural factors that influence behaviour patterns.

Risk-taking behaviours and occupational exposures create direct pathways for increased disease emergence vulnerability through enhanced contact with potential disease reservoirs, vectors, or infected individuals, often in settings where protective measures are inadequate or impractical to implement. Occupations involving direct animal contact, such as farming, veterinary work, wildlife management, hunting, and meat processing, create regular opportunities for zoonotic disease transmission, often occurring in settings with limited biosafety protections or inadequate personal protective equipment. Similarly, occupations that require travel to diverse geographic regions, work in crowded conditions, or involve frequent interpersonal contact can increase exposure to novel pathogens while facilitating their geographic spread through mobile worker populations. Recreational activities such as hunting, camping, ecotourism, and adventure travel can create exposure opportunities in natural settings where contact with wildlife disease reservoirs is more likely to occur, while often involving individuals who may have limited experience with appropriate protective behaviours or risk assessment.

Health-seeking behaviour patterns significantly influence disease emergence outcomes through their effects on early detection, treatment initiation, and secondary transmission prevention, creating differential individual and community-level impacts based on healthcare utilisation patterns. Delays in seeking healthcare following symptom onset can result in more severe individual outcomes while extending the period during which infected individuals can transmit disease to family members, coworkers, and community contacts before appropriate isolation or treatment measures are implemented. Multiple interconnected factors, including symptom recognition and interpretation, risk perception and health beliefs, healthcare accessibility and affordability, past experiences with healthcare systems, and cultural preferences for different types of care, influence healthcare-seeking behaviour. Cultural factors, including preferences for traditional healing practices or religious healing approaches, can delay engagement with formal healthcare systems. However, these approaches can also provide valuable therapeutic options that should be integrated into comprehensive care approaches, rather than dismissed or discouraged.

Social interaction patterns and mixing behaviours fundamentally shape disease transmission dynamics by determining who encounters whom, under what circumstances, for how long, and with what intensity of contact, creating network structures that can either facilitate or impede disease spread through populations. Age-structured mixing patterns influence which age groups are most likely to acquire and transmit infections, with important implications for vaccination strategies, school closure policies, and targeted intervention approaches during outbreaks. Social gathering patterns, including religious observances, cultural celebrations, recreational activities, and family gatherings, can create super-spreading opportunities where a single infected individual can transmit the disease to many others simultaneously. The size, duration, and characteristics of these gatherings influence the magnitude of the transmission risk. Understanding local social mixing patterns is essential for predicting disease spread patterns and designing targeted interventions that can effectively interrupt transmission chains while minimising social and economic disruption.

Travel and mobility patterns are increasingly important factors in disease emergence and spread, due to the growing connectivity of global transportation networks and the increasing volumes of international travel that can rapidly distribute pathogens across geographic boundaries before their emergence is detected or control measures can be implemented. International travel can introduce exotic pathogens to immunologically naive populations. In contrast, domestic travel can spread locally emerging diseases to distant geographic areas where surveillance systems may not be prepared for early detection. Business travel, tourism, labour migration, and forced displacement due to conflict, natural disasters, or economic crises create distinct patterns of mobility that may influence disease emergence risk in various ways, necessitating tailored approaches to risk assessment and prevention. The speed of modern transportation networks means that pathogens can spread globally within days or hours of emergence, emphasising the importance of global disease surveillance systems and rapid response capacity that can detect and respond to emerging threats before they become pandemic.

Adherence to preventive behaviours and public health recommendations during disease outbreaks significantly influences transmission dynamics and outbreak outcomes, resulting in differential impacts based on population-level compliance with recommended protective measures. Preventive behaviour adoption is influenced by complex interactions among risk perception, self-efficacy, social norms, trust in public health authorities, and practical barriers to implementation, creating patterns of compliance that may vary significantly across different population groups and change over time during extended outbreaks. Behavioural fatigue can reduce adherence to prevention measures over time, particularly when interventions require sustained behaviour change or impose significant social or economic costs on individuals or communities. Communication strategies must be carefully designed to maintain motivation for adopting preventive behaviour while addressing legitimate concerns and barriers that may impede compliance, including economic hardship, social isolation, and conflicting information from different sources.

Food consumption patterns and agricultural practices create specific pathways for disease emergence through their influence on foodborne pathogen transmission and human-animal-environment interfaces that can facilitate zoonotic spillover events. Consumption of undercooked meat, raw dairy products, or contaminated produce can reduce the transmission of zoonotic diseases. At the same time, intensive animal agriculture can amplify pathogen loads and contribute to the development of antimicrobial resistance through the overuse of antibiotics in food production. Traditional food preparation and preservation methods may protect against some pathogens while potentially creating risks for others, requiring careful assessment of trade-offs and culturally appropriate modification strategies that respect traditional practices while reducing disease risks. The globalisation of food systems creates opportunities for the rapid international spread of foodborne pathogens while potentially disrupting traditional food safety practices that have evolved within specific local contexts and may be more appropriate for local conditions than standardised international approaches.

10.6. Ecosystem Disruption and Health Consequences

Ecosystem disruption represents a fundamental driver of disease emergence, as it affects biodiversity, ecological relationships, and environmental services that historically provided natural barriers to pathogen spillover and transmission. This disruption creates novel environmental conditions that can facilitate disease emergence while reducing the capacity of natural systems to regulate pathogen populations (Ostfeld, 2009). Healthy ecosystems maintain complex predator-prey relationships, competitive interactions, and environmental conditions that can regulate pathogen populations and limit opportunities for cross-species transmission through multiple interconnected mechanisms, including host dilution effects, vector control through natural predators, and environmental barriers to pathogen survival and transmission. Human activities that disrupt these natural systems create novel ecological conditions that can facilitate disease emergence while simultaneously reducing the capacity of natural systems to provide ecosystem services that support human Health and well-being. This requires comprehensive approaches to ecosystem management that consider health implications alongside other environmental and economic concerns.

Biodiversity loss associated with ecosystem disruption can increase the risk of disease emergence through several interconnected mechanisms that alter ecological relationships and reduce natural barriers to pathogen transmission, creating conditions more favourable to disease emergence and spread. The elimination of natural predators that historically controlled disease vector populations can lead to vector population explosions, increasing transmission opportunities while reducing the effectiveness of natural biological control mechanisms. The loss of host species that may serve as less competent reservoirs for zoonotic pathogens can concentrate infection in more competent reservoir species, potentially increasing the probability of spillover events and the efficiency of pathogen transmission. The reduction in ecosystem resilience that accompanies biodiversity loss diminishes the capacity of ecological systems to buffer against environmental perturbations and recover from disturbances, thereby increasing the vulnerability of ecosystems to additional stressors that could further exacerbate disease emergence risks.

The dilution effect, whereby greater host species diversity reduces disease transmission rates by distributing infection across multiple species with varying levels of competence for pathogen amplification and transmission, can be compromised when biodiversity is reduced through habitat destruction, species extinctions, or the introduction of invasive species that alter community composition. Simplified ecosystems with reduced species diversity may be more vulnerable to disease outbreaks and less capable of recovering from disturbances, as they provide fewer opportunities for natural regulation of pathogen populations through ecological mechanisms. However, the relationship between biodiversity and disease risk is complex. It may vary depending on the specific pathogens and ecosystems involved, requiring careful assessment of local ecological conditions and pathogen characteristics when developing conservation strategies for disease prevention.

Deforestation and habitat fragmentation create edge effects that bring human populations into closer contact with wildlife disease reservoirs, while altering microclimatic conditions in ways that may favour specific disease vectors or pathogens and stress wildlife populations, potentially increasing pathogen shedding. Forest edges typically experience elevated temperatures, reduced humidity, increased light penetration, and greater temperature variability compared to intact forest interiors, creating environmental conditions that may be more suitable for some disease vectors while potentially stressing wildlife populations and compromising their immune function. The fragmentation of natural habitats forces wildlife into smaller, more isolated populations, which may be more susceptible to disease outbreaks due to reduced genetic diversity and increased population density. This fragmentation also creates corridors along which pathogens can spread between habitat patches, potentially reaching human settlements.

Wetland drainage and aquatic habitat modification eliminate essential ecosystem services, including natural water filtration, flood control, and habitat for natural vector predators, while creating new environmental conditions that may favour different disease vectors or reservoirs than those present in intact wetland systems. Wetlands serve as natural water treatment systems, removing pathogens and pollutants from water while supporting complex food webs that include fish, amphibians, birds, and other species that consume mosquito larvae and other disease vectors. The conversion of wetlands to agricultural or urban uses eliminates these ecosystem services, while potentially creating artificial water bodies, such as irrigation canals, retention ponds, and drainage ditches, that serve as breeding sites for vectors without the natural predator populations that would control vector numbers in intact ecosystems.

Invasive species introductions can disrupt existing ecological relationships in ways that influence disease emergence risk by introducing novel pathogens, serving as competent reservoirs for existing pathogens, altering host-pathogen dynamics, or modifying environmental conditions in ways that affect disease transmission patterns. Invasive plant species can alter habitat structure, microclimate conditions, and resource availability in ways that favour vector species. Invasive animal species can serve as competent reservoirs for pathogens that may subsequently spill over into native wildlife populations or domestic animal populations. The establishment of invasive species often occurs in conjunction with other forms of ecosystem disruption, creating cumulative impacts that may be greater than the sum of individual stressors and may be particularly difficult to predict or manage effectively.

Pollution and environmental contamination can compromise ecosystem health and function in ways that increase the risk of disease emergence, while directly affecting the Health of human and animal populations through multiple pathways that reduce immune function and alter pathogen-host interactions. Chemical pollutants, including pesticides, heavy metals, and industrial chemicals, can disrupt immune system function in wildlife populations, making them more susceptible to infection and potentially increasing pathogen shedding rates, while altering behaviour patterns that may influence disease transmission dynamics. Nutrient pollution from agricultural runoff and sewage discharge can create eutrophic conditions in aquatic systems, favouring blooms of harmful algae and bacteria while creating oxygen-depleted conditions that stress aquatic species and may favour specific pathogens over others.

Plastic pollution and other forms of environmental contamination can create novel microhabitats that harbour pathogens, affecting the behaviour and Health of wildlife species in ways that could influence disease transmission dynamics through mechanisms that are not yet fully understood. The accumulation of plastic debris in marine and terrestrial environments can provide surfaces for biofilm formation, which may harbour pathogenic microorganisms. Meanwhile, microplastic particles can serve as vectors for pathogen transport or affect immune function in organisms that ingest them. Climate change interactions with ecosystem disruption create synergistic effects that may amplify disease emergence risks beyond what would be expected from either stressor alone, requiring integrated approaches to environmental management that consider multiple stressors simultaneously (Pongsiri et al., 2009). Table 10.2 illustrates the role of ecosystem services in disease prevention.

Conclusion

The emergence and re-emergence of infectious diseases result from complex interactions between environmental and social determinants that create novel opportunities for pathogen spillover, amplification, and transmission across human populations, requiring comprehensive understanding and integrated intervention approaches that address multiple risk factors simultaneously. Environmental changes, including deforestation, urbanisation, climate change, and ecosystem disruption, fundamentally alter ecological relationships and create new interfaces between humans, animals, and pathogens that natural barriers have historically separated. In contrast, social determinants, including poverty, inequality, healthcare access, and human behaviour patterns, create differential patterns of vulnerability that disproportionately affect marginalised populations and exacerbate existing health inequities. The interconnected nature of these environmental and social determinants means that effective disease emergence prevention requires comprehensive approaches that recognise the complex feedback relationships between human Health, animal health, and ecological Health while addressing root causes of vulnerability rather than focusing solely on biomedical responses to individual disease threats.

Table 10.2. Ecosystem services and their role in disease prevention

Ecosystem Service	Natural Disease Prevention Function	Human Activities Causing Disruption	Health Consequences of Loss	Restoration/Conservation Strategies
Biodiversity Maintenance	Dilution effect, natural vector control, pathogen regulation	Habitat destruction, fragmentation, and pollution	Increased spillover risk, vector population growth	Protected area networks, habitat corridors, species reintroduction
Water Filtration & Purification	Pathogen removal, water quality maintenance	Wetland drainage, urban development, and industrial pollution	Waterborne disease outbreaks, contaminated water supplies	Wetland restoration, constructed wetlands, watershed protection
Climate Regulation	Temperature and humidity moderation	Deforestation, urbanisation, and industrial emissions	Extended vector seasons, heat stress, extreme weather	Forest conservation, urban green infrastructure, carbon sequestration
Natural Pest Control	Vector population regulation, disease vector predation	Pesticide use, habitat loss, and monoculture agriculture	Vector-borne disease emergence, pesticide resistance	Integrated pest management, habitat restoration, and organic farming
Soil Formation & Nutrient Cycling	Pathogen decomposition, nutrient availability for healthy ecosystems	Intensive agriculture, soil erosion, and chemical fertilisers	Compromised ecosystem resilience, pathogen persistence	Sustainable agriculture, soil conservation, and organic matter enhancement

Table 10.3. Sustainable development goals and disease emergence prevention integration

SDG Target	Specific Relevance to Disease Emergence	Key Performance Indicators	Implementation Strategies for Disease Prevention	Cross-Sectoral Partnerships Required
SDG 3.3: End epidemics of AIDS, tuberculosis, malaria and other communicable diseases	Direct focus on infectious disease control and epidemic prevention	Disease incidence reduction, mortality rates, and health system preparedness indicators	Strengthened surveillance systems, universal health coverage, and rapid response capacity	Health, education, social services, and international cooperation
SDG 6.1: Universal access to safe and affordable drinking water	Prevention of waterborne diseases and elimination of vector breeding sites elimination	Water quality testing, access coverage, and sanitation facility availability	Infrastructure investment, community-based water management, and water quality monitoring	Health, water management, urban planning, rural development
SDG 11.1: Adequate, safe and affordable housing for all	Reduction of overcrowding and improvement of living conditions that facilitate disease transmission	Slum population percentages, housing quality indices, and access to basic services	Integrated urban planning, affordable housing programs, and slum upgrading initiatives	Urban planning, housing, Health, and social services
SDG 13.1: Strengthen resilience and adaptive capacity to climate-related hazards	Climate change adaptation for health systems and disease prevention	Climate vulnerability assessments, adaptation measures implemented, and early warning system coverage	Climate-sensitive disease surveillance, ecosystem-based adaptation, resilient infrastructure	Environment, Health, disaster risk reduction, meteorology
SDG 15.1: Ensure conservation, restoration and sustainable use of terrestrial and inland freshwater ecosystems	Prevention of zoonotic disease spillover through ecosystem conservation	Forest cover percentage, protected area coverage, and biodiversity indices	Protected area establishment, sustainable forest management, habitat restoration	Environment, forestry, agriculture, and indigenous affairs

Table 10.4. Evidence-based interventions for addressing disease emergence determinants across implementation levels

Implementation Level	Environmental Health Interventions	Social Determinants Interventions	Behavioural Change Interventions	Expected Health Outcomes	Primary Implementation Challenges
Individual/Household	Household vector control, water treatment, sanitation improvement, and reduced animal contact	Health education, economic support programs, improved housing, and healthcare access facilitation	Risk communication, behaviour change counselling, community engagement	Reduced exposure risk, improved health-seeking behaviour, enhanced personal protection	Behaviour change, sustainability, resource constraints, cultural acceptability
Community/Local	Community-based disease surveillance, ecosystem restoration, and vector control programs	Social cohesion building, community health programs, and local healthcare capacity strengthening	Community mobilisation, peer education, social norm change	Enhanced early detection, collective efficacy, and improved community resilience	Community engagement complexity, coordination challenges, and resource allocation
National/Regional	Protected area establishment, environmental regulation, urban planning, and infrastructure development	Universal health coverage, poverty reduction programs, and education system strengthening	National health communication campaigns, policy-level behaviour change	System-wide risk reduction, improved health equity, enhanced preparedness	Political will requirements, competing priorities, and resource mobilisation
Global/International	Climate change mitigation, biodiversity conservation, and international environmental agreements	International health cooperation, technology transfer, and capacity building support	Global health communication, knowledge sharing, and coordination mechanisms	Reduced global emergence risk, enhanced pandemic preparedness, improved international cooperation	Coordination complexity, sovereignty concerns, and resource allocation challenges

The global nature of disease emergence risks necessitates international cooperation and coordination to address transboundary environmental changes and social inequities that create conditions conducive to pandemic threats. This emphasises the importance of multilateral action to address climate change, biodiversity loss, and ecological degradation that transcend national boundaries. Global trade, travel, and communication networks mean that disease emergence in one region can rapidly spread to affect populations worldwide, highlighting the interconnected nature of disease risks and the need for global health security approaches that recognise shared vulnerability to emerging threats. Achieving sustainable disease emergence prevention will require addressing fundamental social and environmental justice issues that create differential vulnerability patterns across populations, including systemic inequalities in income, education, housing, and access to healthcare, which form the basis of fundamental vulnerability to health threats.

The COVID-19 pandemic has demonstrated both the devastating potential of emerging infectious diseases and the critical importance of addressing underlying environmental and social determinants that contribute to disease emergence and spread. It has also revealed how social inequities amplify disease risks and create differential impacts across populations. Moving forward, investments in pandemic preparedness and prevention must address these underlying determinants through integrated One Health approaches that bring together expertise from human Health, veterinary medicine, environmental science, and social sciences to develop effective and sustainable prevention strategies (World Health Organisation, 2021). Future research and intervention priorities should focus on developing a better understanding of the mechanisms through which environmental and social determinants interact to influence disease emergence while creating evidence-based strategies for addressing these drivers effectively through early warning systems, community-based interventions, and policy frameworks that integrate health considerations into decisions about land use, development, and environmental management. Table 10.3 shows the integration of sustainable development goals and disease emergence prevention.

The goal of addressing environmental and social determinants of disease emergence extends beyond preventing specific diseases to creating healthier, more equitable, and more sustainable communities that demonstrate resilience to multiple health threats while promoting human well-being and environmental sustainability. This requires transformative approaches that address root causes of vulnerability while building capacity for adaptation and response to novel health challenges that will inevitably emerge as global environmental and social systems continue to change. By addressing social and ecological determinants comprehensively through integrated approaches that recognise the interconnections between human Health, animal health, and environmental Health, we can work toward a future where disease emergence risks are minimised and, when outbreaks do occur, their impacts are distributed more equitably and managed more effectively across all populations (Pike et al., 2014).

Figure 16 shows A comprehensive systems diagram illustrating the complex interconnections between environmental drivers (climate change, deforestation, urbanisation, ecosystem disruption, pollution), social determinants (poverty, education, healthcare access, housing quality, social cohesion), and disease emergence pathways (zoonotic spillover, vector-borne transmission, human-to-human spread). The framework illustrates how environmental changes create ecological conditions that favour pathogen emergence, while social determinants create differential vulnerability patterns across populations. Bidirectional arrows show feedback loops where disease emergence can exacerbate environmental degradation and social inequities. Multiple intervention points are identified at individual, community, national, and global levels, emphasising One Health approaches that integrate human, animal, and environmental health considerations. The diagram includes specific examples of successful interventions at each level. It illustrates how achieving the Sustainable Development Goals contributes to the prevention of the emergence of comprehensive diseases by addressing underlying determinants rather than focusing solely on disease-specific responses.

Table 10.4 above presents evidence-based interventions for addressing determinants of disease emergence.

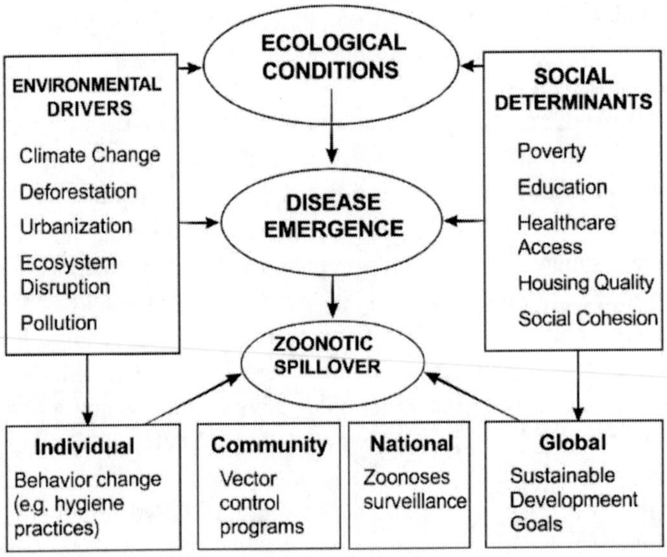

Figure 16. Integrated Framework for Environmental and Social Determinants of Disease Emergence.

Acknowledgments

The authors would like to extend our appreciation to those who offered helpful commentary during the drafting process of this manuscript. We also acknowledge the role Nova Science Publishers played in enabling the work described herein.

References

Altizer, S., Ostfeld, R. S., Johnson, P. T., Kutz, S., & Harvell, C. D. (2013). Climate change and infectious diseases: from evidence to a predictive framework. *Science*, 341(6145), 514-519. https://doi.org/10.1126/science.1239401.

Bambra, C., Gibson, M., Sowden, A., Wright, K., Whitehead, M., & Petticrew, M. (2010). Tackling the wider social determinants of health and health inequalities: evidence from systematic reviews. *Journal of Epidemiology and Community Health*, 64(4), 284-291. https://doi.org/10.1136/jech.2008.082743.

Funk, S., Salathé, M., & Jansen, V. A. (2010). Modelling the influence of human behaviour on the spread of infectious diseases: a review. *Journal of the Royal Society Interface*, 7(50), 1247-1256. https://doi.org/10.1098/rsif.2010.0142.

Gottdenker, N. L., Streicker, D. G., Faust, C. L., & Carroll, C. R. (2014). Anthropogenic land use change and infectious diseases: a review of the evidence. *EcoHealth*, 11(4), 619-632. https://doi.org/10.1007/s10393-014-0941-z.

Jones, K. E., Patel, N. G., Levy, M. A., Storeygard, A., Balk, D., Gittleman, J. L., & Daszak, P. (2008). Global trends in emerging infectious diseases. *Nature*, 451(7181), 990-993. https://doi.org/10.1038/nature06536.

Keiser, J., Utzinger, J., Caldas de Castro, M., Smith, T. A., Tanner, M., & Singer, B. H. (2005). Urbanisation in sub-Saharan Africa and implication for malaria control. *American Journal of Tropical Medicine and Hygiene*, 71(2), 118-127.

McMichael, A. J. (2004). Environmental and social influences on emerging infectious diseases: past, present and future. *Philosophical Transactions of the Royal Society B*, 359(1447), 1049-1058. https://doi.org/10.1098/rstb.2004.1480.

Neiderud, C. J. (2015). How urbanisation affects the epidemiology of emerging infectious diseases. *Infection Ecology & Epidemiology*, 5(1), 27060. https://doi.org/10.3402/iee.v5.27060.

Ostfeld, R. S. (2009). Biodiversity loss and the rise of zoonotic pathogens. *Clinical Microbiology and Infection*, 15(S1), 40-43. https://doi.org/10.1111/j.1469-0691.2008.02691.x.

Patz, J. A., Daszak, P., Tabor, G. M., Aguirre, A. A., Pearl, M., Epstein, J., ... & Bradley, D. J. (2004). Unhealthy landscapes: policy recommendations on land use change and infectious disease emergence. *Environmental Health Perspectives*, 112(10), 1092-1098. https://doi.org/10.1289/ehp.6877.

Pike, J., Bogich, T., Elwood, S., Finn, I. R., & Daszak, P. (2014). Economic optimisation of a global strategy to address the pandemic threat. *Proceedings of the National Academy of Sciences*, 111(52), 18519-18523. https://doi.org/10.1073/pnas.1412661112.

Pongsiri, M. J., Roman, J., Ezenwa, V. O., Goldberg, T. L., Koren, H. S., Newbold, S. C., ... & Salkeld, D. J. (2009). Biodiversity loss affects global disease ecology. *BioScience*, 59(11), 945-954. https://doi.org/10.1525/bio.2009.59.11.6.

Semenza, J. C., & Menne, B. (2009). Climate change and infectious diseases in Europe. *The Lancet Infectious Diseases*, 9(6), 365-375. https://doi.org/10.1016/S1473-3099(09)70104-5.

World Health Organization. (2021). *Tripartite and UNEP support OHHLEP's definition of "One Health"*. World Health Organization. https://www.who.int/news/item/01-12-2021-tripartite-and-unep-support-ohhlep-s-definition-of-one-health.

Woolhouse, M. E., & Gowtage-Sequeria, S. (2005). Host range and emerging and reemerging pathogens. *Emerging Infectious Diseases*, 11(12), 1842-1847. https://doi.org/10.3201/eid1112.050995.

Chapter 11

Antimicrobial Resistance: A Global One Health Crisis

Maajid Mohi Ud Din Malik[1,*], PhD
and Shweta Chougule[2]

[1]Department of Radiology and Imaging Technology, Dr. D. Y. Patil School of Allied Health Sciences, Dr. D. Y. Patil Vidyapeeth Pune (Deemed to be University), Sant Tukaram Nagar, Pimpri, Pune, India
[2]Dr. D. Y. Patil School of Allied Health Sciences, Dr. D. Y. Patil Vidyapeeth Pune (Deemed to be University), Sant Tukaram Nagar, Pimpri, Pune, India

Abstract

Antimicrobial resistance (AMR) represents one of the most pressing global health security threats of the 21st century, fundamentally challenging our ability to treat infectious diseases and threatening to reverse decades of medical progress. This multifaceted crisis emerges from the complex interplay between biological mechanisms of resistance development, widespread antimicrobial use and misuse across human medicine, veterinary practice, and agriculture, and the rapid transmission of resistance genes through interconnected human, animal, and environmental pathways. The mechanisms driving AMR include spontaneous mutations, horizontal gene transfer, and selective pressure from antimicrobial exposure that favours resistant organisms while eliminating susceptible competitors. Inappropriate prescribing practices in healthcare settings, the prophylactic use in livestock production, and agricultural applications create selection pressures that accelerate the development and spread of resistance. The economic burden of AMR is substantial, with projections indicating potential costs exceeding $100 trillion globally by 2050 if current trends continue, while attributable deaths could reach 10 million annually. Addressing this crisis requires coordinated One Health approaches that recognise the interconnected nature of human, animal, and environmental Health, and implementing comprehensive stewardship programs across all relevant sectors. National and international action plans, including the Global Action Plan on Antimicrobial Resistance, provide frameworks for coordinated responses to antimicrobial resistance. Still, implementation remains challenging due to resource constraints, regulatory gaps, and the need for sustained political commitment. Success in combating AMR demands integrated surveillance systems, responsible antimicrobial use policies, investment in research and development, and recognition of AMR as a critical component of Sustainable Development Goal 3 for ensuring healthy lives and promoting well-being for all.

---

* Corresponding Author's Email: maajid.malik@dpu.edu.in

In: Advances in the One Health Approach
Editors: Maajid Mohi Ud Din Malik, Abhay Saraf, Harshal Tukaram Pandve et al.
ISBN: 979-8-90134-202-2

Keywords: antimicrobial resistance, antibiotic resistance, One Health, stewardship, global health security, horizontal gene transfer, healthcare-associated infections, agricultural antimicrobials, Sustainable Development Goal 3, infectious disease control

Introduction

Antimicrobial resistance represents a paradigmatic One Health crisis that exemplifies the complex interconnections between human Health, animal health, and environmental Health, requiring coordinated global action across multiple sectors to address effectively (World Health Organisation, 2021). The phenomenon of microorganisms developing resistance to antimicrobial agents that were once effective against them threatens to return humanity to a pre-antibiotic era, where simple infections could prove fatal and routine medical procedures become prohibitively dangerous due to the risks of infection. The development and spread of antimicrobial resistance occurs through natural evolutionary processes that are accelerated by human activities, including the widespread use and misuse of antimicrobial agents in human medicine, veterinary practice, and agricultural production systems. These activities create selective pressures that favour the survival and proliferation of resistant organisms while eliminating susceptible competitors, leading to the emergence of multidrug-resistant pathogens that pose significant threats to patient safety and public Health. The interconnected nature of modern global systems means that resistance genes can spread rapidly between humans, animals, and environmental reservoirs through direct contact, food chains, water systems, and international travel and trade networks. Understanding antimicrobial resistance as a One Health issue is essential because resistance genes do not respect species boundaries or geographic borders, requiring comprehensive approaches that address all sources of selective pressure while implementing coordinated surveillance and response systems across human, animal, and environmental health sectors. The challenge of antimicrobial resistance intersects directly with Sustainable Development Goal 3, which calls for ensuring healthy lives and promoting well-being for all people at all ages, as the loss of effective antimicrobial agents threatens progress toward universal health coverage and could undermine achievements in reducing maternal and child Mortality, controlling infectious diseases, and improving health outcomes globally.

11.1. Mechanisms and Drivers of Antimicrobial Resistance

Antimicrobial resistance arises through fundamental biological mechanisms that enable microorganisms to survive exposure to antimicrobial agents that would normally inhibit their growth or kill them, involving complex molecular processes that can occur through spontaneous genetic mutations, acquisition of resistance genes from other organisms, or modification of cellular structures and metabolic pathways (Holmes et al., 2016). The primary mechanisms of resistance include enzymatic inactivation of antimicrobial agents, modification of target sites to reduce drug binding, efflux pump systems that actively remove antimicrobials from bacterial cells, and altered metabolic pathways that bypass the antimicrobial's intended target. These mechanisms can develop independently in individual organisms through random mutations that provide survival advantages when antimicrobial agents are present, or they can be acquired through horizontal gene transfer processes, which enable the rapid spread of resistance traits across different bacterial species and genera.

Enzymatic inactivation represents one of the most clinically significant resistance mechanisms, involving the production of enzymes that chemically modify antimicrobial agents, rendering them ineffective against their intended targets. Beta-lactamases exemplify this mechanism by cleaving the beta-lactam ring structure, which is essential for the activity of penicillins, cephalosporins, and related antibiotics. Extended-spectrum beta-lactamases (ESBLs) and carbapenemases represent particularly concerning developments that confer resistance to broad classes of antibiotics, including those considered last-resort treatments. Aminoglycoside-modifying enzymes similarly inactivate necessary antibiotics through acetylation, adenylation, or phosphorylation reactions, which prevent these drugs from binding to bacterial ribosomes and thereby inhibiting protein synthesis.

Target site modification involves genetic changes that alter the structure of cellular components to which antimicrobial agents normally bind or interact, thereby reducing the drugs' effectiveness without necessarily eliminating their activity. Penicillin-binding protein modifications in methicillin-resistant Staphylococcus aureus (MRSA) exemplify this mechanism by creating altered target sites that have reduced affinity for beta-lactam antibiotics while maintaining their essential cellular functions. Similarly, mutations in DNA gyrase and topoisomerase IV confer resistance to fluoroquinolone antibiotics by altering the structure of the target enzymes while preserving their crucial role in DNA replication and repair processes.

Efflux pump systems actively transport antimicrobial agents out of bacterial cells before they can reach effective intracellular concentrations, often conferring resistance to multiple drug classes simultaneously and contributing to multidrug resistance phenotypes. These pump systems can be constitutively expressed or induced in response to antimicrobial exposure, and their overexpression can result from mutations in regulatory genes that usually control pump production. The broad substrate specificity of many efflux pumps means that increased pump activity can confer resistance to structurally unrelated antimicrobials, complicating treatment decisions and potentially limiting therapeutic options.

The drivers of antimicrobial resistance are multifaceted and operate across human, animal, and environmental domains, creating complex feedback loops that accelerate the development and spread of resistance (Prestinaci et al., 2015). Selective pressure from antimicrobial use represents the primary driver of resistance development, as the presence of antimicrobial agents creates environmental conditions that favour resistant organisms while eliminating susceptible competitors. This selective pressure operates regardless of whether antimicrobial use is appropriate or inappropriate; however, the magnitude and duration of the selective pressure can be influenced by factors such as dose, treatment duration, choice of agent, and adherence to treatment regimens.

Inappropriate antimicrobial prescribing in healthcare settings contributes significantly to resistance development through several pathways, including prescription of antimicrobials for viral infections where they provide no benefit, selection of broad-spectrum agents when narrow-spectrum alternatives would be effective, inadequate dosing that creates suboptimal drug concentrations, and prolonged treatment courses that extend selective pressure beyond necessary durations. Multiple factors, including diagnostic uncertainty, time pressures in clinical settings, patient expectations, defensive medicine practices, and gaps in knowledge about optimal antimicrobial use principles, drive these practices.

Healthcare-associated factors that promote the development of resistance include high antimicrobial use intensity in hospital settings, inadequate infection prevention and control practices that facilitate the transmission of resistant organisms between patients, and the use of medical devices that provide pathways for infection and create sites for biofilm formation where resistance can develop. Immunocompromised patient populations in healthcare settings are particularly vulnerable to infections with resistant organisms and may require extended antimicrobial treatment courses, which can further select for the development of resistance. Table 11.1 shows central mechanisms of antimicrobial resistance.

11.2. Use and Misuse in Human Medicine, Veterinary Practice, and Agriculture

The patterns of antimicrobial use across human medicine, veterinary practice, and agricultural production create interconnected selection pressures that drive the development and spread of antimicrobial resistance through complex pathways that link these traditionally separate domains (Laxminarayan et al., 2013). Understanding the scope and nature of antimicrobial use in each sector is essential for developing effective interventions that can reduce inappropriate use while preserving the effectiveness of these critically essential agents for legitimate therapeutic applications. The volume of antimicrobial use varies significantly between sectors, with global estimates suggesting that agricultural use accounts for most of the total antimicrobial consumption in many regions, followed by human medicine and veterinary practice for companion animals.

In human medicine, antimicrobial use patterns are characterised by significant variations across healthcare settings, patient populations, and geographic regions, reflecting differences in disease burden, prescribing practices, regulatory frameworks, and healthcare system characteristics (Van Boeckel et al., 2014). Hospital settings typically demonstrate high antimicrobial use intensity due to the concentration of severely ill patients with severe infections, the prevalence of invasive procedures that increase infection risk, and the presence of immunocompromised populations who may require prophylactic antimicrobial treatment. However, studies consistently demonstrate substantial inappropriate use in hospital settings, including excessive use of broad-spectrum agents when narrow-spectrum alternatives would be effective, prolonged treatment durations beyond evidence-based recommendations, and inadequate adherence to antimicrobial stewardship guidelines.

Outpatient antimicrobial prescribing accounts for the most significant volume of human antimicrobial use in most healthcare systems and exhibits particularly high rates of inappropriate use, especially for respiratory tract infections, where viral etiologies are common. Still, bacterial infections are often presumed without adequate diagnostic confirmation. Primary care settings face unique challenges in antimicrobial prescribing due to diagnostic uncertainty, time constraints, patient expectations for antimicrobial treatment, and limited access to rapid diagnostic tests that could guide treatment decisions. The phenomenon of defensive prescribing, where clinicians prescribe antimicrobials to avoid potential adverse outcomes rather than based on clinical evidence of bacterial infection, contributes significantly to inappropriate use patterns. Self-medication with antimicrobials represents a significant contributor to inappropriate use in many regions, particularly where antimicrobials are available without prescription or where regulatory enforcement is inadequate. The over-the-counter availability of antimicrobials enables patients to self-diagnose and self-treat conditions that may not require antimicrobial treatment, often resulting in insufficient dosing, inappropriate drug selection, and premature treatment discontinuation, which can promote the development of resistance. Internet pharmacies and informal drug markets further complicate efforts to control the inappropriate access and use of antimicrobials.

Veterinary antimicrobial use encompasses both therapeutic applications for treating sick animals and prophylactic or metaphylactic use to prevent disease in healthy animals or control the spread of disease in animal populations (Van Boeckel et al., 2015). Therapeutic use in veterinary medicine generally follows principles similar to those in human medicine, involving the diagnosis of bacterial infections and the selection of appropriate antimicrobial agents based on pathogen susceptibility and pharmacokinetic considerations. However, veterinary practice faces unique challenges, including limited diagnostic capacity in some settings, economic constraints that may discourage extensive diagnostic testing, and the need to treat multiple animals simultaneously in outbreak situations.

Food animal production systems represent the largest single category of antimicrobial use globally, with applications including growth promotion, disease prevention, and treatment of clinical infections in livestock and poultry populations. Growth promotion use, which involves administration of subtherapeutic doses of antimicrobials to enhance feed conversion efficiency and weight gain, has been identified as particularly problematic for resistance development due to the prolonged exposure periods and suboptimal drug concentrations involved. Many countries have implemented restrictions or bans on the use of growth promoters, but the implementation and enforcement vary significantly.

Prophylactic and metaphylactic use in food animal production involves the administration of antimicrobials to healthy animals to prevent disease occurrence or to control disease spread when some animals in a population are affected. These practices are often considered necessary for animal welfare and economic reasons, particularly in intensive production systems where high animal density and stress factors increase disease susceptibility. However, the mass medication approaches typically employed can create significant selective pressure for the development of resistance, while potentially exposing large numbers of animals to antimicrobial agents.

Aquaculture represents a rapidly growing sector of antimicrobial use, with unique challenges related to drug delivery in aquatic environments, limited treatment options for fish diseases, and the potential for antimicrobial residues to persist in these environments, where they may continue to exert selective pressure for the development of resistance. The intensive nature of many aquaculture operations, combined with environmental stress factors and high stocking densities, creates conditions that are favourable to disease outbreaks, which may require antimicrobial intervention.

Agricultural crop production involves the use of antimicrobials for plant disease control, particularly for bacterial and fungal pathogens that can cause significant economic losses in the production of fruits, vegetables, and ornamental crops. While the volumes involved are generally smaller than those used in animal production, the environmental application of antimicrobials in agricultural settings can contribute to the development of resistance in environmental bacterial populations. It may affect non-target organisms, including beneficial microorganisms that contribute to soil health and plant nutrition. Table 11.2 shows antimicrobial use patterns and resistance drivers across human and animal health sectors.

Table 11.1. Major Mechanisms of antimicrobial resistance and clinical examples

Resistance Mechanism	Molecular Basis	Key Examples	Affected Drug Classes	Clinical Impact	Detection Methods
Enzymatic Inactivation	β-lactamases, aminoglycoside-modifying enzymes	ESBL-producing Enterobacteriaceae, Carbapenem-resistant Enterobacteriaceae (CRE)	β-lactams, aminoglycosides, carbapenems	Treatment failures, increased Mortality, and healthcare costs	Phenotypic tests, PCR, and whole genome sequencing
Target Site Modification	Altered penicillin-binding proteins, DNA gyrase mutations	MRSA, fluoroquinolone-resistant gram-negatives	β-lactams, fluoroquinolones	Limited treatment options, prolonged infections	Susceptibility testing, molecular diagnostics
Efflux Pump Overexpression	Multidrug resistance pumps, regulatory mutations	Pseudomonas aeruginosa, Acinetobacter baumannii	Multiple classes (fluoroquinolones, β-lactams)	Multidrug resistance, therapeutic challenges	Efflux pump inhibitor assays, genetic analysis
Reduced Permeability	Porin loss, altered membrane composition	Carbapenem-resistant P. aeruginosa	β-lactams, carbapenems	Reduced drug effectiveness, treatment complications	Permeability assays, structural analysis
Bypass Pathways	Alternative metabolic routes	Trimethoprim-sulfamethoxazole resistance	Folate synthesis inhibitors	Persistent infections, treatment limitations	Metabolic pathway analysis, resistance gene detection

Table 11.2. Antimicrobial use patterns and resistance drivers across human and animal health sectors

Sector/Setting	Primary Use Categories	Volume Estimates (Global)	Key Resistance Drivers	Regulatory Frameworks	Intervention Priorities
Human Healthcare - Hospitals	Treatment, prophylaxis	15-20% of total human use	High-intensity use, broad-spectrum selection, transmission	Prescription requirements, stewardship programs	Diagnostic stewardship, narrow-spectrum selection, and infection control
Human Healthcare - Outpatient	Respiratory infections, urinary tract infections	80-85% of total human use	Inappropriate viral prescribing, incomplete courses	Professional regulation, clinical guidelines	Point-of-care diagnostics, patient education, prescriber training
Food Animal Production	Growth promotion, prevention, treatment	60-80% of global antimicrobial use	Subtherapeutic dosing, mass medication	Varying restrictions globally	Growth promoter bans, alternatives development, surveillance
Companion Animal Veterinary	Treatment, prophylaxis	5-10% of veterinary use	High-potency drug use, client compliance	Veterinary oversight required	Owner education, stewardship guidelines, and diagnostic use
Aquaculture	Disease treatment, prevention	2-5% of agricultural use	Environmental persistence, biofilm formation	Limited regulatory oversight	Alternative therapies, ecological monitoring

11.3. Resistance Gene Transmission Pathways

The transmission of antimicrobial resistance genes occurs through complex pathways that connect human, animal, and environmental reservoirs, enabling the rapid spread of resistance traits across different bacterial species, ecosystems, and geographic regions through both vertical and horizontal gene transfer mechanisms (Munita & Arias, 2016). Understanding these transmission pathways is crucial for developing effective interventions to limit the spread of resistance and for implementing surveillance systems that can detect and track the emergence and dissemination of resistance. The interconnected nature of modern global systems, including food production and distribution networks, international travel and trade, and shared environmental resources, creates multiple opportunities for the transmission of resistance genes between traditionally separate domains.

Horizontal gene transfer represents the primary mechanism by which resistance genes spread rapidly between bacterial populations, involving the transfer of genetic material between organisms that are not in a parent-offspring relationship and enabling resistance traits to cross species boundaries that would not be traversable through vertical inheritance alone. The three primary mechanisms of horizontal gene transfer are conjugation, transformation, and transduction, each of which can occur under varying environmental conditions and transfer different types of genetic elements, including those carrying resistance genes. Conjugation involves direct cell-to-cell contact through pili structures, which enable the transfer of plasmids carrying resistance genes. This process can occur between diverse bacterial species and in various environmental conditions, including human and animal gastrointestinal tracts, soil, water, and biofilm communities.

Plasmids represent significant vehicles for the transmission of resistance genes because they can carry multiple resistance genes simultaneously, enabling the rapid acquisition of multidrug resistance phenotypes through single transfer events. Large conjugative plasmids can carry resistance genes that affect numerous antimicrobial classes, along with other advantageous traits, including virulence factors, heavy metal resistance, and metabolic capabilities, which provide fitness advantages in various environmental niches. The ability of plasmids to replicate independently of the host chromosome enables them to be maintained in bacterial populations even in the absence of continuous antimicrobial selective pressure. However, their retention may be influenced by metabolic costs associated with plasmid maintenance.

Integrons and transposons represent additional genetic elements that facilitate the mobility of resistance genes by enabling the movement of resistance genes between different genetic contexts, including chromosomes, plasmids, and bacteriophages. Class 1 integrons are particularly prevalent in clinical isolates and environmental bacteria and can capture and express resistance gene cassettes through site-specific recombination mechanisms. The modular nature of integron-mediated resistance gene capture enables bacteria to accumulate multiple resistance genes over time and to lose genes that are no longer advantageous under changed selective conditions.

Environmental reservoirs play a crucial role in the transmission of resistance genes by serving as mixing vessels where bacteria from different sources can interact and exchange genetic material, and by providing selective conditions that favour the maintenance and spread of resistance genes (Davies & Davies, 2010). Soil environments contain diverse bacterial communities with extensive networks of gene exchange. Antimicrobial residues from agricultural use, sewage application, and pharmaceutical manufacturing can create selective pressures that favour resistant organisms in soil microbial communities. Aquatic environments, including surface water bodies, groundwater, and marine systems, receive antimicrobial residues and resistant bacteria from multiple sources, including sewage treatment plant effluents, agricultural runoff, and aquaculture operations.

Sewage treatment systems represent critical interfaces for the transmission of resistance genes because they concentrate bacteria from human and animal sources, along with antimicrobial residues, creating conditions that promote horizontal gene transfer while potentially failing to eliminate resistant organisms before they are discharged into receiving waters. Conventional sewage treatment processes may reduce, but not eliminate, antimicrobial residues and resistant bacteria. Additionally, some treatment processes may promote horizontal gene transfer through concentration effects and environmental stress that induces bacterial competence for DNA uptake.

Food production and distribution systems provide pathways for the transmission of resistance genes from animal reservoirs to human populations through the consumption of contaminated food products, with concerns related to meat and dairy products from animals treated with antimicrobials. Resistant bacteria can contaminate carcasses during slaughter and processing, survive food preservation processes, and reach consumers through inadequately cooked products. Cross-contamination during food preparation can spread resistant bacteria to other food items and environmental surfaces, creating opportunities for human exposure and gut colonisation with resistant organisms.

Healthcare environments represent high-risk settings for the transmission of resistance genes due to the concentration of vulnerable patients, intensive antimicrobial use, and the presence of medical devices that can harbour biofilm communities, where horizontal gene transfer can occur. Healthcare-associated transmission can occur through direct patient-to-patient contact, contaminated environmental surfaces, medical equipment, and the hands of healthcare workers. The selection pressure created by high antimicrobial use intensity in healthcare settings favours the persistence and spread of resistant organisms once they are introduced.

International travel and trade networks facilitate the rapid global dissemination of resistance genes through the movement of people, animals, and products that carry resistant bacteria. Air travel can transport resistant organisms across continents within hours, and travellers may acquire resistant bacteria during their travels and take them to new geographic regions upon return. International trade in live animals, animal feed, and food products can disseminate resistant bacteria and residual antimicrobials across national boundaries, potentially introducing novel resistance genes to naive bacterial populations.

Figure 17 shows A comprehensive flow diagram illustrating the interconnected pathways through which antimicrobial resistance genes spread between human, animal, and environmental compartments. The diagram illustrates humans, livestock, companion animals, wildlife, and ecological reservoirs (soil, water, and sewage) as interconnected nodes, with bidirectional arrows indicating the flow of resistance genes. Specific transmission mechanisms are labelled, including direct contact between humans and animals, food chain transmission from livestock to humans, environmental contamination through sewage and agricultural runoff, horizontal gene transfer in ecological settings, and global dissemination through travel and trade. The diagram emphasises key interface points such as healthcare settings, farms, food processing facilities, sewage treatment plants, and international transportation hubs. Selective pressures from antimicrobial use in each compartment are depicted as driving forces that promote the development and spread of resistance. The figure includes examples of specific resistance genes (such as mcr-1, NDM-1, ESBL genes) and their documented transmission routes between sectors.

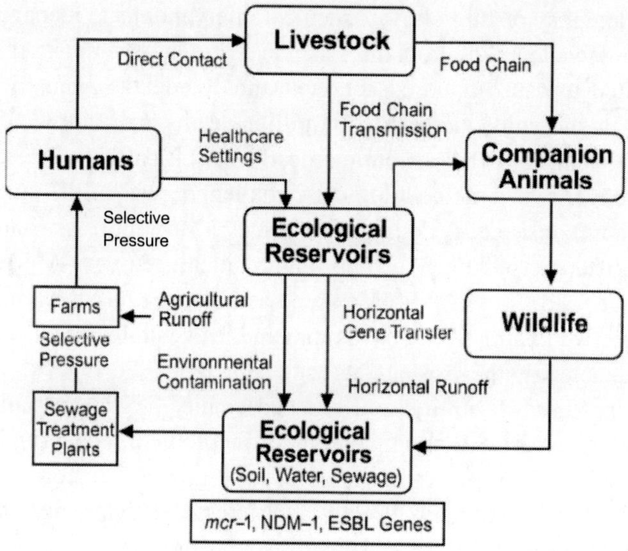

Figure 17. Antimicrobial resistance gene transmission pathways in One Health systems.

11.4. Economic and Health Impacts

The economic and Health impacts of antimicrobial resistance represent a growing crisis that threatens to undermine decades of medical progress while imposing substantial costs on healthcare systems, agricultural sectors, and broader economies worldwide (Cassini et al., 2019). The magnitude of these impacts is difficult to quantify precisely due to the complexity of attributing outcomes directly to resistance versus underlying diseases. Still, available evidence suggests that the costs are already substantial and are projected to increase dramatically if current trends continue unchecked. Economic analyses must consider both direct costs associated with treating resistant infections and indirect costs related to productivity losses, reduced quality of life, and broader societal impacts, including effects on medical procedures that depend on effective antimicrobial prophylaxis.

Direct healthcare costs associated with antimicrobial resistance arise from multiple sources, including prolonged hospitalisation, increased need for intensive care, use of more expensive second- and third-line antimicrobial agents, additional diagnostic testing, and management of treatment complications and adverse events. Patients with resistant infections typically require more extended hospital stays compared to those with susceptible infections, with studies documenting increases ranging from several days to several weeks, depending on the pathogen and infection site. These extended stays not only increase direct medical costs but also occupy hospital beds that could otherwise be used for other patients, potentially creating capacity constraints that affect the overall efficiency of the healthcare system.

The use of reserve antimicrobials for treating resistant infections often involves drugs that are significantly more expensive than first-line agents, with costs potentially differing by orders of magnitude between standard and last-resort treatments. Beyond drug acquisition costs, reserve antimicrobials may require more intensive monitoring for adverse effects, specialised administration procedures, and additional laboratory testing to guide dosing and assess treatment response. Some reserve antimicrobials have significant toxicity profiles that require careful monitoring and may result in further medical interventions to manage adverse effects.

Mortality attributable to antimicrobial resistance represents the most severe health impact. It has been estimated to cause hundreds of thousands of deaths annually worldwide, with projections suggesting this could increase to 10 million deaths per year by 2050 if no additional action is taken (O'Neill, 2016). Attributing deaths specifically to resistance rather than underlying disease severity is a methodologically challenging task. Still, studies using various analytical approaches consistently demonstrate excess Mortality associated with resistant infections across different pathogen groups and clinical settings. Mortality impacts are particularly pronounced for invasive diseases such as bloodstream infections and pneumonia, where delays in effective treatment can have rapid and irreversible consequences.

Morbidity associated with resistant infections extends beyond Mortality to include prolonged illness, increased disability, and reduced quality of life for patients who survive resistant infections but experience complications or incomplete recovery. Treatment failures may result in chronic infections, recurrent episodes, or progression to more severe disease states that might have been prevented with effective antimicrobial treatment. Some patients may experience permanent disability or organ damage as a result of treatment delays or inadequate treatment effectiveness associated with antimicrobial resistance.

Economic productivity losses associated with antimicrobial resistance occur through multiple pathways, including work absences during prolonged illness, permanent disability that reduces earning capacity, premature mortality that eliminates future productive capacity, and caregiving responsibilities that prevent family members from participating in economic activities. These productivity losses affect not only individuals and families but also employers and broader economic sectors, particularly in regions or occupations where resistant infections are more common.

The healthcare system's impacts extend beyond direct patient care costs to include effects on medical procedures that depend on effective antimicrobial prophylaxis, such as surgery, cancer chemotherapy, organ transplantation, and other interventions that compromise immune function or create infection risks. As resistance reduces the effectiveness of prophylactic antimicrobials, these procedures may become more hazardous or may require modifications that increase costs or compromise their effectiveness. Some procedures may become prohibitively risky in settings with high rates of antimicrobial resistance, potentially limiting access to essential medical interventions.

The agricultural economic impacts of antimicrobial resistance include reduced livestock productivity, increased animal mortality, higher veterinary treatment costs, and potential trade restrictions on products from regions with high rates of resistance (Gandra et al., 2014). Food animal production may face increased costs for alternative disease prevention strategies, enhanced biosecurity measures, and more expensive antimicrobial treatments in the event of infections. Consumer concerns about antimicrobial use and resistance in food production may affect market demand and pricing for animal products, potentially creating economic incentives for production changes but also imposing transition costs on producers.

Table 11.3. Economic and health impact indicators of antimicrobial resistance by healthcare setting and pathogen category

Healthcare Setting	Excess Length of Stay (Days)	Additional Cost per Case (USD)	Attributable Mortality (%)	Key Resistant Pathogens	Economic Burden Drivers
Intensive Care Units	8-15 days	$18,000-$30,000	15-30%	MRSA, CRE, carbapenem-resistant P. aeruginosa	Prolonged ICU stay, expensive therapeutics, and organ support
General Medical Wards	4-10 days	$8,000-$15,000	5-15%	ESBL-producing Enterobacteriaceae, C. difficile	Extended hospitalisation, isolation precautions
Surgical Services	5-12 days	$10,000-$25,000	8-20%	MRSA, resistant gram-negatives	Surgical site infection complications, reoperation
Outpatient Settings	Variable	$1,000-$5,000	<5%	Resistant Streptococcus pneumoniae, MRSA	Treatment failures, multiple antibiotic courses
Long-term Care Facilities	Variable	$2,000-$8,000	10-25%	C. difficile, carbapenem-resistant organisms	Outbreak management, infection control measures

Global economic modelling exercises have projected that the cumulative economic impact of antimicrobial resistance could reach $100 trillion by 2050 if current trends continue, representing a substantial fraction of global economic output and potentially affecting economic growth rates worldwide. These projections incorporate both healthcare costs and broader economic impacts, including productivity losses. Still, they also involve substantial uncertainties due to the difficulty of predicting future resistance trends, technological developments, and policy responses. Table 11.3 shows economic and Health impact indicators of antimicrobial resistance.

The development of novel antimicrobials and alternative therapies requires substantial research and development investments that may not be economically attractive to pharmaceutical companies due to the relatively short treatment courses typical of antimicrobial therapy and the expectation that new drugs will be held in reserve to preserve their effectiveness. This market failure in antimicrobial development represents a significant economic challenge that may require public sector intervention, innovative financing mechanisms, or alternative research and development models to ensure an adequate pipeline of new treatments.

Infection prevention and control measures necessary to limit the spread of resistant organisms impose additional costs on healthcare systems, including infrastructure modifications, enhanced surveillance systems, isolation precautions, personal protective equipment, and specialised cleaning and disinfection procedures. While these investments can provide positive returns by preventing resistant infections, they require upfront costs and ongoing operational expenses that may strain healthcare budgets, particularly in resource-limited settings where resistance rates may be highest but resources for prevention are most limited.

11.5. National and International Action Plans

National and international action plans for addressing antimicrobial resistance have emerged as essential policy frameworks for coordinating multisectoral responses to this complex global health security threat, providing structured approaches for implementing evidence-based interventions across human Health, animal health, and environmental sectors (World Health Organisation, 2021). The development of comprehensive action plans reflects a growing recognition that antimicrobial resistance cannot be addressed effectively through isolated sectoral responses. Instead, it requires coordinated approaches that address all sources of selective pressure while strengthening surveillance, stewardship, and research capacities across interconnected domains.

The Global Action Plan on Antimicrobial Resistance, adopted by the World Health Assembly in 2015, established a framework for national and international responses built around five strategic objectives: improving awareness and understanding of antimicrobial resistance through effective communication, education and training; strengthening the knowledge and evidence base through surveillance and research; reducing the incidence of infection through adequate sanitation, hygiene and infection prevention measures; optimising the use of antimicrobial medicines in human and animal health; and developing the economic case for sustainable investment that takes account of the needs of all countries and increases investment in new drugs, diagnostic tools, vaccines and other interventions. This framework has provided the foundation for developing national action plans and has been complemented by sector-specific guidance documents and implementation support tools.

National action plan development processes typically involve multistakeholder consultations that bring together representatives from human Health, animal health, agriculture, environment, trade, and other relevant sectors to develop comprehensive strategies that address the full scope of antimicrobial resistance challenges within specific country contexts. These processes must balance global best practices with local priorities, resource constraints, and implementation capacity while ensuring that interventions address the most significant resistance threats and sources of selective pressure within national boundaries. Successful national action plans require a high-level political commitment, adequate resource allocation, clear governance structures, and mechanisms for monitoring and evaluating implementation progress.

The implementation of national action plans faces significant challenges, including limited financial resources, competing health priorities, fragmented governance structures that span multiple ministries and agencies, insufficient technical capacity, and resistance to change from stakeholders who may perceive interventions as a threat to their interests or practices. Many countries have successfully developed national action plans but have struggled with implementation due to these challenges, highlighting the importance of realistic planning, phased implementation approaches, and sustained political and financial commitment over extended time periods.

Surveillance systems are critical components of national action plans, necessitating coordination among human health, animal health, and environmental monitoring systems to provide comprehensive data on resistance trends, antimicrobial use patterns, and the effectiveness of interventions. Establishing robust surveillance systems requires substantial investments in laboratory capacity, information systems, training, and quality assurance programs. Ongoing operation, however, requires sustained funding and technical support. Many national action plans have identified surveillance as a priority area, but have faced challenges in securing adequate resources and technical expertise for implementation.

Regulatory frameworks for antimicrobial access and use represent another essential component of national action plans, requiring coordination between agencies responsible for drug regulation, healthcare oversight, agricultural regulation, and environmental protection. Strengthening regulatory frameworks may involve implementing prescription-only requirements for antimicrobials, establishing quality standards for antimicrobial products, controlling importation of substandard products, and developing guidelines for appropriate use across different sectors. Regulatory strengthening must strike a balance between maintaining the proper use of antimicrobials and ensuring access to essential antimicrobials for legitimate therapeutic purposes.

International cooperation mechanisms play a crucial role in supporting the implementation of national action plans through technical assistance, capacity building, resource mobilisation, and knowledge-sharing platforms that enable countries to learn from each other's experiences and adopt successful interventions. Organisations, including the World Health Organisation, the Food and Agriculture Organisation, and the World Organisation for Animal Health, provide guidance, training, and support for the development and implementation of national action plans. Meanwhile, regional networks facilitate cooperation between neighbouring countries facing similar challenges.

Global initiatives, such as the Global Antimicrobial Resistance and Use Surveillance System (GLASS) and the Global Database for Tracking Antimicrobial Resistance in Food and Agriculture, provide platforms for international data sharing and collaborative surveillance that support national decision-making while contributing to a global understanding of resistance trends and the effectiveness of interventions. These initiatives require standardised methodologies, quality assurance systems, and sustainable funding mechanisms to ensure their continued operation and expansion.

Trade and international commerce considerations represent essential components of global cooperation on antimicrobial resistance, as resistance genes and resistant organisms can spread rapidly across borders through the movement of people, animals, food products, and other goods. International standards for antimicrobial use in food production, requirements for resistance testing and reporting, and harmonised approaches to risk assessment and management can help prevent international trade from undermining national efforts to address antimicrobial resistance while avoiding unnecessary trade barriers.

Research and development coordination at the international level is essential for ensuring adequate investment in new antimicrobials, diagnostic tools, vaccines, and alternative therapies, while avoiding duplication of effort and ensuring that research priorities address the most critical needs for combating antimicrobial resistance globally. International research partnerships, funding mechanisms, and knowledge-sharing platforms can help overcome market failures that limit private sector investment in antimicrobial research, while ensuring that new tools are accessible to countries and populations that need them most.

11.6. Stewardship Programs Across Sectors

Antimicrobial stewardship programs represent systematic interventions designed to optimise antimicrobial use patterns while preserving the effectiveness of these critical agents for current and future generations. This requires implementation across the human healthcare, veterinary medicine, and agricultural sectors to address all sources of selective pressure that drive the development and spread of resistance (Ventola, 2015). Effective stewardship programs integrate multiple intervention strategies, including clinical decision support, prescriber education, formulary management, utilisation monitoring, and outcome evaluation, to promote appropriate antimicrobial use while minimising unintended consequences, such as treatment failures or adverse events.

Healthcare stewardship programs have evolved from early initiatives focused primarily on controlling costs and reducing adverse drug events to comprehensive programs that address antimicrobial resistance as a primary objective while maintaining clinical effectiveness and patient safety. Core components of healthcare stewardship programs include prospective audit and feedback systems where trained pharmacists or infectious diseases specialists review antimicrobial prescriptions and provide recommendations for optimisation, formulary restrictions that limit access to broad-spectrum or high-risk agents to appropriate clinical situations, clinical guidelines and protocols that standardise antimicrobial selection and duration decisions, and educational interventions that improve prescriber knowledge and decision-making skills.

Hospital-based stewardship programs typically employ multidisciplinary teams, including infectious disease physicians, clinical pharmacists, microbiologists, infection preventionists, and information technology specialists, who work together to implement evidence-based interventions tailored to local resistance patterns, prescribing practices, and organisational culture. Successful programs require strong leadership support, adequate resources for staff time and technology infrastructure, and integration with existing clinical workflows to minimise burden on prescribers while maximising intervention effectiveness. Outcome measurement is essential for program evaluation and continuous improvement, with metrics including antimicrobial utilisation rates, resistance trends, patient outcomes, and economic impacts.

Outpatient stewardship programs face unique challenges due to the distributed nature of care delivery, limited time for complex decision-making, and reduced access to diagnostic testing and specialist consultation. Effective outpatient interventions include clinical decision support tools integrated into electronic health records, patient and prescriber education programs, rapid diagnostic testing to guide treatment decisions, and delayed prescribing strategies that enable patients to fill prescriptions only if symptoms persist or worsen. Community-wide stewardship initiatives may involve coordination between multiple healthcare organisations, public health agencies, and community groups to implement population-level interventions.

Veterinary stewardship programs encompass both companion animal practice and food animal production systems, with interventions adapted to the specific challenges and opportunities within each context (Tang et al., 2017). Companion animal stewardship parallels human healthcare approaches, with an emphasis on selecting appropriate antimicrobials based on culture and susceptibility testing when feasible, adhering to treatment guidelines, and providing client education to ensure completion of prescribed treatment courses. Veterinary stewardship programs may involve collaboration between veterinarians, veterinary pharmacists, and animal health organisations to develop guidelines, provide education, and monitor antimicrobial use patterns.

Food animal stewardship programs focus on optimising antimicrobial use in production systems while maintaining animal health and welfare, involving interventions such as veterinary oversight requirements for antimicrobial use decisions, restrictions on growth promotion applications, development of alternatives to antimicrobial interventions, and implementation of comprehensive animal health management programs that reduce disease occurrence and antimicrobial need. Successful food animal stewardship necessitates collaboration among producers, veterinarians, nutritionists, and other animal health professionals to implement integrated approaches that address multiple factors influencing animal health and antimicrobial use.

Agricultural stewardship for crop production involves optimising antimicrobial applications to control plant diseases while minimising environmental impact and the development of resistance in farming ecosystems. Interventions include integrated pest management approaches that combine antimicrobial applications with other disease control strategies, application timing and methods that maximise effectiveness while minimising exposure duration, and monitoring systems that track antimicrobial use and resistance development in agricultural settings.

Technology solutions play increasingly essential roles in stewardship program implementation across all sectors, including electronic health record systems that provide clinical decision support and utilisation monitoring, laboratory information systems that facilitate rapid communication of culture results, mobile applications that provide treatment guidance and patient education, and data analytics platforms that enable population-level monitoring and evaluation. Artificial intelligence and machine learning technologies show promise for enhancing stewardship programs through improved prediction of infection risk, optimisation of treatment recommendations, and automated monitoring of prescribing patterns.

Quality improvement methodologies offer frameworks for implementing and sustaining stewardship programs through systematic approaches that identify improvement opportunities, test interventions, measure outcomes, and scale successful practices. These methodologies emphasise the importance of understanding local context, engaging stakeholders in intervention design and implementation, and using data to guide continuous refinement of stewardship approaches.

International collaboration in stewardship program development and implementation enables the sharing of successful practices, harmonisation of approaches across different healthcare systems and countries, and development of global standards and guidelines that can be adapted to local contexts. Professional organisations, academic institutions, and international agencies play crucial roles in facilitating knowledge exchange and providing technical assistance for stewardship program development, particularly in resource-constrained settings where local expertise and resources may be limited.

Evaluation of stewardship program effectiveness requires comprehensive measurement approaches that assess both process indicators, such as program implementation fidelity and reach, and outcome indicators, including antimicrobial utilisation changes, resistance trends, clinical outcomes, and economic impacts (Llor & Bjerrum, 2014). Long-term evaluation is essential because the implications of stewardship interventions on resistance may not become apparent for months or years, and sustained implementation is required to maintain benefits over time.

Conclusion

Antimicrobial resistance represents a paradigmatic One Health crisis demanding coordinated global action across human health, animal health, and environmental sectors to address complex biological, social, and economic drivers perpetuating this growing global health security threat. Resistance development mechanisms operate through natural evolutionary processes accelerated by the widespread use of antimicrobials across healthcare, agricultural, and environmental settings, creating selection pressures that favour resistant organisms while facilitating the rapid transmission of resistance genes through horizontal transfer mechanisms that transcend species and geographic boundaries.

Economic and health impacts are already substantial, projected to exceed $100 trillion globally by 2050 while causing millions of preventable deaths annually. These impacts extend beyond healthcare systems to affect agricultural productivity, international trade, and broader economic development, particularly in low- and middle-income countries where resistance rates are often highest but resources are most limited. The disproportionate impact on vulnerable populations exacerbates existing health inequities, threatening progress toward Sustainable Development Goal 3.

National and international action plans provide essential coordination frameworks, but implementation remains challenging due to resource constraints, competing priorities, and fragmented governance structures. Antimicrobial stewardship programs represent critical interventions for optimising antimicrobial use patterns while preserving the effectiveness of antimicrobial agents. New antimicrobial development, diagnostic tools, vaccines, and alternative therapies are crucial; however, current market incentives are insufficient to ensure adequate private sector investment, necessitating innovative financing mechanisms and public-private partnerships (Woolhouse & Farrar, 2014).

Infection prevention through vaccination, infection control, and sanitation represents critical components in reducing antimicrobial treatment needs. Addressing antimicrobial resistance as a global health security threat requires recognising that no country can solve this problem alone—international cooperation is essential for surveillance, research, capacity building, and coordinated policy responses that prevent resistance development and spread across borders.

Acknowledgments

The authors would like to extend our appreciation to those who offered helpful commentary during the drafting process of this manuscript. We also acknowledge the role Nova Science Publishers played in enabling the work described herein.

References

Cassini, A., Högberg, L. D., Plachouras, D., Quattrocchi, A., Hoxha, A., Simonsen, G. S., ... & Monnet, D. L. (2019). Attributable deaths and disability-adjusted life-years caused by infections with antibiotic-resistant bacteria in the EU and European Economic Area in 2015: a population-level modelling analysis. *The Lancet Infectious Diseases*, 19(1), 56-66. https://doi.org/10.1016/S1473-3099(18)30605-4.

Davies, J., & Davies, D. (2010). Origins and evolution of antibiotic resistance. *Microbiology and Molecular Biology Reviews*, 74(3), 417-433. https://doi.org/10.1128/MMBR.00016-10.

Gandra, S., Barter, D. M., & Laxminarayan, R. (2014). Economic burden of antibiotic resistance: how much do we really know? *Clinical Microbiology and Infection*, 20(10), 973-980. https://doi.org/10.1111/1469-0691.12798.

Holmes, A. H., Moore, L. S., Sundsfjord, A., Steinbakk, M., Regmi, S., Karkey, A., ... & Piddock, L. J. (2016). Understanding the mechanisms and drivers of antimicrobial resistance. *The Lancet*, 387(10014), 176-187. https://doi.org/10.1016/S0140-6736(15)00473-0.

Laxminarayan, R., Duse, A., Wattal, C., Zaidi, A. K., Wertheim, H. F., Sumpradit, N., ... & Cars, O. (2013). Antibiotic resistance—the need for global solutions. *The Lancet Infectious Diseases*, 13(12), 1057-1098. https://doi.org/10.1016/S1473-3099(13)70318-9.

Llor, C., & Bjerrum, L. (2014). Antimicrobial resistance: risk associated with antibiotic overuse and initiatives to reduce the problem. *Therapeutic Advances in Drug Safety*, 5(6), 229-241. https://doi.org/10.1177/2042098614554919.

Munita, J. M., & Arias, C. A. (2016). Mechanisms of antibiotic resistance. *Microbiology Spectrum*, 4(2), 4-2. https://doi.org/10.1128/microbiolspec.VMBF-0016-2015.

O'Neill, J. (2016). *Tackling drug-resistant infections globally: final report and recommendations*. The Review on Antimicrobial Resistance. https://amr-review.org/sites/default/files/160525_Final%20paper_with%20cover.pdf.

Prestinaci, F., Pezzotti, P., & Pantosti, A. (2015). Antimicrobial resistance: a global multifaceted phenomenon. *Pathogens and Global Health*, 109(7), 309-318. https://doi.org/10.1179/2047773215Y.0000000030.

Tang, K. L., Caffrey, N. P., Nóbrega, D. B., Cork, S. C., Ronksley, P. E., Barkema, H. W., ... & Ghali, W. A. (2017). Restricting the use of antibiotics in food-producing animals and its associations with antibiotic resistance in food-producing animals and human beings: a systematic review and meta-analysis. *The Lancet Planetary Health*, 1(8), e316-e327. https://doi.org/10.1016/S2542-5196(17)30141-9.

Van Boeckel, T. P., Brower, C., Gilbert, M., Grenfell, B. T., Levin, S. A., Robinson, T. P., ... & Laxminarayan, R. (2015). Global trends in antimicrobial use in food animals. *Proceedings of the National Academy of Sciences*, 112(18), 5649-5654. https://doi.org/10.1073/pnas.1503141112.

Van Boeckel, T. P., Gandra, S., Ashok, A., Caudron, Q., Grenfell, B. T., Levin, S. A., & Laxminarayan, R. (2014). Global antibiotic consumption 2000 to 2010: an analysis of national pharmaceutical sales data. *The Lancet Infectious Diseases*, 14(8), 742-750. https://doi.org/10.1016/S1473-3099(14)70780-7.

Ventola, C. L. (2015). The antibiotic resistance crisis: part 1: causes and threats. *Pharmacy and Therapeutics*, 40(4), 277-283.

Woolhouse, M., & Farrar, J. (2014). Policy: An intergovernmental panel on antimicrobial resistance. *Nature*, 509(7502), 555-557. https://doi.org/10.1038/509555a.

World Health Organization. (2021). *Global action plan on antimicrobial resistance*. World Health Organization. https://www.who.int/publications/i/item/9789241509763.

Chapter 12

Food Safety and Foodborne Disease Prevention

Quazi Syed Zahiruddin[1], PhD, MD
and Maajid Mohi Ud Din Malik[2,*], PhD

[1]Directorate of Research and Innovations, Datta Meghe Institute of Higher Education and Research (DMIHER), India
[2]Department of Radiology and Imaging Technology, Dr. D. Y. Patil School of Allied Health Sciences, Dr. D. Y. Patil Vidyapeeth· Pune (Deemed to be University), Sant Tukaram Nagar, Pimpri, Pune, India

Abstract

Food safety represents a critical global health challenge that affects billions of people worldwide through foodborne diseases caused by pathogenic microorganisms, chemical contaminants, and other hazards present in food systems. The global burden of foodborne diseases is substantial, with an estimated 600 million cases occurring annually, resulting in 420,000 deaths and significant economic losses that disproportionately affect vulnerable populations in low- and middle-income countries. Food production systems present multiple contamination risks throughout the farm-to-fork continuum, from primary production through processing, distribution, preparation, and consumption, requiring comprehensive approaches that address biological, chemical, and physical hazards at each stage. Modern food systems are becoming increasingly complex and globalised, presenting new challenges for ensuring food safety while also providing opportunities for the rapid international spread of foodborne pathogens and contamination events. Effective food safety systems require robust regulatory frameworks, science-based standards, comprehensive surveillance and outbreak response capabilities, and coordinated approaches that integrate human Health, animal health, and environmental considerations consistent with One Health principles. Consumer education and behaviour change are essential components of comprehensive food safety strategies, as many foodborne illnesses result from unsafe food handling practices in both domestic and commercial settings. Addressing food safety challenges is integral to achieving Sustainable Development Goal 3, which aims to ensure healthy lives and promote well-being for all, while also contributing to Goals 2 and 12, related to ending hunger and ensuring sustainable consumption and production patterns. Success in preventing foodborne diseases requires integrated approaches that address food system vulnerabilities while building capacity for

* Corresponding Author's Email: maajid.malik@dpu.edu.in

In: Advances in the One Health Approach
Editors: Maajid Mohi Ud Din Malik, Abhay Saraf, Harshal Tukaram Pandve et al.
ISBN: 979-8-90134-202-2

prevention, detection, and response across the entire food chain from production to consumption.

Keywords: food safety, foodborne disease, food systems, One Health, farm-to-fork, food security, HACCP, outbreak investigation, consumer education, Sustainable Development Goal 3, global Health

Introduction

Food safety represents a fundamental prerequisite for human Health and well-being, intersecting with multiple dimensions of sustainable development, including nutrition security, economic growth, and environmental protection. This exemplifies the interconnected nature of human, animal, and ecological Health that defines One Health approaches (World Health Organisation, 2015). The safety of food supplies affects every person on Earth and represents one of the most basic requirements for survival and Health. Yet, foodborne diseases continue to impose substantial burdens on individuals, families, communities, and national economies worldwide. The complexity of modern food systems, characterised by global supply chains, intensive production methods, and diverse processing and distribution networks, creates both opportunities for improving food safety through technological innovations and standardised practices, and new challenges related to the rapid international spread of contamination events and emerging food safety hazards. Understanding food safety as a One Health issue is essential because foodborne pathogens often originate from animal reservoirs, can be influenced by environmental conditions, and require coordinated responses across human Health, veterinary medicine, agriculture, and environmental management sectors. The prevention of foodborne diseases requires comprehensive approaches that address risks throughout the entire food chain, from primary production through consumption, while recognising that food safety is not only a technical challenge but also involves social, economic, and cultural factors that influence food system practices and consumer behaviours. Achieving food safety objectives is directly linked to Sustainable Development Goal 3, which aims to ensure healthy lives and promote well-being for all, while also contributing to achieving food security goals and sustainable food system objectives that recognise the interconnections between human Health, environmental sustainability, and economic development in food production and consumption systems.

12.1. Foodborne Disease Burden and Trends

The global burden of foodborne diseases represents a significant public health challenge that affects an estimated 600 million people annually, resulting in approximately 420,000 deaths worldwide and imposing substantial economic costs on individuals, healthcare systems, and national economies (World Health Organisation, 2015). These estimates, developed through comprehensive efforts by the World Health Organisation and its international partners, represent the most systematic attempt to quantify the global impact of foodborne diseases. However, they likely underestimate the actual burden due to underreporting, diagnostic limitations, and surveillance gaps in many regions. The burden of foodborne diseases is unevenly distributed globally, with the highest rates of illness and death occurring in low- and middle-income countries where food safety systems may be less developed, environmental conditions favour pathogen survival and transmission, and vulnerable populations have limited access to safe food and healthcare services.

Foodborne diseases encompass a diverse range of illnesses caused by ingestion of contaminated food or water, including infections caused by bacteria, viruses, parasites, and fungi, as well as poisoning from chemical contaminants, natural toxins, and other hazardous substances. Bacterial pathogens are the leading cause of foodborne illness globally, with major contributors including nontyphoidal Salmonella species, Campylobacter species, enteropathogenic Escherichia coli, and Clostridium perfringens, each causing millions of cases annually and posing significant public health concerns across various geographic regions and food systems (Scallan et al., 2011). Viral pathogens, particularly norovirus, also significantly contribute to the global foodborne disease burden, often causing large outbreaks associated with contaminated food handlers or water used in food production and preparation.

The epidemiological patterns of foodborne diseases vary significantly across different regions and populations, reflecting differences in food production systems, dietary patterns, environmental conditions, socioeconomic factors, and access to healthcare. High-income countries typically report higher rates of specific foodborne pathogens, such as Campylobacter and Salmonella, which may reflect better surveillance systems rather than necessarily more accurate incidence rates. They also experience outbreaks associated with fresh produce, processed foods, and complex food supply chains. Low- and middle-income countries often experience higher burdens of enteric diseases that may include substantial foodborne transmission components, along with higher rates of illness and death from foodborne diseases due to factors including malnutrition, limited healthcare access, and environmental conditions that favour pathogen transmission.

Emerging trends in foodborne diseases reflect the changing nature of food systems, shifting consumer preferences, the impact of climate change, and evolving pathogen characteristics, all of which create new challenges for food safety management (Havelaar et al., 2015). The globalisation of food systems has enabled the rapid international spread of foodborne pathogens and contamination events, with single production facilities potentially affecting consumers across multiple countries and continents. Fresh produce has emerged as an increasingly important vehicle for foodborne disease transmission, with outbreaks associated with leafy greens, sprouts, berries, and other products that are often consumed without cooking steps that would eliminate pathogens.

Climate change is creating new food safety challenges through multiple pathways, including altered environmental conditions that affect pathogen survival and transmission, extreme weather events that can compromise food production and processing infrastructure, and changing agricultural practices that may introduce new contamination risks. Rising temperatures and changing precipitation patterns can alter the geographic distribution and seasonal patterns of foodborne pathogens, leading to shifts in their prevalence. At the same time, extreme weather events, such as floods and droughts, can create conditions that increase the risk of contamination or compromise food safety control systems.

Antimicrobial resistance represents an emerging concern for foodborne disease prevention and treatment, as resistant pathogens can spread through food systems and cause infections that are more difficult to treat when they occur in humans. The use of antimicrobials in food animal production contributes to the development of resistance. It can result in resistant bacteria entering the food chain, creating risks for consumers who may acquire resistant infections through foodborne transmission pathways or experience treatment failures when resistant pathogens cause illness.

Demographic and social changes are influencing foodborne disease patterns through factors such as urbanisation, changing dietary patterns, increased consumption of convenience foods and ready-to-eat products, and growing populations of immunocompromised individuals who may be at a higher risk for severe foodborne illnesses. An ageing global population creates larger numbers of people who may be more susceptible to foodborne diseases due to age-related changes in immune function. Meanwhile, medical advances that enable the survival of people with compromised immune systems create populations that require special consideration in food safety planning. Table 12.1 shows the global burden of major foodborne diseases by pathogen and region.

The economic impact of foodborne diseases extends far beyond direct healthcare costs to include productivity losses, trade impacts, and broader economic consequences that can affect entire sectors and regions. Individual cases of foodborne illness can result in medical expenses, lost wages, and reduced quality of life. In contrast, severe cases may require hospitalisation, long-term care, or result in permanent disability or death. Healthcare systems incur substantial costs for treating foodborne diseases, including emergency department visits, hospitalisations, diagnostic testing, and treatment of complications, with costs varying significantly based on the pathogen, severity, and characteristics of the healthcare system.

Foodborne disease outbreaks can have significant economic impacts on food producers, processors, and retailers, including product recalls, facility closures, legal liability, and loss of consumer confidence, which can persist long after the immediate resolution of the outbreak. Large outbreaks associated with widely distributed products can impact entire industries and result in substantial economic losses that extend throughout the food supply chain. International trade in food products can be significantly affected by foodborne disease outbreaks, leading to import restrictions, increased inspection requirements, and a loss of market access, which may have lasting economic consequences for exporting countries and industries.

The development of surveillance systems for foodborne diseases requires substantial investments in laboratory capacity, reporting systems, epidemiological expertise, and coordination mechanisms. However, these investments provide essential information for prevention and control efforts, enabling early detection and response to outbreaks. Enhanced surveillance systems in many countries have improved the detection and characterisation of foodborne disease outbreaks, leading to a better understanding of disease patterns and more effective prevention and control measures. However, significant surveillance gaps remain in many regions where resources are limited.

12.2. Food Production Systems and Contamination Risks

Modern food production systems encompass complex networks of primary production, processing, distribution, and preparation activities that present multiple opportunities for contamination with pathogenic microorganisms, chemical hazards, and other substances that can cause foodborne illness when consumed (Newell et al., 2010). Understanding contamination risks throughout food production systems requires a comprehensive assessment of hazard sources, transmission pathways, and control points that can be targeted for intervention to reduce food safety risks. The diversity of food production systems, ranging from small-scale traditional operations to extensive industrial facilities, creates different risk profiles and requires tailored approaches to hazard identification and control that consider system-specific characteristics and constraints.

Primary food production represents the foundation of food systems. It includes agricultural crop production, livestock raising, aquaculture, and wild food harvesting activities that can introduce various contamination sources into food supplies. Agricultural production systems face contamination risks from multiple sources, including animal waste used as fertiliser, contaminated irrigation water, wildlife intrusion, and environmental contamination from industrial or urban sources that can introduce pathogenic microorganisms, chemical residues, or other hazards into food crops (Grace, 2015). Livestock production systems pose risks for microbial contamination through the faecal shedding of pathogenic organisms, cross-contamination between animals, and environmental factors that can promote pathogen survival and transmission within production facilities.

Intensive animal agriculture systems create challenges for food safety due to high animal density, shared air and water systems, and practices such as antimicrobial use that can influence pathogen ecology and resistance patterns. Pathogenic organisms such as Salmonella, Campylobacter, and enterohemorrhagic E. coli can colonise food animals without causing apparent illness, creating asymptomatic carriers that can contaminate carcasses during slaughter and processing. The concentration of large numbers of animals in confined spaces can facilitate rapid transmission of pathogens between animals while creating environmental conditions that may promote pathogen survival and amplification.

Aquaculture production systems face unique food safety challenges related to water quality, feed contamination, and environmental conditions that can promote the growth of pathogenic organisms or the accumulation of chemical contaminants. Fish and shellfish can bioaccumulate ecological pollutants, including heavy metals, pesticides, and industrial chemicals, while also serving as hosts for parasites and other pathogens that can cause illness in consumers. Shellfish present risks because they filter large volumes of water during feeding and can concentrate pathogens from contaminated water sources. They are often consumed raw or lightly cooked in ways that may not eliminate these pathogens.

Food processing operations transform raw agricultural products into finished food products through various manufacturing processes that can either reduce or increase food safety risks, depending on the specific processes involved and the effectiveness of control measures implemented. Heat treatment processes, such as pasteurisation, sterilisation, and cooking, can effectively eliminate vegetative pathogens when appropriately applied. Still, they may not destroy bacterial spores, some viruses, or chemical contaminants that require different control approaches. Minimal processing operations that preserve the fresh characteristics of foods may provide limited pathogen reduction while creating products with extended shelf life and distribution, which can amplify the impact of contamination events.

Processing environments can serve as sources of contamination when pathogenic organisms establish in facility infrastructure, equipment, or environmental niches where they can persist and contaminate products over extended periods. Listeria monocytogenes poses a particular concern in processing environments due to its ability to survive and multiply under refrigeration conditions, as well as establish persistent environmental contamination in processing facilities.

Table 12.1. Global burden of major foodborne diseases by pathogen and region

Pathogen Category	Annual Cases (Millions)	Annual Deaths (Thousands)	Primary Disease Syndromes	High-Burden Regions	Key Food Vehicles	Case Fatality Rate (%)
Nontyphoidal Salmonella	78.7	59.3	Gastroenteritis, bacteremia, typhoid-like illness	Sub-Saharan Africa, South Asia	Eggs, poultry, produce, dairy	0.075
Campylobacter spp.	95.6	21.8	Gastroenteritis, Guillain-Barré syndrome	Global distribution	Poultry, dairy, water	0.023
Enteropathogenic E. coli	79.2	94.4	Diarrhoea, haemolytic uremic syndrome	Sub-Saharan Africa, South Asia	Beef, produce, water	0.119
Norovirus	125.0	35.0	Acute gastroenteritis	Global distribution	Shellfish, produce, contaminated water	0.028
Shigella spp.	50.2	64.3	Dysentery, reactive arthritis	South Asia, Sub-Saharan Africa	Water, produce, person-to-person	0.128
Clostridium perfringens	43.2	2.4	Food poisoning, necrotising enterocolitis	Global distribution	Meat, poultry, and gravies	0.006
Hepatitis A virus	13.2	27.7	Acute hepatitis	Low-income regions	Shellfish, produce, water	0.210
Typhoid fever (S. Typhi)	12.5	149.0	Enteric fever	South Asia, Sub-Saharan Africa	Water, produce, dairy	1.192

Table 12.2. Contamination sources and risk factors across food production systems

Production Stage	Primary Contamination Sources	Key Risk Factors	Major Pathogens of Concern	Critical Control Points	Prevention Strategies
Primary Production - Crops	Irrigation water, soil amendments, wildlife, and worker hygiene	Water quality, manure application timing, and harvest practices	E. coli O157:H7, Salmonella, Cyclospora	Water treatment, composting, and field sanitation	Good Agricultural Practices, water testing, and worker training
Primary Production - Livestock	Faecal contamination, feed, water, and environmental persistence	Animal density, stress factors, and antimicrobial use	Salmonella, Campylobacter, STEC	Feed quality, water treatment, animal health	Biosecurity, vaccination, antimicrobial stewardship
Food Processing	Environmental harborage, cross-contamination, and ingredient contamination	Facility design, sanitation efficacy, temperature control	Listeria monocytogenes, Salmonella, Clostridium botulinum	Heat treatment, environmental monitoring, and sanitation	HACCP, ecological sampling, facility design
Food Distribution	Temperature abuse, cross-contamination, pest contamination	Cold chain maintenance, storage conditions, handling practices	Pathogen growth, toxin production	Temperature monitoring, storage separation	Cold chain management, pest control, hygiene training
Food Service/ Retail	Cross-contamination, temperature abuse, and poor hygiene	Food handler practices, equipment sanitation, time-temperature	Norovirus, Salmonella, Clostridium perfringens	Cooking temperatures, cooling procedures, and hand hygiene	Food handler training, monitoring systems, and equipment maintenance

Cross-contamination between raw and processed products poses a significant food safety risk in processing operations, necessitating the strict segregation of raw and finished product areas, along with comprehensive sanitation and hygiene programs. Table 12.2 shows contamination sources and risk factors across the food production system.

Food distribution and storage systems pose additional contamination risks through temperature abuse, cross-contamination, pest infestation, and handling practices that can introduce pathogens or exacerbate existing contamination during transport and storage. Cold chain maintenance is crucial for preventing the growth of pathogenic organisms in perishable foods. Still, temperature excursions during transport and storage are typical and can create conditions that facilitate the rapid multiplication of pathogens. Cross-contamination during distribution can occur through shared transport vehicles, storage facilities, and handling equipment that meet multiple food products without adequate cleaning and sanitisation.

The globalisation of food systems has created complex supply chains that span multiple countries and continents, presenting new challenges for ensuring food safety throughout extended distribution networks while enabling the rapid international spread of contamination events. Traceability systems are essential for allowing the rapid identification and removal of contaminated products from commerce. However, many food systems lack adequate traceability capabilities, particularly for fresh produce and other minimally processed products that often pass through multiple intermediaries before reaching consumers.

Emerging technologies in food production and processing create both opportunities for improving food safety through better hazard control and new risks that may not be fully understood or adequately controlled. Novel food processing technologies, such as high-pressure processing, pulsed electric fields, and irradiation, can provide pathogen reduction while preserving food quality characteristics; however, they require careful validation and control to ensure their effectiveness. Genetically modified foods and novel ingredients require safety assessment and regulatory oversight to ensure they do not introduce new food safety risks while potentially providing benefits such as enhanced nutritional content or reduced need for pesticide applications.

Climate change is creating new food safety challenges throughout food production systems through altered environmental conditions that affect pathogen ecology, extreme weather events that can compromise infrastructure and control systems, and changing agricultural practices that may introduce new contamination risks (Uyttendaele et al., 2016). Rising temperatures can impact the survival and growth of pathogens in food and food production environments, while changing precipitation patterns can affect water quality and availability for food production and processing operations. Extreme weather events, such as floods, can contaminate food production areas and compromise food safety infrastructure, while droughts can concentrate pathogens and contaminants in limited water sources.

12.3. Farm-to-Fork Approach to Food Safety

The farm-to-fork approach to food safety represents a comprehensive strategy that recognises food safety as a shared responsibility requiring coordinated action across all stages of the food system, from primary production through consumption, to prevent, eliminate, or reduce food safety hazards that could harm consumer health (Painter et al., 2013). This integrated approach acknowledges that food safety cannot be assured through interventions at any single point in the food chain, but requires systematic attention to hazard prevention and control throughout the entire food system. Each stage builds upon the efforts of previous stages, preparing foods for safe handling in subsequent phases. The farm-to-fork concept emphasises the importance of traceability, communication, and coordination between different actors in the food system to ensure that food safety measures are effective and that problems can be rapidly identified and addressed when they occur.

Primary production represents the foundation of farm-to-fork food safety systems. It involves implementing Good Agricultural Practices (GAPs) and Good Animal Husbandry Practices that minimise contamination risks during crop and livestock production while establishing the basis for safe food production throughout the remainder of the food chain. Effective primary production food safety programs address multiple risk factors, including water quality for irrigation and animal drinking, soil amendments and fertiliser application practices, pest and disease management approaches, worker health and hygiene, and facility and equipment sanitation. These programs must be tailored to specific production systems and local conditions while adhering to science-based principles that effectively reduce contamination risks.

Water management represents a critical component of primary production food safety, as contaminated water used for irrigation, pesticide application, or animal consumption can introduce pathogenic microorganisms into food production systems and subsequently contaminate food products. Water sources must be evaluated for microbial quality and chemical contamination, with treatment systems implemented as necessary to ensure the water meets the appropriate quality standards for its intended uses. The timing of irrigation applications relative to harvest is crucial for fresh produce, allowing for pathogen die-off and minimising direct contamination of edible portions of crops.

Soil amendment practices, including the use of manure, compost, and other organic materials to enhance soil fertility and structure, necessitate careful management to prevent the introduction of pathogenic microorganisms while providing agronomic benefits. Raw manure applications must follow appropriate timing and application method requirements to allow for pathogen reduction before harvest. At the same time, composting processes must achieve adequate temperatures and holding times to eliminate pathogens before the compost is used. Synthetic fertilisers and other agricultural inputs must be used according to label directions and regulatory requirements to prevent chemical residues that could pose food safety risks.

Processing and manufacturing operations build upon primary production food safety efforts by implementing Hazard Analysis and Critical Control Points (HACCP) systems and other science-based food safety management approaches that systematically identify hazards, establish critical control points, and monitor and verify the effectiveness of control measures (Heiman et al., 2015). HACCP principles provide a framework for food processors to analyse their operations, identify points where hazards can be prevented, eliminated, or reduced to acceptable levels, and establish monitoring and corrective action procedures that ensure consistent implementation of control measures. Prerequisite programs, including sanitation standard operating procedures, pest control, personnel hygiene, and facility maintenance, provide the foundation upon which HACCP systems operate effectively.

Thermal processing represents one of the most effective methods for eliminating vegetative pathogens in foods. It requires careful validation and monitoring to ensure that target organisms are consistently eliminated while maintaining food quality and nutritional characteristics.

Process validation studies must demonstrate that heating processes achieve sufficient time-temperature combinations to reduce target pathogens to safe levels. Ongoing monitoring ensures that processes continue to operate within the validated parameters. Alternative processing technologies, such as high-pressure processing, irradiation, and chemical sanitisers, can provide pathogen reduction for foods that cannot tolerate conventional thermal processing but require similar validation and monitoring approaches.

Distribution and storage systems must maintain the integrity of food safety measures implemented during production and processing while preventing contamination and pathogen growth during transport and storage. Temperature control is particularly critical for perishable foods that can support pathogen growth, requiring validated cold chain systems that maintain appropriate temperatures from processing through retail. Packaging systems must protect food from contamination while providing suitable barrier properties and durability for the intended distribution and storage conditions. Traceability systems enable rapid identification and removal of contaminated products from distribution channels when problems are identified, requiring documentation and record-keeping systems that track product movement throughout the supply chain.

Retail and food service operations represent critical control points where food undergoes final preparation before consumption, and where contamination or temperature abuse can compromise the safety of foods that were safely produced and distributed. Food handlers in retail and food service operations must be trained in safe food handling practices, including personal hygiene, temperature control, preventing cross-contamination, and cleaning and sanitising procedures. Food service operations must implement food safety management systems that address receiving, storage, preparation, cooking, holding, and service of foods while maintaining documentation and monitoring systems that verify compliance with food safety requirements.

Consumer education and behaviour change represent essential components of comprehensive farm-to-fork food safety systems, as many foodborne illnesses result from unsafe food handling practices in domestic kitchens and consumer settings. Consumers must understand basic food safety principles, including safe food purchasing, storage, preparation, and handling of leftovers, to prevent contamination and pathogen growth in their home environments. Educational programs must be tailored to the needs of different audiences and cultural contexts, while addressing common misconceptions and barriers that prevent the adoption of safe food handling practices.

Emergency response and outbreak management systems provide critical capabilities for the rapid detection, investigation, and control of foodborne disease outbreaks and food contamination events, necessitating coordination among food safety authorities, public health agencies, and food industry stakeholders. Rapid response capabilities enable the quick identification of contaminated products and their removal from the market, while epidemiological investigations identify the sources of outbreaks and inform preventive measures. Communication systems must provide timely and accurate information to consumers, industry, and other stakeholders while avoiding unnecessary panic or economic disruption.

Continuous improvement processes are essential for maintaining and enhancing farm-to-fork food safety systems as new hazards emerge, production systems evolve, and scientific understanding advances. Performance monitoring systems track key indicators of food safety system effectiveness while providing feedback for system improvements. Research and development efforts identify new hazards, develop improved control technologies, and evaluate the effectiveness of existing control measures under changing conditions.

12.4. Regulatory Frameworks and Standards

Regulatory frameworks for food safety provide the legal and institutional foundation for ensuring that food systems operate in ways that protect public Health while facilitating efficient food production, processing, and distribution that meet consumer needs and economic objectives (Hoffmann et al., 2017). Effective food safety regulatory systems establish science-based standards, implement risk assessment and management processes, provide oversight and enforcement mechanisms, and facilitate international trade through harmonised approaches that recognise equivalent levels of protection across different regulatory systems. The complexity of modern food systems requires sophisticated regulatory approaches that address diverse hazards, production methods, and distribution channels while remaining practical and achievable for regulated entities ranging from small-scale producers to large multinational corporations.

International food safety standards, primarily developed by the Codex Alimentarius Commission, provide globally harmonised guidance for food safety regulation while respecting national sovereignty and the right of countries to establish food safety measures appropriate for their specific circumstances and risk profiles. Codex standards address a wide range of food safety topics, including microbiological criteria, chemical residue limits, food additives, labelling requirements, and food hygiene practices. This provides a scientific foundation for national regulatory systems while facilitating international trade through reduced technical barriers. The development of Codex standards involves extensive scientific review, stakeholder consultation, and consensus-building processes that ensure standards reflect current scientific knowledge while being practical for implementation across diverse food systems and regulatory contexts.

National regulatory frameworks must translate international standards and guidance into enforceable domestic requirements that address local food safety priorities, production systems, and institutional capabilities while maintaining consistency with international trade obligations and bilateral agreements. Regulatory systems typically comprise multiple agencies with distinct responsibilities for various aspects of food safety, necessitating coordination mechanisms that ensure comprehensive coverage without gaps or overlaps that could compromise effectiveness. Food safety agencies must have adequate authority, resources, and technical capacity to fulfil their regulatory responsibilities while maintaining independence from commercial interests that could compromise their public health mission.

Risk assessment processes provide the scientific foundation for regulatory decision-making by systematically evaluating the likelihood and severity of adverse health effects from food safety hazards under specific exposure conditions (Gould et al., 2013). Quantitative microbial risk assessment methods enable regulators to estimate the public health impact of various food safety interventions and establish performance standards that achieve the desired levels of public health protection. Chemical risk assessment approaches evaluate the safety of food additives, pesticide residues, environmental contaminants, and other chemical substances that may be present in foods, establishing safe exposure levels and regulatory limits that protect consumer health while allowing beneficial uses of these substances.

Hazard Analysis and Critical Control Points (HACCP) requirements represent a cornerstone of modern food safety regulations, requiring food businesses to implement systematic approaches to hazard identification, risk assessment, and control measure implementation tailored to their specific operations and products. Regulatory HACCP requirements typically include mandatory elements such as hazard analysis, critical control point identification, critical limit establishment, monitoring procedures, corrective actions, verification activities, and record-keeping, while allowing flexibility in how these elements are implemented to accommodate different types of operations and products. HACCP regulations must be supported by inspection and audit programs that verify the effectiveness of implementation while providing technical assistance to help regulated entities achieve compliance.

Microbiological criteria and performance standards establish regulatory limits for pathogenic organisms and indicator organisms in foods, providing measurable targets for food safety control systems while enabling enforcement actions when standards are exceeded. Performance standards typically focus on pathogen reduction rather than absolute absence, recognising that complete elimination may not be feasible or necessary for all foods and that risk-based approaches can achieve public health protection while maintaining food system efficiency. Sampling and testing programs must be statistically valid and practical for implementation while providing reliable information about compliance with established criteria.

Food facility registration and inspection systems provide regulatory oversight of food production, processing, and distribution facilities through licensing requirements, periodic inspections, and compliance monitoring, which verify the implementation of food safety requirements. Inspection programs must be risk-based, focusing resources on higher-risk facilities and operations while maintaining coverage of all regulated entities at frequencies appropriate for their risk profiles. Inspector training and standardisation programs ensure consistent application of regulatory requirements while providing technical assistance to help regulated entities achieve compliance.

Product approval and notification systems regulate the introduction of new foods, food ingredients, and food technologies to ensure safety assessment before market introduction while avoiding unnecessary barriers to innovation and product development. Pre-market safety assessment requirements must be proportionate to the potential risks, while providing an adequate scientific review of safety data. Post-market surveillance systems monitor the safety of approved products and enable rapid response when safety concerns arise after market introduction.

Import control systems ensure that imported foods meet domestic food safety requirements while facilitating efficient international trade through risk-based approaches that focus resources on higher-risk products and suppliers. Import requirements may include facility registration, product certification, laboratory testing, and inspection programs that verify compliance with domestic standards and regulations. Mutual recognition agreements and equivalence determinations can reduce regulatory burden on international trade while maintaining food safety protection through recognition of equivalent foreign regulatory systems. Enforcement mechanisms provide regulatory agencies with tools to address non-compliance and ensure that food safety violations are corrected promptly to protect public

Health. Enforcement tools typically include warning letters, civil penalties, product recalls, facility suspensions, and criminal prosecutions for serious violations, with penalties graduated according to the severity of the violation and the history of non-compliance. Recall systems enable rapid removal of unsafe products from commerce while providing public notification of food safety risks and corrective actions being taken.

12.5. Outbreak Investigation and Source Tracking

Foodborne disease outbreak investigation and source tracking represent critical components of food safety systems that enable the rapid identification, characterisation, and control of foodborne disease clusters, while providing essential information for the prevention of similar outbreaks in the future (Kirk et al., 2015). Effective outbreak investigation requires close collaboration between epidemiologists, laboratory scientists, environmental health specialists, and regulatory authorities to detect outbreaks rapidly, identify contaminated foods and their sources, implement control measures, and communicate findings to stakeholders and the public. The complexity of modern food systems, with their global supply chains and widely distributed products, creates both challenges and opportunities for outbreak investigation. This requires sophisticated investigative methods and international cooperation to trace the sources of contamination and prevent continued exposure.

Outbreak detection typically begins with the recognition of illness clusters through surveillance systems that monitor reports of foodborne diseases from healthcare providers, laboratories, and other sources. These systems utilise statistical methods and outbreak detection algorithms to identify increases in disease incidence that may indicate common source exposures. Enhanced surveillance systems that integrate clinical, laboratory, and epidemiological data can improve the sensitivity and timeliness of outbreak detection while reducing false alarms that could trigger unnecessary investigations. Syndromic surveillance approaches monitor illness patterns based on symptoms rather than confirmed diagnoses, potentially enabling earlier detection of outbreaks before laboratory confirmation is available.

Laboratory methods for outbreak investigation have been revolutionised by molecular subtyping techniques, particularly whole-genome sequencing, that enable the precise characterisation of outbreak-associated pathogens and the identification of genetic relationships between isolates from patients, food, and environmental sources. Pulsed-field gel electrophoresis (PFGE) provided the foundation for molecular outbreak investigation for many years and continues to be used for rapid initial characterisation, while whole genome sequencing offers superior resolution and is becoming the standard method for outbreak investigation. Molecular characterisation enables investigators to distinguish outbreak-associated cases from sporadic cases, identify the geographic scope of outbreaks, and link human cases to contaminated foods and environmental sources.

Epidemiological investigation methods seek to identify common exposures among outbreak cases through interviews, questionnaires, and analytical studies that compare exposures between cases and controls or between cases with different exposure patterns. Hypothesis-generating interviews explore the full range of potential exposures experienced by cases. At the same time, analytical studies test specific hypotheses about outbreak sources using statistical methods that quantify associations between exposures and illness. Traceback investigations follow the distribution chain of implicated foods backwards from points of consumption to identify familiar sources and potential points of contamination. Table 12.3 illustrates the methods and applications of foodborne outbreak investigations.

Environmental investigation involves inspection of food production, processing, and distribution facilities implicated in outbreaks to identify contamination sources, evaluate control measures, and collect samples for laboratory analysis. Environmental sampling programs aim to isolate outbreak pathogens from foods, food contact surfaces, and facility environments, utilising molecular characterisation to link environmental isolates to human cases. Root cause analysis methods systematically examine facility operations, control systems, and management practices to identify factors that contributed to the occurrence of contamination and outbreaks.

Traceback investigations follow the movement of implicated foods through distribution channels to identify standard suppliers, processors, and production sources that could be responsible for contamination. Modern supply chains often involve multiple intermediaries and complex distribution networks, which can make traceback investigations challenging and time-consuming, particularly for fresh produce and other minimally processed foods that may pass through numerous handlers before reaching consumers. Traceability systems that maintain records of product movement and supplier relationships can facilitate more rapid and accurate traceback investigations in the event of outbreaks.

Source attribution methods utilise epidemiological, laboratory, and traceback evidence to identify the most likely source of outbreak-associated contamination, while also quantifying uncertainty in source identification. Microbial forensic approaches compare genetic characteristics of outbreak isolates with databases of isolates from potential source environments to identify likely contamination sources and transmission pathways. Statistical methods can integrate multiple types of evidence to provide probabilistic assessments of different source attribution hypotheses while accounting for uncertainty and data limitations.

International outbreak investigations require coordination between the public health and food safety agencies of multiple countries when contaminated products are distributed internationally or when illness cases occur in various countries. International networks, such as the Global Foodborne Infections Network, facilitate communication and collaboration between countries investigating multinational outbreaks, while providing technical assistance and standardised protocols. Bilateral and multilateral agreements establish frameworks for information sharing and coordinated response to international food safety emergencies.

Communication during outbreak investigations must strike a balance between the need for timely public health action and the importance of accuracy, while also avoiding unnecessary economic harm to food industries and producers. Risk communication strategies must provide clear and accurate information about the outbreak's scope, implicated foods, protective actions for consumers, and the progress of the investigation, while acknowledging uncertainty and avoiding speculation that could mislead the public or cause unnecessary alarm. Media relations and social media monitoring are crucial components of outbreak communication strategies in today's information environment.

Outbreak investigation findings contribute to prevention by identifying risk factors, control measure failures, and system vulnerabilities that can be addressed through regulatory action, industry guidance, or research initiatives (Pires et al., 2021).

Table 12.3. Foodborne outbreak investigation methods and applications

Investigation Component	Primary Methods	Key Applications	Strengths	Limitations	Technology Trends
Outbreak Detection	Surveillance systems, statistical algorithms	Early outbreak recognition	Automated detection, population coverage	Reporting delays, underascertainment	Real-time surveillance, machine learning
Case Finding	Healthcare provider networks, laboratory reporting	Case identification and recruitment	Active surveillance, laboratory confirmation	Resource-intensive, consent issues	Electronic health records, mobile apps
Laboratory Characterisation	Whole genome sequencing, serotyping	Pathogen subtyping and comparison	High resolution, source attribution	Technical complexity, cost	Portable sequencing, rapid diagnostics
Epidemiological Analysis	Cohort studies, case-control studies	Exposure assessment and hypothesis testing	Statistical rigour, multiple hypothesis testing	Recall bias, confounding	Web-based surveys, GIS mapping
Environmental Investigation	Food sampling, facility inspections	Contamination source identification	Direct evidence, root cause analysis	Sample degradation, access limitations	Environmental genomics, rapid testing
Traceback Investigation	Supply chain analysis, record review	Product source identification	Product-specific information	Complex supply chains, incomplete records	Blockchain, digital traceability

After-action reviews and lessons learned processes systematically evaluate outbreak investigation performance and identify opportunities for improvement in detection systems, investigation methods, and response procedures. Long-term follow-up studies can determine the effectiveness of prevention measures implemented in response to outbreak investigations, while also monitoring for the recurrence of similar problems.

12.6. Consumer Education and Behaviour Change

Consumer education and behaviour change are crucial components of comprehensive food safety systems, as many foodborne illnesses stem from unsafe food handling practices in domestic kitchens where regulatory oversight is limited and individuals must take responsibility for implementing safe food practices (Thomas et al., 2013). Effective consumer education programs must address knowledge gaps about food safety risks and safe handling practices, while considering the behavioural, social, and environmental factors that influence food safety practices in real-world settings.

Food safety knowledge varies widely across populations, with studies consistently identifying significant gaps in understanding basic principles, including safe cooking temperatures, proper refrigeration practices, cross-contamination prevention, and recognising food spoilage. Common misconceptions include the belief that foods are safe if they look and smell normal, the notion that freezing kills all pathogens, and the assumption that natural or organic foods are inherently safer.

Behaviour change theory provides frameworks for understanding the factors influencing consumer food safety practices and designing educational interventions that promote behaviour change beyond simple knowledge transfer. The Theory of Planned Behaviour suggests that attitudes, subjective norms, and perceived behavioural control influence behavioural intentions. Social Cognitive Theory emphasises the importance of observational learning and environmental factors.

Risk perception plays a crucial role in determining whether consumers adopt recommended practices. However, consumer risk perceptions often differ significantly from scientific risk assessments, which are influenced by media coverage, personal experiences, and cultural beliefs. Consumers frequently overestimate the risks associated with food additives and pesticide residues, while underestimating the risks of microbial contamination.

Demographic and socioeconomic factors influence both food safety knowledge and practices, with disparities reflecting differences in educational opportunities, resource availability, and cultural food practices. Cultural and ethnic factors significantly influence food handling practices through traditional cooking methods, food preferences, and beliefs that may differ from mainstream recommendations.

Educational intervention strategies encompass a wide range of approaches, including mass media campaigns, community-based education programs, school-based curricula, healthcare provider counselling, and digital platforms that reach different audiences through various communication channels. Digital technologies offer new opportunities through mobile applications, social media platforms, interactive websites, and other digital tools, providing personalised guidance and just-in-time information.

Evaluation of consumer education effectiveness requires measurement approaches that assess not only knowledge acquisition but also behaviour change, sustained practice adoption, and health outcomes when possible (Foodborne Disease Burden Epidemiology Reference Group, 2015). Process evaluation measures program reach, implementation fidelity, and participant satisfaction, while outcome evaluation assesses changes in knowledge, attitudes, behavioural intentions, and reported practices.

Conclusion

Food safety represents a fundamental public health challenge that requires comprehensive, coordinated approaches across the entire food system to prevent a substantial foodborne disease burden affecting hundreds of millions globally each year, while imposing significant economic costs. The complexity of the modern food system, characterised by global supply chains, diverse production methods, and rapidly evolving technologies, creates unprecedented challenges and opportunities for implementing innovative hazard prevention and control approaches. Understanding food safety as a One Health issue, which connects human health, animal health, and environmental health, is essential for developing effective strategies.

The global burden of foodborne diseases, with an estimated 600 million annual cases and 420,000 deaths, represents substantial public health challenges disproportionately affecting vulnerable populations in low- and middle-income countries. The farm-to-fork approach provides a framework for systematic hazard prevention and control throughout the food chain, recognising that food safety requires coordinated action from primary production through consumption.

Regulatory frameworks and standards provide legal and institutional foundations for food safety systems, establishing science-based requirements, oversight mechanisms, and enforcement tools. International harmonisation facilitates trade while maintaining public health protection; however, implementation remains challenging due to resource constraints and institutional limitations (Lake et al., 2012).

Outbreak investigation and source tracking capabilities are essential for rapid detection and control. Consumer education and behaviour change are crucial components in addressing knowledge gaps and the behavioural factors that influence food handling practices. The intersection of food safety with broader development objectives—such as food security, nutrition, and sustainable development—requires integrated approaches. Achieving Sustainable Development Goals 2, 3, and 12 depends on safe and nutritious food systems.

Future challenges include emerging pathogens, evolving food production technologies, climate change impacts, and shifting consumer expectations that require adaptive approaches. Success requires sustained commitment from all stakeholders, with adequate resources, technical capacity, and political will, to implement comprehensive food safety systems that protect public health while supporting sustainable food systems and economic development.

Acknowledgments

The authors would like to extend our appreciation to those who offered helpful commentary during the drafting process of this manuscript. We also acknowledge the role Nova Science Publishers played in enabling the work described herein.

References

Foodborne Disease Burden Epidemiology Reference Group. (2015). WHO methodology for estimation of the global burden of foodborne diseases. *Food Control*, 57, 328-338. https://doi.org/10.1016/j.foodcont.2015.03.042.

Gould, L. H., Walsh, K. A., Vieira, A. R., Herman, K., Williams, I. T., Hall, A. J., & Cole, D. (2013). Surveillance for foodborne disease outbreaks—United States, 1998-2008. *MMWR Surveillance Summaries*, 62(2), 1-34.

Grace, D. (2015). Food safety in low and middle income countries. *International Journal of Environmental Research and Public Health*, 12(9), 10490-10507. https://doi.org/10.3390/ijerph120910490.

Havelaar, A. H., Kirk, M. D., Torgerson, P. R., Gibb, H. J., Hald, T., Lake, R. J., ... & Speybroeck, N. (2015). World Health Organisation global estimates and regional comparisons of the burden of foodborne disease in 2010. *PLoS Medicine*, 12(12), e1001923. https://doi.org/10.1371/journal.pmed.1001923.

Heiman, K. E., Mody, R. K., Johnson, S. D., Griffin, P. M., & Gould, L. H. (2015). Escherichia coli O157 outbreaks in the United States, 2003-2012. *Emerging Infectious Diseases*, 21(8), 1293-1301. https://doi.org/10.3201/eid2108.141364.

Hoffmann, S., Devleesschauwer, B., Aspinall, W., Cooke, R., Corrigan, T., Havelaar, A., ... & Morris, J. G. (2017). Attribution of global foodborne disease to specific foods: Findings from a World Health Organization structured expert elicitation. *PLoS One*, 12(9), e0183641. https://doi.org/10.1371/journal.pone.0183641.

Kirk, M. D., Pires, S. M., Black, R. E., Caipo, M., Crump, J. A., Devleesschauwer, B., ... & Angulo, F. J. (2015). World Health Organization estimates of the global and regional disease burden of 22 foodborne bacterial, protozoal, and viral diseases, 2010: a data synthesis. *PLoS Medicine*, 12(12), e1001921. https://doi.org/10.1371/journal.pmed.1001921.

Lake, R. J., Cressey, P. J., Campbell, D. M., & Oakley, E. (2012). Risk ranking for foodborne microbial hazards in New Zealand: burden of disease estimates. *Risk Analysis*, 32(5), 743-752. https://doi.org/10.1111/j.1539-6924.2011.01690.x.

Newell, D. G., Koopmans, M., Verhoef, L., Duizer, E., Aidara-Kane, A., Sprong, H., ... & Kruse, H. (2010). Foodborne diseases—the challenges of 20 years ago still persist while new ones continue to emerge. *International Journal of Food Microbiology*, 139, S3-S15. https://doi.org/10.1016/j.ijfoodmicro.2010.01.021.

Painter, J. A., Hoekstra, R. M., Ayers, T., Tauxe, R. V., Braden, C. R., Angulo, F. J., & Griffin, P. M. (2013). Attribution of foodborne illnesses, hospitalisations, and deaths to food commodities by using outbreak data, United States, 1998-2008. *Emerging Infectious Diseases*, 19(3), 407-415. https://doi.org/10.3201/eid1903.111866.

Pires, S. M., Fischer-Walker, C. L., Lanata, C. F., Devleesschauwer, B., Hall, A. J., Kirk, M. D., ... & Black, R. E. (2021). Aetiology-specific estimates of the global and regional incidence and mortality of diarrhoeal diseases commonly transmitted through food. *PLoS One*, 10(12), e0142927. https://doi.org/10.1371/journal.pone.0142927.

Scallan, E., Hoekstra, R. M., Angulo, F. J., Tauxe, R. V., Widdowson, M. A., Roy, S. L., ... & Griffin, P. M. (2011). Foodborne illness acquired in the United States—major pathogens. *Emerging Infectious Diseases*, 17(1), 7-15. https://doi.org/10.3201/eid1701.P11101.

Thomas, M. K., Murray, R., Flockhart, L., Pintar, K., Pollari, F., Fazil, A., ... & Marshall, B. (2013). Estimates of the burden of foodborne illness in Canada for 30 specified pathogens and unspecified agents, circa 2006. *Foodborne Pathogens and Disease*, 10(7), 639-648. https://doi.org/10.1089/fpd.2012.1389.

Uyttendaele, M., Jaykus, L. A., Amoah, P., Chiodini, A., Cunliffe, D., Jacxsens, L., ... & Rao Jasti, P. (2016). Microbial hazards in irrigation water: Standards, norms, and testing to manage use of water in fresh produce primary production. *Comprehensive Reviews in Food Science and Food Safety*, 15(6), 1003-1028. https://doi.org/10.1111/1541-4337.12219.

World Health Organization. (2015). *WHO estimates of the global burden of foodborne diseases: Foodborne disease burden epidemiology reference group 2007-2015*. World Health Organization. https://www.who.int/publications/i/item/9789241565165.

Chapter 13

Zoonotic Diseases in a Changing World

Abhay Saraf[1], MD
and Maajid Mohi Ud Din Malik[2,*], PhD
[1]Dr. D. Y. Patil School of Allied Health Sciences, Dr. D. Y. Patil Vidyapeeth· Pune (Deemed to be University), Sant Tukaram Nagar, Pimpri, Pune, India
[2]Department of Radiology and Imaging Technology, Dr. D. Y. Patil School of Allied Health Sciences, Dr. D. Y. Patil Vidyapeeth· Pune (Deemed to be University), Sant Tukaram Nagar, Pimpri, Pune, India

Abstract

Zoonotic diseases, defined as infections naturally transmitted between vertebrate animals and humans, represent approximately 75% of emerging infectious diseases and pose increasingly complex challenges in our rapidly changing global environment. Major zoonotic diseases, including rabies, brucellosis, leptospirosis, avian influenza, and coronaviruses, cause millions of human infections annually while imposing substantial economic burdens on healthcare systems, agricultural sectors, and broader economies worldwide. The expansion of the global wildlife trade, estimated to be worth billions of dollars annually, creates unprecedented opportunities for pathogen spillover through increased human-wildlife contact and the international movement of potentially infected animals and animal products. Domestic animals and livestock serve as critical interfaces between wildlife pathogen reservoirs and human populations, with intensive agricultural practices and changing husbandry methods influencing transmission dynamics and emergence risks. Rapid urbanisation has created novel ecological interfaces where urban wildlife species interact closely with dense human populations, facilitating new transmission pathways and creating unique challenges for disease surveillance and control. Climate change is fundamentally altering the geographic distribution, seasonal patterns, and transmission dynamics of zoonotic diseases through effects on vector ecology, host distribution, pathogen survival, and human behaviour patterns. These changing patterns require adaptive surveillance systems and flexible control strategies that can respond to evolving threats. Effective control of zoonotic diseases demands integrated One Health approaches that coordinate human Health, veterinary medicine, wildlife management, and environmental health sectors while addressing the social, economic, and ecological drivers that create conditions for disease emergence and spread. Success in preventing and controlling zoonotic diseases is essential for achieving Sustainable Development Goal 3, which aims to ensure healthy lives and promote well-being for all, while also contributing

* Corresponding Author's Email: maajid.malik@dpu.edu.in

In: Advances in the One Health Approach
Editors: Maajid Mohi Ud Din Malik, Abhay Saraf, Harshal Tukaram Pandve et al.
ISBN: 979-8-90134-202-2

to goals related to sustainable cities, climate action, and life on land that address the broader determinants of zoonotic disease risk.

Keywords: zoonotic diseases, One Health, wildlife trade, disease emergence, spillover, climate change, urban wildlife, livestock, disease surveillance, Sustainable Development Goal 3, pandemic prevention

Introduction

Zoonotic diseases represent a defining challenge of the modern era, accounting for approximately 60% of all human infectious diseases and 75% of emerging infectious diseases, while demonstrating the fundamental interconnectedness of human Health, animal health, and environmental Health that forms the core of One Health approaches to global health security (Jones et al., 2008). The term zoonosis encompasses a vast array of infections that are naturally transmitted between vertebrate animals and humans, ranging from ancient scourges such as rabies and plague, which have shaped human history, to newly emerged threats like SARS, MERS, and COVID-19, which have transformed our understanding of pandemic risk and global vulnerability. The increasing frequency and impact of zoonotic disease emergence reflect the intensification of human interactions with animal populations through activities such as agricultural expansion, wildlife exploitation, urbanisation, and global trade, which create novel pathways for pathogen transmission while amplifying the consequences when spillover events occur. Understanding zoonotic diseases requires recognising that pathogen spillover from animal reservoirs to human populations is not a random process, but is driven by specific ecological, social, and economic factors that can be identified, monitored, and potentially modified to reduce the emergence risk. The complexity of zoonotic disease systems involves multiple host species, diverse transmission pathways, environmental factors that influence pathogen survival and transmission, and human behaviours that determine exposure risk and disease outcomes when infections occur. Climate change is adding new dimensions to zoonotic disease challenges by altering the geographic distribution and abundance of vector and reservoir species, changing environmental conditions that affect pathogen survival and transmission, and influencing human activities and settlement patterns in ways that may increase contact with infected animals. The prevention and control of zoonotic diseases exemplifies the need for integrated approaches that address not only immediate disease threats but also the underlying drivers of emergence and the broader systems that determine human vulnerability to infectious disease risks, making zoonotic disease prevention a critical component of achieving Sustainable Development Goal 3 and other development objectives that depend on healthy and resilient communities.

13.1. Major Zoonotic Diseases and Their Impacts

The landscape of major zoonotic diseases encompasses a diverse array of pathogens that cause significant morbidity and mortality in human populations while imposing substantial economic burdens on healthcare systems, agricultural sectors, and broader economies worldwide. These diseases represent some of the most significant infectious disease threats facing humanity, with several zoonoses ranking among the leading causes of infectious disease mortality globally. In contrast, others pose substantial risks for pandemic emergence that could affect billions of people (Taylor et al., 2001). Understanding the epidemiology, impact, and control challenges associated with major zoonotic diseases is essential for developing effective prevention and response strategies that can reduce disease burden while building resilience against future emergence events.

Rabies represents one of the oldest known zoonotic diseases. It continues to cause an estimated 59,000 human deaths annually, primarily in Asia and Africa, where dog-mediated transmission accounts for over 95% of human cases. Despite being entirely preventable through vaccination, rabies continues to have a devastating impact due to limited access to post-exposure prophylaxis in resource-limited settings, inadequate dog vaccination coverage, and the persistence of wildlife reservoirs that can reintroduce the virus into domestic animal populations. The economic burden of rabies extends beyond direct healthcare costs to encompass substantial investments in prevention programs, livestock losses, and broader impacts on communities, where fear of rabies influences human-animal interactions and economic activities.

Brucellosis affects more than 500,000 people annually worldwide. It represents one of the most common occupational diseases globally, particularly affecting people who work directly with livestock or consume unpasteurised dairy products from infected animals. The chronic, debilitating nature of brucellosis creates substantial individual and societal costs through prolonged illness, reduced productivity, and long-term health complications that may persist even after successful treatment. The agricultural impacts of brucellosis include reproductive losses in affected livestock herds, decreased milk production, and trade restrictions that can significantly impact entire regional economies.

Leptospirosis causes an estimated 1.03 million cases and 58,900 deaths annually worldwide, with the highest burden occurring in tropical regions where environmental conditions favour pathogen survival and transmission. Urban leptospirosis outbreaks associated with flooding and poor sanitation demonstrate how ecological factors and infrastructure limitations can create conditions that facilitate zoonotic disease transmission while disproportionately affecting vulnerable populations. The broad range of mammalian reservoir hosts and diverse transmission pathways make leptospirosis particularly challenging to control through single interventions.

Avian influenza viruses pose ongoing concerns for both the endemic disease burden and the potential for pandemic emergence. Highly pathogenic strains cause substantial economic losses in poultry industries, while low-pathogenic strains maintain transmission in wild bird populations, which serve as genetic mixing vessels for viral evolution. Human infections with novel influenza viruses, including H5N1 and H7N9, as well as other strains, underscore the ongoing risk of influenza pandemics that could rival or surpass the impact of the 1918 pandemic. The global nature of poultry production and wild bird migration creates conditions that allow locally emerging influenza variants to spread rapidly across continents.

Coronaviruses have emerged as major zoonotic threats in the 21st century, with SARS-CoV, MERS-CoV, and SARS-CoV-2 causing three distinct disease emergence events that have resulted in thousands of deaths and trillions of dollars in economic losses. The COVID-19 pandemic highlights the catastrophic potential of zoonotic disease emergence in highly connected modern societies, while also underscoring critical gaps in pandemic preparedness and response capabilities. The diversity of coronavirus species in wildlife reservoirs, particularly bats, suggests continued risk for future coronavirus emergence events.

Vector-borne zoonoses, including Lyme disease, Rocky Mountain spotted fever, and various viral encephalitides, cause substantial disease burdens in many regions, demonstrating how environmental changes can alter disease transmission patterns and expand the geographic ranges of vector-borne diseases. The complex ecological relationships involved in vector-borne zoonoses make these diseases particularly sensitive to environmental changes, creating challenges for predicting and controlling the emergence and spread of disease. Table 13.1 shows major zoonotic diseases.

Foodborne zoonoses represent a significant category of diseases that affect hundreds of millions of people annually through contaminated animal products, including nontyphoidal salmonellosis, campylobacteriosis, and various parasitic infections that are transmitted through inadequately processed meat, dairy, or other animal products. The globalisation of food systems has created opportunities for the rapid international spread of foodborne zoonoses. In contrast, intensive animal production systems may develop conditions that amplify pathogen loads and facilitate the emergence of antimicrobial-resistant strains.

Neglected tropical diseases with zoonotic components, including echinococcosis, cysticercosis, and various leishmaniasis forms, disproportionately affect the world's poorest populations while receiving limited attention and resources for control efforts. These diseases often involve complex life cycles with multiple host species and environmental stages, making control interventions challenging. Their impacts on affected communities may be underestimated due to limited surveillance and diagnostic capacity in endemic areas.

Emerging zoonotic diseases continue to appear with increasing frequency, driven by factors including ecological disruption, climate change, increased human-animal contact, and global connectivity that facilitates rapid spread once emergence occurs (Morse et al., 2012). Recent examples include the Nipah virus, Hendra virus, and the expansion of Rift Valley fever, as well as various tick-borne diseases, which demonstrate the ongoing risk of novel zoonotic disease emergence and the importance of maintaining robust surveillance and response capabilities for unknown threats.

The economic impacts of zoonotic diseases extend far beyond direct healthcare costs to include agricultural losses, trade disruptions, and broader economic consequences that can affect entire regions and financial sectors. Livestock diseases such as foot-and-mouth disease and highly pathogenic avian influenza can result in massive animal culling operations and trade restrictions that impose costs measured in billions of dollars. Human disease impacts include healthcare costs, productivity losses, and reductions in quality of life that may persist long after the resolution of acute illness.

13.2. Wildlife Trade and Disease Risks

The global wildlife trade represents a multibillion-dollar industry that encompasses legal and illegal commerce in live animals, animal parts, and animal products, creating unprecedented opportunities for zoonotic pathogen spillover through increased human contact with diverse wildlife species and international movement of potentially infected animals across geographic boundaries (Karesh et al., 2012). This vast commercial network involves millions of individual animals representing thousands of species that are captured, bred, transported, and sold for various purposes, including food consumption, traditional medicine, pets, entertainment, and research, with each stage of the trade chain creating potential exposure opportunities for workers, consumers, and communities involved in wildlife commerce.

The legal wildlife trade operates under various international and national regulatory frameworks, including the Convention on International Trade in Endangered Species (CITES), which aim to ensure sustainability and prevent overexploitation, while often providing limited oversight of disease risks associated with traded species. Live animal markets, breeding facilities, processing operations, and retail establishments involved in legal wildlife trade create interfaces where humans, domestic animals, and diverse wildlife species may interact in ways that facilitate pathogen transmission between species that might never encounter each other in natural settings. The concentration of multiple species in confined spaces, often under stressful conditions that may compromise immune function, creates ideal conditions for pathogen amplification and cross-species transmission.

Illegal wildlife trafficking represents one of the world's most lucrative illicit activities, with estimated annual values reaching billions of dollars and involving sophisticated international networks that operate outside regulatory oversight and disease surveillance systems. The clandestine nature of the illegal wildlife trade means that diseased animals may be transported across borders without health inspections or quarantine procedures that could detect and prevent the introduction of exotic pathogens into new regions. Law enforcement efforts focused on species conservation and trafficking prevention may not adequately address the disease risks associated with the illegal wildlife trade, creating gaps in disease prevention that could facilitate the introduction and establishment of novel zoonotic diseases.

Traditional medicine practices in various cultures often involve the use of wildlife-derived products, which may pose zoonotic disease risks through direct contact during preparation and consumption, or through contamination of processing equipment and environments. Pangolin scales, rhinoceros horn, bear bile, and numerous other wildlife products used in traditional medicine systems may harbour pathogens that can survive processing and storage conditions, creating exposure opportunities for practitioners, consumers, and communities involved in conventional medicine trade networks. The high economic value of some traditional medicine products creates incentives for continued wildlife harvesting despite potential disease risks.

Bushmeat consumption represents a critical pathway for zoonotic disease transmission in many regions, involving hunting, processing, and consumption of wild animals for protein and income generation, which creates multiple opportunities for human exposure to wildlife pathogens. Hunting activities bring humans into direct contact with wildlife in forests and other natural environments, where exposure to infected animals or contaminated environments can occur through wounds, respiratory exposure, or contact with infected animal tissues and fluids. Processing activities, including butchering, cooking, and preservation of bushmeat, create additional exposure opportunities while potentially spreading contamination to household and community environments.

The exotic pet trade involves the international movement of diverse wildlife species into domestic settings, where they may transmit pathogens to humans through direct contact, environmental contamination, or interaction with domestic animals that serve as bridge hosts for human transmission (Can et al., 2019). Reptiles, amphibians, birds, mammals, and other exotic pets may harbour pathogens that pose minimal risks to their natural hosts but can cause serious illness in humans with different immune systems and no evolutionary exposure to these pathogens. Import regulations and health screening procedures for exotic pets vary widely between countries. They may not adequately address disease risks, particularly for pathogens with long incubation periods or subclinical infection patterns.

Wildlife tourism and recreational hunting create temporary but potentially significant exposure opportunities when people travel to regions with endemic wildlife diseases or participate in activities that involve direct contact with potentially infected animals. Hunting expeditions, wildlife photography, ecotourism activities, and research programs may expose participants to vector-borne diseases, respiratory pathogens, or contact-transmitted infections that they subsequently carry to their home regions, where these pathogens may not be endemic and where healthcare providers may not recognise symptoms or know appropriate treatment protocols.

Captive wildlife facilities, including zoos, wildlife sanctuaries, research facilities, and private collections, create concentrated populations of diverse wildlife species that may facilitate pathogen transmission between species, while also creating occupational exposure risks for workers and potentially exposing visitors to novel pathogens, despite generally higher standards of veterinary care and disease monitoring compared to commercial wildlife trade, captive wildlife facilities have been implicated in several zoonotic disease outbreaks and remain essential considerations for zoonotic disease surveillance and prevention programs. Table 13.2 illustrates the wildlife trade pathways and their associated risks of zoonotic diseases.

International regulatory frameworks for wildlife trade disease prevention remain fragmented and often inadequately implemented, with limited coordination between agencies responsible for species conservation, animal health, and public Health that creates gaps in oversight and prevention efforts. CITES focuses primarily on species conservation rather than disease prevention, while animal health regulations may not adequately address the diversity of pathogens that may be present in traded wildlife species. Public health authorities may not be involved in overseeing wildlife trade, despite the significant disease risks that these activities pose to human populations.

Surveillance and monitoring systems for wildlife trade-associated diseases are generally inadequate, particularly for illegal trade networks that operate outside regulatory oversight and for regions were resource constraints and institutional limitations limit surveillance capacity. Early detection of novel zoonoses associated with wildlife trade requires surveillance systems that monitor both human and animal Health along trade routes while maintaining laboratory capacity for pathogen identification and characterisation. International cooperation and information sharing are crucial for effective surveillance systems across global networks involved in wildlife trade.

Prevention and control interventions for wildlife trade-associated disease risks require integrated approaches that address trade practices, regulatory oversight, surveillance capabilities, and emergency response systems while respecting cultural practices and economic needs of communities involved in wildlife commerce. Education and behaviour change interventions must be tailored to different audiences, including traders, consumers, regulators, and healthcare providers, while providing practical alternatives that address the underlying economic and cultural drivers of risky wildlife trade practices (Johnson et al., 2020).

Table 13.1. Major zoonotic diseases - Epidemiology, impact, and control challenges

Disease	Pathogen	Primary Reservoirs	Annual Human Cases	Annual Deaths	Primary Transmission Routes	Geographic Distribution	Major Control Challenges
Rabies	Rabies virus	Dogs, bats, wild carnivores	~60,000 exposures	~59,000	Bites, scratches, mucous membrane contact	Worldwide, mainly Asia/Africa	Access to post-exposure prophylaxis, dog vaccination coverage
Brucellosis	Brucella species	Cattle, goats, sheep, swine	>500,000	~2,000	Direct contact, unpasteurised dairy	Worldwide, the highest in the Mediterranean/Asia	Occupational exposure, food safety, and animal vaccination
Leptospirosis	Leptospira species	Rodents, livestock, wildlife	~1,000,000	~58,900	Water/soil contact, direct contact	Tropical/subtropical regions	Environmental contamination, multiple reservoirs
Salmonellosis	Nontyphoidal Salmonella	Poultry, cattle, reptiles, and amphibians	~78,000,000	~59,000	Foodborne, direct contact	Worldwide	Food safety, antimicrobial resistance
Q fever	Coxiella burnetii	Goats, sheep, cattle	~40,000	~200	Inhalation, unpasteurised dairy	Worldwide	Environmental persistence, aerosol transmission
Lyme disease	Borrelia burgdorferi	Deer, rodents	~300,000	<100	Tick vectors	North America, Europe, Asia	Vector control, diagnostic challenges
Avian influenza	Influenza A viruses	Wild birds, poultry	Variable	Variable	Respiratory, direct contact	Worldwide	Viral evolution, pandemic potential
MERS	MERS-CoV	Dromedary camels	~2,600	~900	Respiratory, direct contact	Middle East, sporadic global	Limited human-to-human transmission, no vaccine

Table 13.2. Wildlife trade pathways and associated zoonotic disease risks

Trade Category	Species Examples	Primary Activities	Exposure Pathways	Major Pathogen Groups	High-Risk Regions	Risk Mitigation Strategies
Live Animal Markets	Civets, bats, pangolins, birds	Sale, slaughter, consumption	Direct contact, aerosols, contaminated surfaces	Coronaviruses, influenza viruses, paramyxoviruses	Asia, Africa	Market regulation, species restrictions, hygiene protocols
Bushmeat Trade	Primates, ungulates, rodents, bats	Hunting, processing, and consumption	Blood contact, respiratory exposure, ingestion	Filoviruses, simian viruses, and bacterial pathogens	Central/West Africa, Amazon	Hunter education, processing safety, and cooking guidelines
Exotic Pet Trade	Reptiles, birds, and small mammals	Import, breeding, and household keeping	Direct handling, environmental contamination	Salmonella, Chlamydia, and viral pathogens	Global, urban centres	Import screening, owner education, and veterinary oversight
Traditional Medicine	Pangolins, rhinos, bears, various species	Processing, preparation, consumption	Contact during preparation, ingestion	Various bacterial, viral, and parasitic	Asia, some African regions	Product testing, practitioner training, and alternative promotion
Wildlife Tourism	Various species in natural habitats	Viewing, photography, interaction	Vector exposure, respiratory contact	Vector-borne, respiratory pathogens	Tropical/subtropical regions	Traveller education, prophylaxis, protective measures

13.3. Domestic Animal and Livestock Considerations

Domestic animals and livestock represent critical interfaces between wildlife pathogen reservoirs and human populations, serving as amplifying hosts, bridge species, and direct sources of zoonotic pathogen transmission while also providing essential economic, nutritional, and social benefits that make their management a complex challenge requiring careful balance of production objectives with disease prevention goals (Cleaveland et al., 2001). The intensification of livestock production systems, driven by growing global demand for animal products and economic pressures to maximise efficiency, has created new configurations of human-animal-pathogen interactions that may increase risks for zoonotic disease emergence and transmission while also providing opportunities for improved surveillance, prevention, and control interventions through coordinated management of defined animal populations.

Industrial livestock production systems concentrate large numbers of genetically similar animals in confined spaces with high population density, frequent animal movement, and shared air and water systems that can facilitate rapid pathogen transmission within and between facilities while creating conditions that may select for increased pathogen virulence or antimicrobial resistance. These systems often involve complex supply chains with multiple premises, including breeding facilities, growing operations, processing plants, and distribution networks, that create numerous opportunities for pathogen introduction, amplification, and dissemination throughout regional and international markets. The economic scale and integration of modern livestock industries mean that disease emergence events can have rapid and far-reaching consequences, affecting global food security and trade relationships.

Swine production systems pose concerns for zoonotic disease emergence due to the genetic and physiological similarities between pigs and humans that facilitate the adaptation of porcine pathogens for human transmission. Additionally, pigs are susceptible to both human and avian influenza viruses, which enables genetic reassortment and the emergence of pandemic influenza strains. Intensive swine production practices, including high animal density, frequent animal movement, and the use of antimicrobials for growth promotion and disease prevention, create selective pressures that may promote the evolution of pathogens with enhanced transmissibility or virulence. Meanwhile, the use of antibiotics contributes to the development of antimicrobial resistance, complicating the treatment of both animal and human infections.

Poultry production systems face ongoing challenges from avian influenza viruses that can cause devastating outbreaks in poultry populations while posing risks for human infection and pandemic emergence through viral evolution and adaptation. The diversity of influenza virus strains circulating in wild bird populations provides a constant source of novel genetic material that can be introduced into domestic poultry populations through direct contact or environmental contamination. At the same time, intensive production systems may amplify and modify these viruses in ways that enhance their pandemic potential. Highly pathogenic avian influenza outbreaks necessitate massive culling operations, which impose substantial economic costs. In contrast, low-pathogenic strains may circulate undetected in poultry populations and evolve to exhibit increased virulence or adapt to humans.

Dairy cattle operations present zoonotic disease risks through direct contact exposure during milking and animal handling activities, the consumption of unpasteurised dairy products, and environmental contamination that can affect both farm workers and surrounding communities. Brucellosis, tuberculosis, and various other bacterial pathogens can be transmitted from infected dairy cattle to humans through multiple pathways, resulting in significant production losses and necessitating expensive control programs that may involve testing, culling, and movement restrictions. Consuming raw milk, whether for cultural reasons or perceived health benefits, poses particularly high risks for the transmission of enteric pathogens and other zoonotic diseases from dairy animals to consumers.

Small ruminant production systems, including sheep and goat operations, face challenges from zoonotic diseases such as Q fever, brucellosis, and various parasitic infections that can affect both animal health and human Health, while also impacting production efficiency and market access. Sheep and goats may serve as reservoir hosts for pathogens that cause minimal disease in these species but can cause serious illness in humans, creating situations where infected animals may not show obvious signs of disease while remaining capable of transmitting pathogens to humans through direct contact, aerosol transmission, or contaminated environments.

Companion animals, including dogs, cats, and various exotic pets, maintained in household settings, create opportunities for intimate contact between humans and animals that can facilitate the transmission of zoonotic pathogens through direct contact, environmental contamination, and vector-mediated transmission pathways (Robertson et al., 2000). Pet ownership practices, including allowing animals in bedrooms, sharing food and water dishes, and limited veterinary care, may increase exposure risks while providing emotional and social benefits that make risk reduction interventions challenging to implement. Urban and suburban companion animal populations may serve as bridge hosts between wildlife reservoirs and human populations, while also creating pathways for the introduction of exotic pathogens through the international pet trade and travel.

Working animals, including horses, oxen, and various species used for transportation, agriculture, and other purposes, create occupational exposure risks for people who work directly with these animals. They may also serve as sentinels for vector-borne and other environmental zoonoses that can affect both animal and human populations. Equine encephalitis viruses, glanders, and various parasitic infections represent examples of zoonoses associated with working animals that require specialised surveillance and prevention approaches tailored to specific working relationships and exposure patterns. Table 13.3 shows livestock systems and associated zoonotic disease risks.

Antimicrobial use in livestock production poses a significant concern for zoonotic disease prevention, as antibiotic use contributes to the selection of antimicrobial-resistant pathogens that can be transmitted to humans through direct contact, food consumption, and environmental pathways. Subtherapeutic antibiotic use for growth promotion and disease prevention creates selective pressure that favours the development of resistant organisms, while potentially altering gut microbiome composition in ways that may affect susceptibility to pathogens and transmission dynamics. The volume of antimicrobial use in livestock production exceeds human medical use in many countries, creating substantial selective pressure for resistance development that affects both animal and human Health.

Genetic modification and selective breeding practices in livestock production have created animal populations with characteristics that may influence zoonotic disease susceptibility, pathogen carriage, and transmission potential, while providing production benefits such as improved feed conversion, increased growth rates, and enhanced disease resistance.

Table 13.3. Livestock systems and associated zoonotic disease risks

Livestock System	Primary Species	Production Characteristics	Major Zoonotic Pathogens	Transmission Routes	Key Risk Factors	Control Approaches
Industrial Swine	Domestic pigs	High-density, confined systems	Influenza viruses, Streptococcus suis, hepatitis E	Respiratory, direct contact, foodborne	Genetic uniformity, stress, and antimicrobial use	Biosecurity, vaccination, surveillance
Poultry Operations	Chickens, turkeys, ducks	Intensive confinement, rapid turnover	Avian influenza, Salmonella, Campylobacter	Respiratory, direct contact, foodborne	High density, wild bird contact, trade	Compartmentalisation, culling protocols, and processing safety
Dairy Operations	Cattle, goats	Intensive milking, close contact	Brucellosis, tuberculosis, Q fever	Direct contact, unpasteurised products, aerosols	Worker exposure, raw milk consumption	Testing, pasteurisation, worker protection
Beef Cattle	Cattle	Extensive grazing, feedlots	E. coli O157:H7, anthrax, brucellosis	Foodborne, direct contact, environmental	Processing contamination, environmental persistence	Slaughter hygiene, vaccination, surveillance
Small Ruminants	Sheep, goats	Mixed extensive/intensive	Q fever, brucellosis, Rift Valley fever	Aerosols, direct contact, vector-borne	Birthing season exposures, environmental contamination	Reproductive management, vaccination, vector control
Backyard Poultry	Chickens, ducks	Small-scale, mixed species	Salmonella, avian influenza, Newcastle disease	Direct contact, environmental contamination	Limited biosecurity, mixed ages/species	Education, flock management, and veterinary care

Genetic uniformity in livestock populations may increase their vulnerability to disease outbreaks, while also providing opportunities for population-wide interventions, such as vaccination and genetic selection for disease resistance traits. Genetic technologies, including gene editing, may offer new approaches for reducing zoonotic disease risks while raising novel questions about safety and regulatory oversight.

Climate change impacts on livestock systems include altered disease distribution patterns, changes in vector ecology, heat stress effects on animal immune function, and modifications to production practices that may influence zoonotic disease risks in complex ways, which are not yet fully understood. Rising temperatures may expand the geographic range of vector-borne diseases that affect livestock. At the same time, extreme weather events can compromise biosecurity measures and create conditions that facilitate the transmission of pathogens between wildlife and domestic animal populations.

13.4. Urban Wildlife and Disease Transmission

Urbanisation has created novel ecological interfaces where wildlife species adapted to urban environments interact closely with dense human populations, creating unprecedented opportunities for zoonotic disease transmission through direct contact, shared resources, and modified transmission pathways that did not exist in historical human-wildlife relationships (Bradley & Altizer, 2007). Urban wildlife populations often exhibit different disease dynamics compared to their rural counterparts due to factors such as altered nutrition, increased population density, reduced genetic diversity, exposure to pollutants, and modified social behaviours, which can influence pathogen transmission patterns and create new challenges for disease surveillance and control in urban environments.

Urban rodent populations represent one of the most significant urban wildlife disease risks, with rats and mice serving as reservoirs for numerous zoonotic pathogens, including hantaviruses, arenaviruses, Leptospira species, and various bacterial and parasitic agents that can be transmitted to humans through direct contact, aerosol inhalation, contaminated food and water, and arthropod vectors that feed on infected rodents. Urban environments provide abundant food sources, shelter, and breeding sites for rodent populations. At the same time, human activities create disturbance patterns and alter resource availability, which may influence rodent population dynamics and disease transmission patterns. Dense urban housing, inadequate waste management, and ageing infrastructure create conditions that facilitate rodent establishment and proliferation, bringing rodent populations into close contact with human residents.

Urban bird populations, including pigeons, crows, gulls, and various other species that have adapted to urban environments, can serve as reservoirs for numerous zoonotic pathogens, such as Salmonella, Campylobacter, Chlamydia psittaci, and different viral agents that can be transmitted through direct contact, environmental contamination, and aerosol exposure. Bird feeding activities, nesting sites in buildings, and roosting areas create opportunities for human exposure to infected birds and contaminated environments. Urban bird populations may exhibit different disease prevalence and transmission patterns compared to rural populations due to factors such as altered diets, increased stress, and exposure to urban environmental contaminants.

Urban carnivore populations, including foxes, coyotes, raccoons, and various other species that have colonised urban environments, present complex disease risks through their roles as both reservoir hosts for zoonotic pathogens and potential bridge species that can facilitate pathogen transmission between urban wildlife, domestic animals, and human populations. Rabies transmission from urban wildlife to domestic animals and humans remains a significant concern in many urban areas. At the same time, other pathogens, including parasitic agents and bacterial infections, may also be transmitted through carnivore populations. Urban carnivores may exhibit altered behaviour patterns, including a reduced fear of humans and increased contact with domestic animals, which can facilitate disease transmission.

Urban water systems, including stormwater management infrastructure, ornamental water features, and various aquatic habitats created or modified by urban development, can serve as amplification sites for waterborne zoonotic pathogens while providing habitat for reservoir hosts and vectors that may not be present in natural aquatic systems. Leptospirosis transmission associated with urban flooding and contaminated water sources underscores the role of urban infrastructure and water management practices in creating conditions that facilitate zoonotic disease transmission, disproportionately affecting vulnerable populations with limited access to safe housing and sanitation facilities.

Urban green spaces, including parks, gardens, and various naturalised areas within urban environments, create interfaces where humans may encounter wildlife species and vectors that harbour zoonotic pathogens, while providing significant recreational, aesthetic, and ecological benefits. These benefits make risk management interventions complex and potentially controversial. Tick-borne diseases, including Lyme disease and Rocky Mountain spotted fever, may be transmitted in urban green spaces. Various other vector-borne and direct-contact zoonoses may also occur in these settings, depending on local wildlife populations and environmental conditions.

Urban domestic animal populations, including free-roaming cats and dogs, introduce additional complexity into urban wildlife disease ecology through their interactions with both wildlife and human populations, while potentially serving as bridge hosts that facilitate pathogen transmission between these different compartments. Feral cat colonies may serve as reservoirs for Toxoplasma gondii and various other pathogens while also affecting urban bird and small mammal populations through predation pressure that may alter wildlife disease dynamics. Urban dog populations may be exposed to wildlife pathogens through contact with infected animals or contaminated environments while potentially transmitting these pathogens to human owners or other domestic animals.

Urban vector populations, including mosquitoes, ticks, fleas, and various arthropod species that transmit zoonotic pathogens, may exhibit different ecology and disease transmission patterns in urban environments compared to natural settings due to factors including modified breeding sites, altered host availability, microclimate effects of urban heat islands, and exposure to pesticides and other urban environmental factors. Urban mosquito populations may utilise artificial breeding sites, including stormwater systems, ornamental water features, and various containers, which provide breeding habitats. Urban heat island effects may alter seasonal activity patterns and pathogen development rates within vectors.

Urban food systems, including outdoor dining, food trucks, farmers' markets, and various other food service activities, create opportunities for wildlife to meet human food sources while potentially facilitating the transmission of foodborne zoonoses through the contamination of food preparation and service areas by wildlife. Urban agriculture, including community gardens, rooftop farms, and backyard food production, may create additional wildlife-human interfaces while potentially providing benefits for food security and community health. These benefits must be balanced against the potential risks of disease transmission.

Surveillance and monitoring of urban wildlife diseases face unique challenges, including access limitations in private properties, complex jurisdictional responsibilities involving multiple agencies, limited baseline data on urban wildlife disease ecology, and public safety concerns related to wildlife capture and sampling activities. Effective urban wildlife disease surveillance requires collaboration among public health agencies, animal control services, wildlife management agencies, and research institutions, as well as engagement with community stakeholders who may interact with urban wildlife populations.

Prevention and control interventions for urban wildlife diseases must strike a balance between public health protection and wildlife conservation objectives, community preferences for wildlife presence, and practical constraints imposed by urban environments and governance structures. Integrated pest management approaches that combine habitat modification, exclusion techniques, population control methods, and public education may be more effective and acceptable than single-intervention approaches while requiring sustained commitment and coordination between multiple stakeholder groups (Himsworth et al., 2013).

13.5. Climate Change and Shifting Disease Patterns

Climate change is fundamentally altering the epidemiology and geographic distribution of zoonotic diseases through complex mechanisms that affect pathogen survival, vector ecology, reservoir host distribution, human behaviour patterns, and environmental conditions that determine transmission opportunities, creating both predictable changes and novel disease emergence scenarios that challenge existing surveillance and control systems (Altizer et al., 2013). The magnitude and pace of climate change impacts on zoonotic diseases vary significantly between different pathogen systems, geographic regions, and time scales, requiring adaptive management approaches that can respond to both gradual shifts in disease patterns and abrupt changes associated with extreme weather events and ecosystem disruptions.

Temperature increases associated with climate change directly affect the biology and ecology of arthropod vectors that transmit many critical zoonotic diseases. Higher temperatures generally accelerate vector development rates, shorten generation times, and increase reproductive output, while also affecting pathogen development rates within vectors and the duration of pathogen survival in environmental reservoirs. These temperature effects can increase transmission intensity in areas that remain within suitable temperature ranges for vector survival while potentially expanding the geographic range of vector-borne zoonoses into previously temperate regions where vectors could not previously establish sustainable populations. However, extreme temperatures may also exceed the thermal tolerance limits of vectors and pathogens, creating complex non-linear relationships between temperature change and disease transmission that vary by species and local environmental conditions.

Vector-borne zoonoses, including West Nile virus, Lyme disease, Rocky Mountain spotted fever, and various other tick- and mosquito-borne diseases, are experiencing geographic range expansions and altered seasonal transmission patterns associated with the effects of climate change on vector distribution and activity patterns. Warming temperatures are enabling the northward expansion of many vector species, while extending transmission seasons in areas where vectors were previously limited by cold temperatures during the winter months. These changes are creating new areas of risk where human and animal populations may lack immunity to vector-borne pathogens. At the same time, surveillance and control systems may not be prepared for novel disease threats.

Changing precipitation patterns associated with climate change have complex effects on zoonotic disease transmission, influencing vector breeding sites, reservoir host population dynamics, and the survival of environmental pathogens. Increased precipitation and flooding can create new breeding habitats for mosquito vectors, while also facilitating the transmission of water-associated pathogens, including Leptospira species and various other bacterial and parasitic agents that can survive in contaminated water sources. Drought conditions may concentrate vectors and reservoir hosts around limited water sources, potentially intensifying transmission while also affecting host immune function and susceptibility to infection through nutritional stress and other drought-related impacts.

Extreme weather events including hurricanes, floods, droughts, wildfires, and severe storms create acute disruptions to ecological systems and human communities that can trigger zoonotic disease outbreaks through multiple pathways including habitat disruption that forces wildlife into contact with human settlements, breakdown of sanitation and vector control systems, population displacement that may increase exposure to novel pathogens, and stress effects on both human and animal immune systems that may increase susceptibility to infection. Post-disaster environments often feature compromised surveillance and healthcare systems, which may delay detection and response to zoonotic disease outbreaks while creating conditions that favour rapid pathogen transmission.

Wildlife population responses to climate change, including range shifts, phenological changes, and alterations in population dynamics, can significantly affect zoonotic disease ecology through changes in reservoir host distribution, abundance, and contact patterns with human populations. Many wildlife species are shifting their geographic ranges toward higher latitudes and elevations in response to warming temperatures, potentially introducing zoonotic pathogens to new areas while creating novel contact opportunities with human populations that may have limited previous exposure to these pathogens. Changes in wildlife migration timing, breeding patterns, and habitat use can alter seasonal disease transmission patterns while potentially creating new pathways for pathogen introduction and establishment.

Domestic animal and livestock responses to climate change include heat stress effects that may compromise immune function and increase susceptibility to zoonotic pathogens, altered grazing and management patterns that may increase wildlife contact, and modifications to production systems that could impact biosecurity and disease control measures. Heat stress in livestock can reduce vaccine efficacy and increase shedding of foodborne pathogens. At the same time, extreme weather events can compromise biosecurity measures and create opportunities for pathogen introduction from wildlife or other external sources.

Environmental pathogen persistence and survival are influenced by climate change through altered temperature and moisture conditions, which impact pathogen viability in soil, water, and other ecological reservoirs. Some pathogens benefit from warmer, moister conditions, while others may be adversely affected by extreme temperatures or drought conditions. Anthrax spores, for example, may remain viable in soil for extended periods under suitable conditions, but may be affected by extreme environmental conditions associated with climate change. Conversely, various water-associated pathogens may benefit from increased flooding and waterlogging, which create favourable ecological conditions for pathogen survival and transmission. Table 13.4 illustrates the impact of climate change on major zoonotic disease systems.

Human behavioural responses to climate change, including migration patterns, changes in livelihoods, and adaptation strategies, can significantly affect zoonotic disease exposure risks through altered contact patterns with reservoir hosts and vectors, modifications to food production and consumption practices, and adjustments to housing and settlement patterns that may increase or decrease disease transmission opportunities. Climate-induced migration may bring human populations into contact with novel zoonotic pathogens, potentially introducing these pathogens to new areas where they can establish transmission cycles involving local wildlife and domestic animal populations.

Agricultural and land-use adaptations to climate change, including changes in crop selection, modifications to irrigation systems, alterations to livestock systems, and adjustments to settlement patterns, can create new zoonotic disease risks while potentially reducing others. This requires a careful assessment of disease implications when planning climate adaptation strategies. The expansion of irrigation systems may create new breeding habitats for mosquito vectors, while shifts to different livestock species may alter the zoonotic disease risks associated with animal production systems.

Surveillance and early warning systems for climate-sensitive zoonotic diseases require integration of climate monitoring data with disease surveillance information to enable prediction and preparation for disease emergence and expansion events associated with climate variability and change. Seasonal forecasting systems that predict climate conditions related to increased disease transmission can enable proactive prevention and control measures. Meanwhile, long-term monitoring systems can track gradual shifts in disease patterns, which require adaptive management responses.

Climate change adaptation strategies for zoonotic disease prevention must address both direct climate effects on disease transmission and indirect effects mediated through changes in human and animal behaviour, land-use patterns, and socioeconomic conditions that influence disease exposure and vulnerability (Mills et al., 2010). Integrated approaches that address climate adaptation and zoonotic disease prevention simultaneously may be more effective and efficient than separate interventions while providing co-benefits for multiple development objectives, including Health, food security, and environmental sustainability.

13.6. Control Strategies and Challenges

The control of zoonotic diseases requires integrated approaches that address multiple transmission pathways, diverse host species, and complex ecological and social determinants that influence pathogen maintenance and transmission while balancing public health objectives with economic, social, and environmental considerations that affect the feasibility and sustainability of control interventions (Zinsstag et al., 2011). Effective zoonotic disease control strategies must be based on a thorough understanding of transmission cycles, risk factors, and intervention points that offer opportunities for breaking transmission chains or reducing human exposure to infected animals and contaminated environments, while also addressing the underlying drivers that create conditions favourable for zoonotic disease emergence and spread.

Surveillance systems for zoonotic diseases must integrate human health, animal health, and environmental monitoring components to provide comprehensive detection and characterisation capabilities that can identify disease emergence events, track transmission patterns, and evaluate the effectiveness of control interventions across the complex, multi-host systems involved in zoonotic disease maintenance and transmission. One Health surveillance approaches that coordinate surveillance activities across human medicine, veterinary medicine, wildlife management, and environmental health sectors can provide more complete situational awareness than sector-specific surveillance while enabling more rapid detection and response to zoonotic disease threats. However, implementing integrated surveillance systems requires substantial coordination mechanisms, standardised protocols, information-sharing systems, and sustained funding, which may be challenging to achieve and maintain.

Vaccination strategies for zoonotic disease control may target human populations, animal reservoirs, or both, depending on the specific disease system, available vaccines, and the feasibility of reaching target populations with vaccination interventions. Human vaccination against zoonotic diseases is available for a limited number of diseases, including rabies post-exposure prophylaxis, yellow fever, and Japanese encephalitis. Most human zoonotic disease vaccines are used for high-risk populations, such as laboratory workers, veterinarians, or travellers to endemic areas, rather than for population-wide prevention programs. Animal vaccination programs can be highly effective for certain zoonotic diseases, with notable successes including the control of rabies in domestic dogs and wildlife populations, the control of brucellosis in livestock, and the reduction of various other diseases where animal vaccination can eliminate or reduce pathogen circulation in reservoir populations.

Wildlife vaccination programs present unique technical and logistical challenges, including difficulties accessing wild animal populations, the need for oral or other remote delivery systems, concerns about vaccine safety for non-target species, and environmental impacts of vaccine distribution methods. Oral rabies vaccination programs for wildlife populations have achieved significant success in eliminating rabies from large geographic areas while demonstrating the potential for wildlife vaccination approaches when appropriate technologies and delivery systems are available. However, most zoonotic diseases lack effective wildlife vaccines or practical delivery systems that would enable population-level vaccination of wildlife reservoirs.

Vector control interventions can be effective for vector-borne zoonoses but require sustained implementation and community engagement to achieve lasting impact while addressing environmental and Health concerns associated with pesticide use and other vector control methods. Integrated vector management approaches that combine multiple control methods, including habitat modification, biological control agents, targeted pesticide applications, and personal protective measures, may be more effective and sustainable than single-method approaches, while reducing reliance on chemical pesticides that may have adverse environmental and Health effects. Community-based vector control programs that engage local communities in vector control activities can be more sustainable and cost-effective than top-down programs, while providing education and capacity-building benefits that contribute to the long-term sustainability of control.

Environmental management interventions address habitat and environmental factors that influence pathogen survival, vector breeding, and contact opportunities between humans and infected animals or vectors, offering opportunities for sustainable zoonotic disease prevention through modifications to land use, water management, waste management, and other environmental factors. Habitat modification to reduce vector breeding sites, improve drainage, and eliminate wildlife harborage near human settlements can provide lasting benefits for zoonotic disease prevention while potentially providing co-benefits for other Health and environmental objectives. However, environmental management interventions may require substantial upfront investments and long-term maintenance, while potentially creating conflicts with other land-use objectives or ecological conservation goals.

Livestock and domestic animal interventions, including improved husbandry practices, biosecurity measures, disease surveillance and control programs, and antimicrobial stewardship, can reduce zoonotic disease risks while potentially providing production benefits that create economic incentives for adoption. Good agricultural practices that address animal health, food safety, and worker safety can reduce exposure risks throughout the food production chain while improving product quality and market access for producers. However, implementing livestock interventions requires technical knowledge, financial resources, and regulatory support that may not be available in all production systems. At the same time, market incentives may not always align with public health objectives.

Regulatory and policy interventions provide frameworks for zoonotic disease prevention through food safety regulations, import/export controls, wildlife trade oversight, occupational safety requirements, and other legal and regulatory mechanisms that can address specific risk factors and create incentives for adoption of prevention measures. International regulations, including CITES, OIE standards, and Codex Alimentarius, provide harmonised approaches to particular aspects of zoonotic disease prevention. At the same time, national and local rules can address location-specific risks and priorities. However, regulatory interventions require enforcement capacity, technical expertise, and political support that may be limited, potentially creating economic costs that could impact compliance and effectiveness. Table 13.5 presents zoonotic disease control strategies, including approaches, applications, and implementation challenges.

Education and behaviour change interventions target human behaviours that affect zoonotic disease exposure risk, including occupational safety practices, food handling behaviours, wildlife contact patterns, and healthcare-seeking behaviours, which can significantly influence disease transmission and outcomes when infections occur. Effective education programs must be tailored to specific audiences and cultural contexts, while addressing practical barriers that may prevent the adoption of recommended behaviours, even when knowledge levels are adequate. Community-based education programs that engage local leaders and organisations may be more effective than top-down approaches, as they provide opportunities for two-way communication that can improve program relevance and effectiveness.

International cooperation and coordination are crucial for addressing zoonotic diseases that cross national boundaries through wildlife migration, international trade, travel, and other pathways, which can rapidly spread pathogens across continents before local control measures can be implemented. Global surveillance networks, international laboratory networks, and rapid response mechanisms enable countries to share information, coordinate investigations, and enforce harmonised control measures that can be more effective than isolated national responses. However, international cooperation requires sustained political commitment, adequate funding, and technical harmonisation that may be challenging to achieve and maintain across diverse countries and regions with different priorities and capabilities.

Table 13.4. Climate change impacts on major zoonotic disease systems

Disease System	Primary Climate Drivers	Geographic Impact Patterns	Seasonal Changes	Transmission Intensity Effects	Vulnerable Populations	Adaptation Requirements
Vector-borne (Lyme, West Nile)	Temperature, precipitation	Northward expansion, elevation shifts	Extended seasons, earlier onset	Increase in suitable areas	Outdoor workers, endemic residents	Vector surveillance, prevention education
Water-associated (Leptospirosis)	Precipitation, flooding, temperature	Urban areas, flood-prone regions	Rainy season intensification	Outbreak potential increased	Urban poor, agricultural workers	Flood management, sanitation infrastructure
Rodent-borne (Hantavirus)	Precipitation, temperature, extreme events	Variable by region	Seasonal host population dynamics	Periodic outbreak increases	Rural residents, outdoor recreationalists	Rodent control, risk communication
Livestock-associated (Rift Valley fever)	Precipitation cycles, flooding	Pastoral regions, irrigation areas	Rainy season emergence	Epidemic amplification	Pastoralists, veterinary workers	Livestock vaccination, movement control
Wildlife-associated (Rabies)	Temperature, habitat disruption	Range shifts of reservoir species	Modified wildlife behaviour	Contact pattern changes	Rural communities, animal handlers	Wildlife surveillance, pet vaccination
Foodborne (Salmonellosis)	Temperature, extreme events	Heat-affected regions, supply chains	Summer amplification	Processing/storage challenges	Food service workers, consumers	Cold chain, processing safety

Table 13.5. Zoonotic disease control strategies - Approaches, applications, and implementation challenges

Control Strategy	Primary Applications	Target Population/Setting	Implementation Requirements	Effectiveness Factors	Major Challenges	Success Examples
Human Vaccination	High-risk occupations, post-exposure	Healthcare workers, veterinarians, travellers	Vaccine availability, delivery systems	Coverage rates, vaccine efficacy	Limited vaccine availability, access barriers	Rabies post-exposure prophylaxis, yellow fever
Animal Vaccination	Reservoir control, herd immunity	Livestock, pets, wildlife	Vaccine development, delivery logistics	Population coverage, duration of immunity	Wildlife access, vaccine cold chain	Livestock brucellosis, wildlife rabies programs
Vector Control	Vector-borne disease prevention	Endemic communities, outbreak areas	Technical capacity, community engagement	Vector population reduction, resistance management	Insecticide resistance, environmental concerns	Malaria control programs, arbovirus prevention
Environmental Management	Habitat modification, exposure reduction	Communities, production systems	Planning, implementation resources	Sustainability, multiple benefit integration	Competing land uses, maintenance requirements	Urban rat control, wetland management
Surveillance Systems	Early detection, monitoring	Multisectoral, integrated systems	Laboratory capacity, coordination mechanisms	Timeliness, sensitivity, representativeness	Resource constraints, coordination complexity	Global surveillance networks, laboratory networks
Regulatory Controls	Risk reduction, prevention standards	International trade, food systems	Legal frameworks, enforcement capacity	Compliance rates, standard effectiveness	Enforcement challenges, economic impacts	CITES implementation, food safety regulations

Resource mobilisation for zoonotic disease control faces challenges, including competing health priorities, a limited understanding of the economic benefits from prevention investments, and difficulties in securing sustained funding for long-term control programs that may require decades to achieve lasting impact. Economic analyses of zoonotic disease control interventions often demonstrate favourable cost-benefit ratios; however, benefits may accrue to different sectors than those bearing the intervention costs, while long-term benefits may not provide adequate incentives for short-term investment decisions. Innovative financing mechanisms, including global health security funding, international development assistance, and public-private partnerships, may help address funding gaps while ensuring adequate resources for comprehensive zoonotic disease prevention and control programs.

Conclusion

Zoonotic diseases represent one of the most complex and significant global health challenges, accounting for most emerging infectious diseases, while demonstrating the fundamental interconnectedness of human health, animal health, and environmental health, defining One Health approaches. The increasing frequency and impact reflect the intensification of human-animal-environment interactions through agricultural expansion, wildlife exploitation, urbanisation, and climate change, creating novel pathogen spillover pathways while amplifying the consequences of emergence events.

The diversity of zoonotic disease systems—ranging from ancient scourges like rabies and plague to newly emerged threats like SARS, MERS, and COVID-19—illustrates both the persistent nature and evolving character of these threats. Major zoonotic diseases continue causing millions of human infections and hundreds of thousands of deaths annually while imposing substantial economic burdens extending beyond direct healthcare costs.

The global expansion of the wildlife trade represents a particularly significant driver of disease risk, creating unprecedented spillover opportunities through increased human contact with diverse wildlife species and the international movement of potentially infected animals. Domestic animals and livestock serve as critical interfaces between wildlife pathogen reservoirs and human populations, with intensive production systems creating new configurations of human-animal-pathogen interactions.

Urbanisation has created novel ecological interfaces where urban-adapted wildlife species interact closely with dense human populations. Climate change fundamentally alters the epidemiology and geographic distribution of zoonotic diseases through its effects on vector ecology, pathogen survival, host distribution, and human behaviour patterns.

Control requires integrated One Health approaches that coordinate surveillance, prevention, and response activities across sectors, while addressing complex ecological and social determinants. Future challenges include emerging pathogens with pandemic potential, antimicrobial resistance, climate change impacts, demographic shifts, and economic changes that influence human-animal interactions.

COVID-19 demonstrated both the devastating potential of zoonotic disease emergence and the critical importance of prepared, coordinated, and adequately resourced systems. Success requires unprecedented international cooperation, sustained political commitment, and recognition that zoonotic disease prevention is a critical component of global security, economic stability, and sustainable development.

Acknowledgments

The authors would like to extend our appreciation to those who offered helpful commentary during the drafting process of this manuscript. We also acknowledge the role Nova Science Publishers played in enabling the work described herein.

References

Altizer, S., Ostfeld, R. S., Johnson, P. T., Kutz, S., & Harvell, C. D. (2013). Climate change and infectious diseases: from evidence to a predictive framework. *Science*, 341(6145), 514-519. https://doi.org/10.1126/science.1239401.

Bradley, C. A., & Altizer, S. (2007). Urbanisation and the ecology of wildlife diseases. *Trends in Ecology & Evolution*, 22(2), 95-102. https://doi.org/10.1016/j.tree.2006.11.001.

Can, Ö. E., D'Cruze, N., Guclu, O., Ransom, C., Takhar, J., & Macdonald, D. W. (2019). Dealing in deadly pathogens: Taking stock of the legal trade in live wildlife and potential risks to human Health. *Global Ecology and Conservation*, 17, e00515. https://doi.org/10.1016/j.gecco.2018.e00515.

Cleaveland, S., Laurenson, M. K., & Taylor, L. H. (2001). Diseases of humans and their domestic mammals: pathogen characteristics, host range and the risk of emergence. *Philosophical Transactions of the Royal Society B*, 356(1411), 991-999. https://doi.org/10.1098/rstb.2001.0889.

Himsworth, C. G., Parsons, K. L., Jardine, C., & Patrick, D. M. (2013). Rats, cities, people, and pathogens: a systematic review and narrative synthesis of literature regarding the ecology of rat-associated zoonoses in urban centers. *Vector-Borne and Zoonotic Diseases*, 13(6), 349-359. https://doi.org/10.1089/vbz.2012.1195.

Johnson, C. K., Hitchens, P. L., Pandit, P. S., Rushmore, J., Evans, T. S., Young, C. C., & Doyle, M. M. (2020). Global shifts in mammalian population trends reveal key predictors of virus spillover risk. *Proceedings of the Royal Society B*, 287(1924), 20192736. https://doi.org/10.1098/rspb.2019.2736.

Jones, K. E., Patel, N. G., Levy, M. A., Storeygard, A., Balk, D., Gittleman, J. L., & Daszak, P. (2008). Global trends in emerging infectious diseases. *Nature*, 451(7181), 990-993. https://doi.org/10.1038/nature06536.

Karesh, W. B., Dobson, A., Lloyd-Smith, J. O., Lubroth, J., Dixon, M. A., Bennett, M., ... & Heymann, D. L. (2012). Ecology of zoonoses: natural and unnatural histories. *The Lancet*, 380(9857), 1936-1945. https://doi.org/10.1016/S0140-6736(12)61678-X.

Mills, J. N., Gage, K. L., & Khan, A. S. (2010). Potential influence of climate change on vector-borne and zoonotic diseases: a review and proposed research plan. *Environmental Health Perspectives*, 118(11), 1507-1514. https://doi.org/10.1289/ehp.0901389.

Morse, S. S., Mazet, J. A., Woolhouse, M., Parrish, C. R., Carroll, D., Karesh, W. B., ... & Daszak, P. (2012). Prediction and prevention of the next pandemic zoonosis. *The Lancet*, 380(9857), 1956-1965. https://doi.org/10.1016/S0140-6736(12)61684-5.

Robertson, I. D., Irwin, P. J., Lymbery, A. J., & Thompson, R. C. A. (2000). The role of companion animals in the emergence of parasitic zoonoses. *International Journal for Parasitology*, 30(12-13), 1369-1377. https://doi.org/10.1016/S0020-7519(00)00134-X.

Taylor, L. H., Latham, S. M., & Woolhouse, M. E. (2001). Risk factors for human disease emergence. *Philosophical Transactions of the Royal Society B*, 356(1411), 983-989. https://doi.org/10.1098/rstb.2001.0888.

Zinsstag, J., Schelling, E., Waltner-Toews, D., & Tanner, M. (2011). From "one medicine" to "one health" and systemic approaches to Health and well-being. *Preventive Veterinary Medicine*, 101(3-4), 148-156. https://doi.org/10.1016/j.prevetmed.2010.07.003.

World Health Organization. (2020). *Taking a multisectoral, one health approach: A tripartite guide to addressing zoonotic diseases in countries*. World Health Organization. https://www.who.int/publications/i/item/taking-a-multisectoral-one-health-approach-a-tripartite-guide-to-addressing-zoonotic-diseases-in-countries.

Chapter 14

Ecosystem Health and Human Well-Being

Purnachandra Kawdu Lamghare[1]
and Maajid Mohi Ud Din Malik[2,*]**, PhD**
[2]Department of Radio-Diagnosis, Dr. D. Y. Patil Medical College, Hospital and Research Centre, Dr. D. Y. Patil Vidyapeeth, Pune (Deemed to be University)- Sant Tukaram Nagar, Pimpri, Pune, India
[2]Department of Radiology and Imaging Technology, Dr. D. Y. Patil School of Allied Health Sciences, Dr. D. Y. Patil Vidyapeeth· Pune (Deemed to be University), Sant Tukaram Nagar, Pimpri, Pune, India

Abstract

Ecosystem health and human wellbeing are fundamentally interconnected through complex relationships that determine the capacity of natural systems to provide essential services supporting human survival, Health, and prosperity while maintaining ecological integrity and resilience in the face of global environmental change. Healthy ecosystems provide critical services, including clean air and water, climate regulation, disease control, food security, and mental health benefits, that directly contribute to human well-being. Meanwhile, ecosystem degradation compromises these services, creating conditions that increase human vulnerability to diseases, natural disasters, and other health threats. Biodiversity loss represents a key driver of ecosystem degradation, reducing the natural regulation of disease transmission through mechanisms such as host dilution effects, vector control by natural predators, and the maintenance of ecological barriers that prevent pathogen spillover from wildlife to human populations. Environmental pollution from industrial, agricultural, and urban sources compromises both ecosystem health and human Health through multiple pathways, including air and water contamination, soil degradation, and disruption of ecological processes that support ecosystem services. One Health and conservation medicine approaches provide frameworks for understanding and addressing the interconnections between ecosystem health, animal health, and human Health through integrated strategies that recognise the shared determinants of Health across human and natural systems. Planetary health concepts emphasise the fundamental dependence of human Health on Earth's natural systems, while highlighting the need for transformative approaches to development that can sustain both human well-being and ecosystem integrity within planetary boundaries. Achieving Sustainable Development Goals related to Health, environmental sustainability, and poverty reduction requires integrated approaches that address ecosystem health as a fundamental determinant of human wellbeing while

* Corresponding Author's Email: maajid.malik@dpu.edu.in

In: Advances in the One Health Approach
Editors: Maajid Mohi Ud Din Malik, Abhay Saraf, Harshal Tukaram Pandve et al.
ISBN: 979-8-90134-202-2

implementing development strategies that enhance rather than compromise ecosystem services and natural capital.

Keywords: ecosystem health, ecosystem services, biodiversity, planetary Health, One Health, conservation medicine, sustainable development, environmental Health, Sustainable Development Goals, natural capital

Introduction

Ecosystem health and human well-being are inextricably linked through complex relationships that have evolved over millennia but are now being fundamentally altered by the scale and pace of human activities that affect Earth's natural systems (Millennium Ecosystem Assessment, 2005). The concept of ecosystem health encompasses the capacity of natural systems to maintain their structure, function, and resilience while providing essential services that support life on Earth, including the regulation of climate, water cycles, and biogeochemical processes that create conditions suitable for human habitation and prosperity. Human wellbeing depends on healthy ecosystems through multiple pathways, including direct provisioning services such as food, water, and raw materials, regulating services including climate control and disease prevention, supporting services such as nutrient cycling and primary production, and cultural services including spiritual, recreational, and aesthetic benefits that contribute to mental Health and quality of life. The degradation of ecosystem health through habitat destruction, pollution, overexploitation, and climate change is compromising the capacity of natural systems to provide these essential services while creating conditions that increase human vulnerability to infectious diseases, natural disasters, food insecurity, and other health threats. Understanding these relationships is critical for developing strategies that can sustain both human well-being and ecosystem health in an era of unprecedented global environmental change driven by human activities. The emerging fields of planetary Health, One Health, and conservation medicine provide frameworks for understanding and addressing these interconnections through integrated approaches that recognise the fundamental dependence of human Health on the Health of Earth's natural systems while implementing interventions that can enhance both human wellbeing and ecosystem integrity within planetary boundaries that define safe operating spaces for human civilisation.

14.1. Ecosystem Services and Human Health

Ecosystem services encompass the diverse benefits that humans derive from functioning ecosystems, including provisioning services that directly provide resources, regulating services that control environmental conditions, supporting services that maintain ecosystem function, and cultural services that contribute to human wellbeing through non-material benefits (Butler et al., 2014). These services represent fundamental life support systems that enable human survival and prosperity while operating through complex ecological processes that may be invisible to human perception but are essential for maintaining environmental conditions suitable for human habitation. Understanding the relationships between ecosystem services and human Health is crucial for recognising the health implications of environmental degradation while identifying opportunities for interventions that can enhance both ecosystem health and human wellbeing through synergistic approaches.

Provisioning services provide direct material benefits that support human Health through access to clean water, nutritious food, medical resources, and raw materials needed for shelter, clothing, and other necessities of life. Clean water provisioning through natural filtration and purification processes in wetlands, forests, and groundwater systems represents one of the most critical ecosystem services for human Health, with compromised water quality leading to waterborne diseases that cause millions of deaths annually, particularly among children in low-income countries. Ecosystem-based water treatment through constructed wetlands and natural filtration systems can provide cost-effective alternatives to traditional technological water treatment, while also offering additional benefits, including habitat creation and carbon sequestration, which contribute to multiple environmental and Health objectives.

Food provisioning through agricultural and marine ecosystems supports human nutrition and food security while maintaining genetic diversity in crop and livestock species that provides resilience against pests, diseases, and climate variability. Diverse agricultural ecosystems that support habitat for natural pest predators and pollinators can reduce dependence on pesticides while enhancing crop productivity and food quality. Marine ecosystems provide essential protein and micronutrients for billions of people while serving as sources of omega-3 fatty acids and other nutrients that contribute to cardiovascular Health and brain development. However, overfishing and habitat degradation are compromising the capacity of marine systems to provide these nutritional benefits while reducing the availability of affordable protein for vulnerable populations.

Medicinal resources from natural ecosystems have provided the foundation for traditional medicine systems and continue to serve as sources of pharmaceutical compounds, with an estimated 25% of modern medications derived from plant compounds and many others based on natural products from fungi, bacteria, and other organisms. Biodiversity loss threatens the continued availability of these medicinal resources, potentially eliminating undiscovered compounds that could provide new treatments for diseases such as cancer, antimicrobial-resistant infections, and neurological disorders. Traditional ecological knowledge systems maintained by indigenous communities represent essential repositories of information about medicinal uses of natural resources while demonstrating sustainable approaches to ecosystem management that maintain both biodiversity and human health benefits.

Regulating services control environmental conditions that directly affect human Health through mechanisms including climate regulation, air quality control, disease regulation, and natural hazard mitigation that reduce human exposure to environmental health threats. Climate regulation through carbon sequestration in forests, grasslands, and soil systems moderates temperature increases and weather extremes that can affect human Health through heat stress, extreme weather events, and changes in disease transmission patterns. Forest ecosystems play a vital role in climate regulation, while also providing additional benefits, including improved air quality through the filtration of pollutants and increased oxygen production.

Air quality regulation through the filtration of particulate matter and gaseous pollutants by vegetation reduces human exposure to air pollution, which causes respiratory diseases, cardiovascular disease, and premature mortality, affecting millions of people worldwide, particularly in urban areas with high pollution levels. Urban green spaces, including parks, street trees, and green roofs, can significantly reduce exposure to air pollution while providing additional benefits, such as temperature regulation, noise reduction, and mental health benefits through contact with nature. The economic value of air quality improvements through ecosystem services often exceeds the costs of creating and maintaining urban green infrastructure while providing multiple co-benefits for human Health and environmental quality.

Disease regulation through natural processes, including predator control of disease vectors, host dilution effects that reduce pathogen transmission, and maintenance of ecological barriers that prevent pathogen spillover, represents a critical but often unrecognised ecosystem service that affects human Health through reduced disease transmission and outbreak risks. Wetland ecosystems that support fish and amphibian populations that consume mosquito larvae can provide natural vector control, reducing the transmission of mosquito-borne diseases while eliminating the need for pesticide applications that may have adverse environmental and Health effects. Forest ecosystems that maintain diverse wildlife communities can reduce the risks of zoonotic disease spillover through dilution effects, which minimise contact between humans and highly competent reservoir hosts. Table 14.1 illustrates the linkages between ecosystem services and human Health.

Natural hazard mitigation through ecosystem services, including flood control by wetlands and forests, coastal protection by mangroves and coral reefs, and soil stabilisation by vegetation, reduces human exposure to natural disasters that cause injuries, deaths, and disease outbreaks, while disrupting health services and infrastructure. Coastal ecosystems, including mangroves, salt marshes, and coral reefs, provide natural barriers against storm surges and wave action, thereby reducing damage from tropical cyclones and tsunamis. These ecosystems also support fisheries and tourism activities, which contribute significantly to local economies. However, coastal development and climate change are degrading these natural protective systems while increasing human vulnerability to coastal hazards.

Supporting services maintain the ecological processes that enable all other ecosystem services, providing indirect benefits for human Health through maintaining ecosystem stability and resilience, which ensures the continued provision of health-supporting services. Primary production through photosynthesis offers the foundation for food webs that support provisioning services while maintaining atmospheric oxygen levels that enable human respiration. Nutrient cycling processes maintain soil fertility, which promotes agricultural production while preventing the accumulation of waste products that could compromise environmental quality and human Health.

Cultural services provide non-material benefits that contribute to human Health and wellbeing through psychological, social, and spiritual pathways that may be difficult to quantify but are essential for mental Health and quality of life. Contact with natural environments has been shown to reduce stress, anxiety, and depression, while improving cognitive function and immune system response through mechanisms that may include reduced levels of stress hormones, increased physical activity, and exposure to beneficial microorganisms. Urban green spaces provide opportunities for physical activity and social interaction that contribute to both physical and mental Health while reducing urban heat island effects and air pollution exposure.

Recreation and tourism opportunities provided by natural ecosystems contribute to physical activity, stress reduction, and economic benefits that support community health and wellbeing while creating financial incentives for ecosystem conservation and sustainable management. Ecotourism activities can provide sustainable income for local communities while funding conservation activities that maintain ecosystem services and biodiversity.

However, tourism activities must be carefully managed to prevent ecosystem degradation that could compromise both environmental Health and long-term economic sustainability.

Spiritual and aesthetic values associated with natural ecosystems contribute to cultural identity, social cohesion, and mental health benefits that may be particularly important for indigenous communities and other groups with strong cultural connections to specific landscapes and ecosystems (Myers et al., 2013). Loss of access to culturally significant natural areas can contribute to psychological stress and social disruption, affecting community health and wellbeing while undermining traditional knowledge systems that may contribute to sustainable ecosystem management practices.

14.2. Biodiversity Loss and Disease Emergence

Biodiversity loss represents one of the most significant global environmental changes affecting ecosystem health and human wellbeing, with current rates of species extinction estimated to be 100 to 1,000 times higher than natural background rates, creating unprecedented disruptions to ecological processes that regulate disease transmission and maintain ecosystem services essential for human Health (Cardinale et al., 2012). The relationship between biodiversity and disease emergence operates through complex mechanisms, including dilution effects where diverse host communities reduce pathogen transmission, the maintenance of ecological barriers that prevent pathogen spillover, and the preservation of natural predator-prey relationships that control vector populations and pathogen amplification in natural systems.

The dilution effect represents one of the most important mechanisms through which biodiversity loss affects disease emergence. It occurs when diverse host communities include species with varying competence for pathogen amplification and transmission, such that increased host diversity reduces overall transmission efficiency by distributing pathogen exposure across hosts with different levels of susceptibility and infectiousness. This phenomenon has been documented for numerous disease systems, including Lyme disease, West Nile virus, and hantavirus, where loss of biodiversity through habitat fragmentation and species extinctions leads to communities dominated by highly competent reservoir hosts that efficiently maintain and transmit pathogens to humans and other susceptible species.

Vector control through natural predators represents another critical pathway through which biodiversity affects disease transmission. Diverse predator communities, including fish, amphibians, birds, and invertebrates, consume large quantities of disease vectors, such as mosquitoes, ticks, and other arthropods that transmit pathogens to humans. Wetland ecosystems that support diverse communities of fish and amphibian predators can provide natural mosquito control, reducing the transmission of mosquito-borne diseases while eliminating the need for pesticide applications that may have adverse environmental and Health effects. However, pollution, habitat destruction, and climate change are causing widespread declines in amphibian populations that serve as important predators of mosquito larvae and other disease vectors.

Pathogen regulation through diverse microbial communities represents an emerging area of research, suggesting that biodiversity loss may affect disease emergence by disrupting natural microbial ecosystems that compete with pathogens for resources and habitats, while producing antimicrobial compounds that inhibit pathogen growth and survival. Soil microbial communities that maintain diverse bacterial and fungal populations can suppress soilborne pathogens through competitive exclusion and the production of antibiotics. In contrast, diverse gut microbiomes in wildlife and domestic animals may provide resistance against pathogenic organisms that could otherwise establish infections and be transmitted to humans.

Habitat fragmentation and edge effects created by human activities, including deforestation, agricultural expansion, and urban development, alter ecological conditions in ways that may favour pathogen transmission while bringing humans into closer contact with infected wildlife populations. Forest fragmentation creates edge habitats with altered microclimate conditions that may be more suitable for specific disease vectors, while concentrating wildlife populations in smaller habitat patches that can facilitate the transmission of pathogens between individuals. Additionally, edge habitats bring human populations into closer proximity with wildlife disease reservoirs while creating opportunities for domestic animals to interact with infected wildlife populations.

Agricultural intensification and monoculture production systems represent major drivers of biodiversity loss, which may increase disease risks through multiple pathways, including the elimination of natural habitats for vector predators, the creation of simplified ecosystems that lack natural disease regulation mechanisms, and the concentration of genetically similar crop and livestock species that may be vulnerable to disease outbreaks. Intensive agriculture that relies on pesticides and fertilisers may reduce beneficial insect populations, which provide natural pest control, while creating runoff that pollutes aquatic ecosystems and reduces biodiversity in surrounding natural areas.

Climate change interactions with biodiversity loss create synergistic effects that may accelerate both biodiversity decline and disease emergence through mechanisms including range shifts that disrupt co-evolved host-pathogen relationships, phenological mismatches between species that depend on each other for ecological services, and creation of novel species assemblages with unpredictable disease dynamics. Climate-induced species range shifts may bring together host and pathogen species that have not previously co-evolved, potentially creating new opportunities for pathogen spillover and emergence.

Urban biodiversity loss through development and habitat modification may affect human Health through reduced ecosystem services, including improved air quality, temperature regulation, and mental health benefits associated with contact with diverse natural communities. Urban green spaces that maintain diverse plant and animal communities may offer greater health benefits than simplified landscaping, while supporting wildlife populations that contribute to natural pest control and other essential ecosystem services. Table 14.2 illustrates the mechanisms of biodiversity loss and disease emergence pathways.

Marine biodiversity loss due to overfishing, pollution, and climate change affects human Health through the reduced availability of nutritious seafood, disruption of aquatic ecosystem services, including coastal protection and climate regulation, and the potential emergence of marine pathogens that could impact Health through seafood consumption or recreational water contact. Coral reef degradation reduces coastal protection services and eliminates habitat for fish species that provide significant nutritional benefits to coastal populations. Ocean acidification and warming associated with climate change are causing widespread mortality in marine ecosystems while potentially creating conditions that favour harmful algal blooms and other marine health threats.

Table 14.1. Ecosystem services and human health linkages

Service Category	Specific Services	Health Benefits	Health Risks from Degradation	Vulnerable Populations	Quantification Methods	Policy Interventions
Provisioning	Clean water, food security, and medicinal plants	Nutrition, hydration, and disease treatment	Malnutrition, waterborne disease, and limited healthcare	Rural poor, indigenous communities	Water quality monitoring, nutritional assessments	Protected areas, sustainable agriculture
Regulating	Climate control, air purification, disease regulation	Reduced heat stress, respiratory Health, and infection control	Climate extremes, air pollution, disease outbreaks	Urban populations, children, and the elderly	Air quality indices, disease surveillance	Urban planning, emission controls
Supporting	Nutrient cycling, primary production, habitat provision	Food web stability, resource availability	Ecosystem collapse, resource scarcity	All populations, future generations	Biodiversity indices, productivity measures	Ecosystem restoration, conservation
Cultural	Recreation, spiritual value, aesthetic benefits	Mental Health, physical activity, cultural identity	Psychological stress, social disconnection	Urban populations, marginalised groups	Wellbeing surveys, usage statistics	Access policies, cultural preservation

Table 14.2. Biodiversity loss mechanisms and disease emergence pathways

Mechanism	Ecological Process	Disease Impact	Examples	Geographic Patterns	Prevention Strategies	Evidence Strength
Dilution Effect	Reduced host diversity increases competent reservoir density	Increased transmission efficiency	Lyme disease, West Nile virus	Habitat fragmentation zones	Habitat conservation, restoration	Strong empirical evidence
Vector Predator Loss	Elimination of natural vector control	Increased vector populations	Mosquito-borne diseases, tick-borne diseases	Wetland drainage, amphibian declines	Predator habitat protection	Moderate evidence
Pathogen Competition Loss	Reduced microbial diversity	Reduced natural pathogen suppression	Soilborne diseases, gut pathogen emergence	Agricultural intensification areas	Microbiome conservation	Emerging evidence
Habitat Edge Effects	Altered microhabitat conditions	Modified vector ecology	Forest malaria, leishmaniasis	Deforestation frontiers	Buffer zones, corridor protection	Strong observational evidence
Host Population Density	Concentrated susceptible hosts	Amplified transmission	Rodent-borne diseases	Agricultural conversion areas	Landscape management	Moderate evidence
Genetic Diversity Loss	Reduced disease resistance	Increased outbreak susceptibility	Crop diseases, livestock diseases	Intensive agriculture	Genetic resource conservation	Historical evidence

Pollinator decline represents a specific aspect of biodiversity loss that affects human Health through reduced crop productivity and food security, with implications for nutrition and food access, particularly in regions that depend on insect-pollinated crops for essential nutrients, including vitamins, minerals, and healthy fats. The global decline in bee and other pollinator populations threatens the production of fruits, vegetables, nuts, and oilseeds that provide essential nutrients for human Health while potentially increasing food prices and reducing food access for vulnerable populations.

Conservation strategies that address biodiversity loss while providing human health benefits include habitat protection and restoration that maintain ecosystem services, the creation of wildlife corridors that connect fragmented habitats and facilitate species movement, sustainable agricultural practices that conserve biodiversity while producing food, and urban planning approaches that incorporate biodiversity conservation into development activities. Protected area systems that maintain large, connected habitats can preserve biodiversity while maintaining ecosystem services that support human Health. Still, these systems must be complemented by sustainable management of surrounding landscapes to address edge effects and maintain connectivity.

Restoration activities that re-establish native vegetation and wildlife populations can restore ecosystem services, including disease regulation, while providing additional benefits such as carbon sequestration, improved water quality, and enhanced recreational opportunities. Wetland restoration projects that re-establish diverse aquatic communities can provide natural vector control while improving water quality and flood control services. However, restoration activities must be carefully planned to avoid unintended consequences, including the creation of habitats for disease vectors or reservoir hosts that could increase, rather than decrease, disease risks.

14.3. Pollution and Environmental Health

Environmental pollution represents a significant threat to both ecosystem health and human Health through multiple pathways, including air and water contamination, soil degradation, and disruption of ecological processes that support life-supporting ecosystem services, while creating conditions that may increase vulnerability to infectious diseases and other health threats (Landrigan et al., 2018). The sources of environmental pollution include industrial activities, agricultural practices, transportation systems, waste management, and energy production that release various chemical, biological, and physical contaminants into air, water, and soil systems where they can persist and accumulate while affecting both human and ecological Health through direct toxicity, bioaccumulation, and ecosystem disruption.

Air pollution represents one of the most significant environmental health threats globally, causing an estimated 7 million premature deaths annually through cardiovascular disease, respiratory disease, stroke, and lung cancer, while also affecting ecosystem health through acid deposition, eutrophication, and direct toxicity to vegetation and wildlife. Particulate matter, nitrogen oxides, sulfur dioxide, ozone, and various toxic compounds released from industrial sources, vehicle emissions, and energy production create complex mixtures of air pollutants that affect both human and ecosystem Health while contributing to climate change and other global environmental problems.

Urban air pollution creates particularly severe health impacts due to high population density and concentrated emission sources, with vulnerable populations, including children, elderly individuals, and people with pre-existing health conditions, experiencing disproportionate impacts from air pollution exposure. Delicate particulate matter that can penetrate deep into the lungs and enter the bloodstream causes systemic inflammation and cardiovascular effects, contributing to heart disease, stroke, and other chronic conditions, while also affecting immune function in ways that may increase susceptibility to infectious diseases.

Ecosystem impacts of air pollution include forest decline, reduced crop productivity, eutrophication of aquatic systems, and biodiversity loss, which compromises ecosystem services such as carbon sequestration, water purification, and natural pest control. Acid deposition from sulfur and nitrogen emissions can acidify soils and water bodies while leaching essential nutrients and mobilising toxic metals that affect both plant and animal health. Ground-level ozone formation from nitrogen oxides and volatile organic compounds can damage vegetation while reducing crop yields and forest productivity.

Water pollution from industrial discharges, agricultural runoff, sewage treatment, and urban stormwater affects both human Health and ecosystem health through contamination of drinking water sources, degradation of aquatic habitats, and disruption of marine food webs that support fisheries and other ecosystem services. Chemical contaminants, including heavy metals, pesticides, pharmaceuticals, and industrial chemicals, can persist in aquatic systems while bioaccumulating in fish and other marine organisms that may be consumed by humans or serve as food sources for wildlife.

Nutrient pollution from agricultural fertilisers and animal waste creates eutrophication in lakes, rivers, and coastal waters, which can lead to harmful algal blooms, oxygen depletion, and fish kills that compromise both ecosystem health and human Health through contamination of drinking water and seafood, while eliminating recreational opportunities and ecosystem services. Harmful algal blooms can produce toxins that cause illness in humans through the consumption of contaminated drinking water or recreational water contact, while also causing massive mortality in marine ecosystems and eliminating commercial and recreational fishing opportunities.

Microplastic pollution represents an emerging concern for both ecosystem health and human Health, with plastic particles now found throughout marine and terrestrial food webs, including in seafood, drinking water, and even human tissues. However, the health implications of microplastic exposure are not yet fully understood. Marine plastic pollution affects wildlife through entanglement and ingestion, while potentially providing surfaces for bacterial growth and the transport of chemical contaminants that could impact both the ecosystem and human Health.

Soil contamination from industrial activities, agricultural chemicals, and waste disposal affects ecosystem health through reduced soil fertility, impaired plant growth, and contamination of groundwater systems, while potentially affecting human Health through direct contact, inhalation of contaminated dust, and consumption of contaminated crops. Heavy metals, including lead, mercury, and cadmium, can persist in soils for decades while being taken up by plants and accumulating in food webs, affecting wildlife and human Health. Table 14.3 shows pollution sources, environmental impacts, and health effects.

Table 14.3. Pollution sources, environmental impacts, and health effects

Pollution Type	Primary Sources	Environmental Impacts	Human Health Effects	Vulnerable Ecosystems	Exposed Populations	Control Strategies
Air Pollution	Industry, transportation, energy	Acid rain, ecosystem damage, and climate change	Respiratory disease, cardiovascular disease	Forests, urban areas	Urban populations, children	Emission controls, clean energy
Water Pollution	Industry, agriculture, sewage	Eutrophication, habitat degradation	Waterborne disease, toxic exposure	Freshwater, marine systems	Downstream communities	Treatment systems, source control
Soil Contamination	Industry, mining, agriculture	Reduced fertility, groundwater contamination	Direct contact, food contamination	Agricultural lands, forests	Agricultural workers, residents	Remediation, safe disposal
Chemical Pollution	Manufacturing, agriculture, waste	Bioaccumulation, ecosystem disruption	Endocrine disruption, cancer	Aquatic systems, food webs	Occupational, dietary exposure	Chemical regulation, alternatives
Noise Pollution	Transportation, industry, urban	Wildlife behaviour changes	Sleep disruption, cardiovascular effects	Wildlife habitats	Urban populations	Sound barriers, planning controls
Light Pollution	Urban lighting, industry	Circadian disruption in wildlife	Sleep disorders, health effects	Nocturnal ecosystems	Urban populations	Lighting design, controls

Chemical pollution from industrial processes, agricultural pesticides, and consumer products includes persistent organic pollutants, endocrine-disrupting compounds, and various toxic substances that can accumulate in ecosystems while affecting both wildlife and human Health through multiple exposure pathways. Endocrine-disrupting chemicals that interfere with hormone systems can affect reproduction, development, and immune function in both humans and wildlife, potentially contributing to population declines in sensitive species, such as amphibians and birds.

Pharmaceutical pollution from the use of human and veterinary medicines represents an emerging concern that affects aquatic ecosystems through sewage treatment plant discharges, potentially contributing to the development of antimicrobial resistance in environmental bacteria and impacting reproduction and development in marine organisms. Antibiotics, hormones, and other pharmaceuticals that are not entirely removed by sewage treatment can persist in aquatic environments, potentially affecting ecosystem health and contributing to the spread of antimicrobial resistance genes.

Electronic waste pollution from discarded electronics contains various toxic metals and compounds that can contaminate soils and water, affecting both ecosystems and human Health through informal recycling activities that often occur in low-income communities with limited environmental protection. Heavy metals, including lead, mercury, and cadmium from electronic waste, can persist in the environment while bioaccumulating in food webs and affecting both wildlife and human Health through multiple exposure pathways.

Climate change interactions with pollution create complex synergistic effects that may amplify both environmental and Health impacts through mechanisms including increased temperature effects on chemical toxicity, altered precipitation patterns that affect contaminant transport and persistence, and extreme weather events that can mobilise contaminants while compromising pollution control infrastructure. Rising temperatures can increase the volatilisation and transport of chemical contaminants, potentially enhancing their toxicity to both humans and wildlife.

Prevention and control strategies for pollution-related health impacts require integrated approaches that address pollution sources while protecting both ecosystem and human Health through emission controls, waste treatment systems, safer chemical alternatives, and land use planning that separates pollution sources from sensitive receptors. Pollution prevention approaches that eliminate or reduce contaminant releases at their sources are generally more effective and cost-effective than end-of-pipe treatment approaches while providing benefits for both environmental and human Health.

Regulatory frameworks, including environmental quality standards, emission limits, and chemical safety regulations, provide the legal foundation for pollution control, while requiring monitoring and enforcement systems to ensure compliance and effectiveness. International agreements, including the Stockholm Convention on Persistent Organic Pollutants and the Paris Agreement on Climate Change, provide frameworks for coordinated global action on pollution problems that cross national boundaries and require multilateral solutions (Whitmee et al., 2015).

14.4. One Health and Conservation Medicine

One Health represents a collaborative, multisectoral, and transdisciplinary approach that recognises the interconnection of human, animal, and environmental Health while working locally, nationally, and globally to achieve optimal health outcomes for all three domains through coordinated prevention, surveillance, control, and mitigation of risks and impacts of emerging diseases while addressing broader health challenges that require integration across traditional disciplinary and sectoral boundaries (Zinsstag et al., 2011). Conservation medicine represents a related field that focuses explicitly on the relationships between ecosystem health, wildlife health, and human Health, emphasising how environmental degradation and biodiversity loss affect disease emergence while developing integrated approaches to conservation and Health that can benefit both wildlife populations and human communities.

The conceptual foundations of One Health and conservation medicine recognise that human Health cannot be achieved in isolation from animal health and environmental Health, as these domains share common determinants including environmental quality, biodiversity, climate conditions, and social and economic factors that affect disease emergence and transmission while influencing the capacity of communities and ecosystems to maintain Health and resilience in the face of environmental change. This integrated perspective requires moving beyond traditional biomedical approaches that focus primarily on individual patients to embrace population health approaches that address the social, environmental, and ecological determinants of Health while implementing interventions that can benefit multiple species and ecosystems simultaneously.

Zoonotic disease prevention and control represents one of the most essential applications of One Health approaches, as approximately 75% of emerging infectious diseases have zoonotic origins while requiring coordinated responses across human medicine, veterinary medicine, and wildlife management to address animal reservoirs, environmental factors, and human behavioural factors that contribute to pathogen spillover and transmission. Successful zoonotic disease control programs, including rabies elimination campaigns, brucellosis control programs, and avian influenza surveillance, demonstrate the benefits of integrated approaches that coordinate vaccination, surveillance, and response activities across human and animal health sectors, while addressing environmental and social factors that affect disease transmission.

Antimicrobial resistance represents another critical area where One Health approaches are essential, as resistance genes can move freely between bacteria in human, animal, and environmental settings. In contrast, the use of antimicrobials in any sector can create selection pressures that affect the development and spread of resistance across all industries. Integrated antimicrobial stewardship programs that coordinate use policies, surveillance systems, and research activities across human medicine, veterinary medicine, and agriculture can be more effective than sector-specific approaches while addressing the complex ecological and evolutionary processes that drive resistance development and spread.

Food safety and security applications of One Health approaches address the complex relationships between animal health, environmental quality, and human nutrition that determine both the safety and availability of food supplies while recognising that food production systems affect ecosystem health through land use, water use, and pollution generation that can have feedback effects on food security and safety. An integrated food systems approach that considers environmental sustainability, animal welfare, food safety, and human nutrition simultaneously can identify synergistic interventions that provide benefits across multiple domains while avoiding unintended consequences that might result from narrow sectoral approaches.

Vector-borne disease control represents an area where One Health approaches can integrate human health interventions with wildlife management and environmental management to address the complex ecological factors that determine vector population dynamics and disease transmission patterns. Integrated vector management programs that combine multiple control methods, including habitat modification, biological control, community-based interventions, and targeted chemical applications, can be more effective and sustainable than single-method approaches, while reducing environmental impacts and addressing community preferences and concerns.

Environmental health applications of One Health recognise that environmental quality affects the health of humans, animals, and ecosystems through shared exposure pathways. At the same time, ecological degradation can create conditions that increase disease risks and reduce the capacity of communities and ecosystems to maintain Health and resilience. Air pollution, water contamination, soil degradation, and climate change affect all species while potentially creating synergistic effects that amplify health impacts beyond what would be expected from individual stressors acting alone.

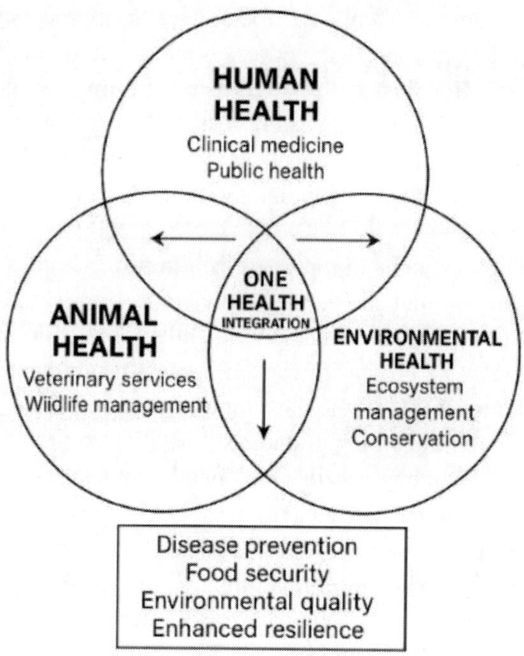

Figure 18. One Health integration framework for ecosystem and human health.

Figure 18 shows A comprehensive systems diagram illustrating the integration of human Health, animal health, and environmental Health within One Health and conservation medicine frameworks. The diagram shows three overlapping circles representing the human health sector (including public Health, clinical medicine, and health policy), the animal health sector (including veterinary medicine, wildlife management, and livestock health), and the environmental health sector (including ecosystem management, environmental science, and conservation). The intersection of all three circles represents collaborative One Health activities, including zoonotic disease surveillance, antimicrobial resistance monitoring, food safety systems, and environmental health assessments. Specific examples are shown around each sector: human Health includes hospitals, public health agencies, and research institutions; animal health includes veterinary services, wildlife agencies, and animal agriculture; environmental Health includes protected areas, environmental monitoring, and ecosystem restoration. The diagram illustrates bidirectional arrows indicating the flow of information, resource sharing, and coordinated interventions between sectors. External factors, including climate change, globalisation, urbanisation, and policy frameworks, are shown to influence all sectors. The bottom of the diagram shows shared outcomes, including reduced disease burden, improved food security, enhanced environmental quality, and increased resilience to global changes.

Surveillance and monitoring systems that integrate One Health approaches can provide more comprehensive detection and characterisation of health threats while enabling coordinated responses that address human, animal, and environmental Health simultaneously. Integrated surveillance systems that share information and coordinate activities between human Health, veterinary, and environmental monitoring systems can detect disease emergence events earlier, providing a better understanding of transmission patterns and risk factors that can inform prevention and control strategies.

Research and development applications of One Health approaches can identify research priorities and develop interventions that address shared health challenges across human, animal, and environmental domains while maximising the impact and efficiency of limited research resources. Transdisciplinary research teams that include expertise from human medicine, veterinary medicine, ecology, social sciences, and other relevant fields can address complex health challenges that cannot be understood or addressed effectively through single-disciplinary approaches.

Education and training programs that prepare health professionals to work in One Health approaches require curricula that integrate knowledge from multiple disciplines while developing skills for collaboration, communication, and systems thinking that enable practical work across sectoral boundaries. Professional development programs for existing practitioners can enhance their capacity for One Health implementation while fostering networks of professionals who can collaborate on integrated health initiatives.

Policy and governance frameworks for One Health implementation require coordination mechanisms that can bring together agencies and organisations with different mandates, priorities, and operating procedures while creating shared objectives and accountability systems that ensure effective collaboration. National One Health strategies and international initiatives, including the One Health Global Network, provide frameworks for coordination while identifying the resources and technical assistance needed for effective implementation.

Economic evaluation of One Health interventions requires methods that can assess costs and benefits across multiple sectors while accounting for the complex interactions and feedback effects that may occur when interventions affect human, animal, and environmental Health simultaneously. Cost-benefit analyses that consider avoided costs from disease prevention, ecosystem service benefits, and broader economic impacts can effectively demonstrate the value of One Health approaches, informing resource allocation decisions and policy development.

Implementation challenges for One Health approaches include institutional barriers that limit collaboration between sectors with different organisational cultures and priorities, funding mechanisms that are organised by industries rather than by shared problems, regulatory frameworks that may not facilitate integrated approaches, and limited capacity for transdisciplinary collaboration among professionals who may lack training and experience in working across sectoral boundaries. Overcoming these challenges requires sustained commitment from leadership in all sectors while developing new institutional arrangements and incentive systems that support integrated approaches.

14.5. Planetary Health Concepts

Planetary Health represents an emerging field that emphasises the fundamental dependence of human Health and civilisation on Earth's natural systems, while recognising that human activities have reached scales that significantly affect the Earth system processes that determine environmental conditions suitable for human Health and wellbeing (Steffen et al., 2015). The planetary health concept builds on earlier frameworks, including ecosystem health and ecological Health, while explicitly addressing the global scale and systemic nature of environmental changes that affect human Health through multiple pathways, including climate change, biodiversity loss, biogeochemical cycle disruption, and pollution, which operate at scales from local to planetary.

The planetary boundaries framework provides a scientific foundation for planetary Health by identifying nine Earth system processes including climate change, biodiversity loss, nitrogen and phosphorus cycles, ocean acidification, land use change, freshwater use, ozone depletion, atmospheric aerosols, and chemical pollution that regulate the stability and resilience of Earth's environment while defining safe operating spaces within which human development can proceed without triggering irreversible environmental changes that could threaten human civilisation. Current evidence suggests that humanity has already crossed planetary boundaries for several of these processes while approaching dangerous thresholds for others, creating unprecedented risks for human Health and wellbeing that require transformative changes in how human societies interact with Earth's natural systems.

Climate change represents the most widely recognised planetary health threat, with human activities including fossil fuel combustion, deforestation, and industrial processes increasing atmospheric greenhouse gas concentrations to levels not experienced for millions of years while triggering temperature increases, precipitation changes, sea level rise, and extreme weather events that affect human Health through direct exposure, food and water security, infectious disease transmission, and social disruption. The health impacts of climate change are already being observed in many regions. In contrast, projected future impacts could affect billions of people through increased heat exposure, water scarcity, food insecurity, and displacement, potentially overwhelming adaptive capacity and compromising health systems.

Biodiversity loss represents another critical planetary health challenge, with current extinction rates far exceeding natural background levels while creating unprecedented disruptions to ecosystem function and stability that affect human Health through reduced ecosystem services, increased disease emergence risks, and loss of genetic resources that provide resilience against environmental changes. The ongoing sixth mass extinction event is eliminating species and ecosystems that have evolved over millions of years, while creating simplified biological communities that may be less stable and resilient than the diverse natural systems they replace.

Biogeochemical cycle disruption, including alterations to nitrogen, phosphorus, and carbon cycles, affects human Health through multiple pathways, including water quality degradation, air pollution, and changes in soil fertility, which have immediate effects that influence food production, environmental quality, and disease transmission patterns. Human activities have approximately doubled the global nitrogen fixation rate while mobilising phosphorus from geological deposits at rates that exceed natural processes by orders of magnitude, creating widespread eutrophication and pollution problems while potentially destabilising biogeochemical cycles that have operated relatively stable for millions of years.

Ocean acidification and marine ecosystem degradation represent planetary-scale changes that affect human Health through the reduced availability of marine protein sources, the compromise of coastal protection services provided by marine ecosystems, and the potential emergence of harmful marine microorganisms that could affect human Health through seafood consumption or recreational water contact. Anthropogenic carbon dioxide emissions are reducing ocean pH, affecting marine organisms such as shellfish, coral reefs, and plankton communities that support marine food webs and provide essential services for human well-being. Table 14.4 illustrates the planetary boundaries and their linkages to human Health.

Freshwater system degradation and water scarcity affect human Health through reduced access to safe drinking water and sanitation, while increasing risks of waterborne diseases and creating conditions for conflict and displacement that can have cascading effects on Health and well-being. Anthropogenic changes to the global hydrological cycle, driven by climate change, land use modification, and direct water extraction, are affecting freshwater availability and quality in many regions, potentially approaching the limits of renewable freshwater resources in some watersheds.

Chemical pollution, including persistent organic pollutants, heavy metals, plastics, and novel synthetic chemicals, represents a planetary-scale change that affects human Health through direct toxicity, endocrine disruption, and ecosystem impacts that can have feedback effects on human Health through compromised ecosystem services. The production and release of synthetic chemicals have increased exponentially over recent decades, while many chemicals persist in the environment and bioaccumulate in food webs, creating global-scale contamination that affects human Health, even in remote regions.

Urban Health represents an essential dimension of planetary Health, as more than half of the global population now lives in urban areas. At the same time, urbanisation continues to accelerate, creating unprecedented concentrations of people and economic activity that can either provide opportunities for improved Health and reduced environmental impact through efficiency gains, or create severe environmental and Health problems through pollution, resource overconsumption, and social inequality. Sustainable urban development that integrates ecological Health, social equity, and economic efficiency represents a critical component of planetary health strategies.

Food system transformation represents a major planetary health priority, as current food production systems are major drivers of climate change, biodiversity loss, water scarcity, and pollution while providing inadequate nutrition for billions of people and contributing to obesity and diet-related diseases in other populations. Sustainable food systems that can provide adequate nutrition for growing populations while operating within planetary boundaries require fundamental changes in agricultural practices, food distribution systems, and consumption patterns that address both environmental sustainability and human Health simultaneously.

Global governance for planetary Health requires international cooperation and coordination on scales that match the planetary scale of environmental changes, while addressing the complex relationships between environmental degradation and human Health that operate across national boundaries and time scales. International agreements, including the Paris Climate Agreement, the Convention on Biological Diversity, and Sustainable Development Goals, provide frameworks for planetary health action while requiring implementation mechanisms that can address the urgent scale and pace of environmental changes affecting human Health.

Transformation pathways for planetary Health require fundamental changes in economic systems, social organisation, and relationship patterns between human societies and natural systems that go beyond incremental improvements in environmental protection or health care delivery to address the root causes of planetary-scale ecological changes that threaten human Health and wellbeing (Watts et al., 2021). These transformations require new models of development that can provide human wellbeing within planetary boundaries while ensuring equitable distribution of benefits and burdens across different populations and regions.

14.6. Sustainable Development Approaches

Sustainable development approaches that integrate environmental sustainability with human Health and wellbeing provide frameworks for addressing ecosystem health and human health challenges simultaneously while recognising the fundamental interdependence of human prosperity and environmental quality in achieving long-term development objectives that can be maintained across generations (Griggs et al., 2013). The Sustainable Development Goals adopted by the United Nations in 2015 provide a comprehensive framework that explicitly recognises these interconnections while establishing specific targets and indicators that address Health, environmental sustainability, and social equity as integrated objectives rather than competing priorities.

Health-focused sustainable development goals, including SDG 3 (Good Health and Well-being), can be achieved without addressing environmental determinants of Health, including clean air and water, safe food systems, stable climate conditions, and healthy ecosystems that provide essential services for human Health and well-being. Conversely, environment-focused goals, including climate action (SDG 13), life below water (SDG 14), and life on land (SDG 15), provide essential foundations for human Health while requiring approaches that consider the health implications of environmental policies and interventions to ensure that ecological protection strategies also support human health objectives.

Integrated approaches to sustainable development require an understanding and addressing of the complex relationships and trade-offs between different development objectives, while identifying synergistic interventions that can advance multiple goals simultaneously through coordinated strategies that optimise benefits across environmental, Health, and social domains. For example, investments in renewable energy systems can simultaneously address climate change, air pollution, and health impacts while providing economic opportunities and energy security that support broader development objectives.

Urban sustainable development represents a critical arena for integrated approaches, as urban areas house more than half of the global population and are responsible for the majority of greenhouse gas emissions, resource consumption, and economic activity worldwide. Sustainable urban development strategies that integrate environmental Health, social equity, and financial efficiency can provide development models that improve human well-being while reducing environmental impact through approaches such as green infrastructure, public transportation, renewable energy systems, and urban agriculture. These approaches

Green infrastructure approaches, including urban forests, parks, green roofs, and constructed wetlands, can provide multiple benefits for urban Health and environmental quality while supporting biodiversity and climate regulation services that contribute to urban resilience and livability. Urban green spaces provide opportunities for physical activity and stress reduction while improving air quality and reducing urban heat island effects that can significantly affect human Health in urban environments. However, green infrastructure must be designed and managed to avoid unintended consequences, including the creation of vector habitats or allergen exposure, which could adversely affect some urban residents.

Sustainable food system development represents another critical area where health and environmental objectives can be integrated through approaches that improve nutrition and food security while reducing the environmental impacts of food production, distribution, and consumption. Sustainable agricultural practices, including agroecology, integrated pest management, and regenerative agriculture, can maintain or improve food production while reducing pesticide use, soil degradation, water pollution, and greenhouse gas emissions that affect both environmental and human Health. Table 14.5 illustrates the integration of Sustainable Development Goals related to Health and the environment.

Nature-based solutions represent innovative approaches to sustainable development that utilise natural systems and processes to address development challenges while providing benefits for human Health, environmental quality, and economic development simultaneously. Examples include wetland restoration for flood control and water treatment, reforestation for climate mitigation and watershed protection, and urban green infrastructure for stormwater management and improving air quality. Nature-based solutions can often provide more cost-effective and resilient alternatives to technological approaches, offering multiple co-benefits that support integrated development objectives.

Circular economy approaches that minimise waste and maximise resource efficiency can reduce environmental impacts while creating economic opportunities and reducing health risks associated with pollution and resource extraction. Circular economy strategies, including industrial symbiosis, product lifecycle extension, and materials recovery, can relieve pressure on natural resources while minimising waste generation and pollution that affect both environmental and human Health.

Community-based approaches to sustainable development recognise that local communities are both the primary beneficiaries and the essential implementers of sustainable development strategies, while ensuring that interventions address regional priorities and conditions, and build local capacity for long-term sustainability. Community-based natural resource management, participatory health programs, and local economic development initiatives can yield more effective and sustainable outcomes than top-down approaches, while respecting cultural values and traditional knowledge systems that contribute to sustainable development objectives.

Table 14.4. Planetary boundaries and human health linkages

Planetary Process	Current Status vs. Boundary	Primary Health Pathways	Health Impact Examples	Vulnerable Regions	Intervention Requirements	Urgency Level
Climate Change	Exceeded (>350 ppm CO2)	Direct exposure, food/water security, disease	Heat illness, malnutrition, vector-borne disease	Small islands, arid regions, and urban areas	Emission reduction, adaptation	Critical
Biodiversity Loss	Far exceeded (>10-100x natural)	Ecosystem services, disease regulation	Reduced natural disease control, loss of medicines	Tropical regions, biodiversity hotspots	Conservation, restoration	Critical
Nitrogen/Phosphorus	Exceeded (>2x natural)	Water quality, air pollution	Waterborne disease, respiratory effects	Agricultural regions, downstream areas	Sustainable agriculture, nutrient management	High
Land Use Change	Approached (>75% ice-free land)	Food security, urban Health	Displacement, food insecurity, disaster risk	Developing countries, coastal areas	Sustainable land management	High
Ocean Acidification	Increasing risk	Marine food security, coastal protection	Protein deficiency, coastal vulnerability	Coastal and island populations	Emission reduction, conservation	High
Freshwater Use	Regional boundaries crossed	Water security, sanitation	Waterborne disease, conflict	Arid regions, megacities	Efficiency, conservation	High
Ozone Depletion	Recovering (policy success)	UV radiation exposure	Skin cancer, immune suppression	High altitude, polar regions	Continued monitoring	Moderate
Atmospheric Aerosols	Poorly quantified	Air quality, climate interactions	Respiratory disease, cardiovascular disease	Urban areas, downwind regions	Emission controls	High
Chemical Pollution	Not quantified	Toxic exposure, ecosystem disruption	Cancer, endocrine disruption	Industrial areas, global	Chemical safety, alternatives	High

Table 14.5. Sustainable development goals - Health and environment integration

SDG	Primary Focus	Health Connections	Environmental Connections	Integration Opportunities	Implementation Challenges	Success Indicators
SDG 3: Good Health	Health and well-being	Direct health outcomes	Environmental Determinants of Health	Healthy environments, disease prevention	Resource constraints, health system capacity	Disease burden reduction, life expectancy
SDG 6: Clean Water	Water and sanitation	Waterborne disease prevention	Watershed protection, aquatic ecosystems	Integrated water management	Infrastructure costs, governance	Universal access, water quality
SDG 11: Sustainable Cities	Urban development	Urban Health, air quality	Urban biodiversity, resource efficiency	Green cities, compact development	Planning capacity, financing	Urban sustainability indices
SDG 13: Climate Action	Climate change mitigation	Climate-sensitive health outcomes	Ecosystem-based adaptation	Nature-based solutions	International cooperation, costs	Emission reduction, adaptation measures
SDG 14: Life Below Water	Marine conservation	Marine food security	Ocean health, biodiversity	Sustainable fisheries, marine protected areas	International governance, enforcement	Marine biodiversity, fisheries sustainability
SDG 15: Life on Land	Terrestrial conservation	Zoonotic disease prevention	Biodiversity, forest conservation	Protected areas, sustainable land use	Land use conflicts, enforcement	Forest cover, species protection

Gender equality and social inclusion are essential dimensions of sustainable development that impact both health outcomes and environmental sustainability through their influence on access to resources, decision-making authority, and vulnerability to environmental changes. Women and marginalised groups often bear disproportionate burdens from ecological degradation while having limited access to resources and decision-making power needed to address environmental challenges. Gender-responsive and socially inclusive approaches to sustainable development can enhance both equity and effectiveness, ensuring that the benefits and burdens of development are distributed fairly across different population groups.

Financing mechanisms for integrated sustainable development require innovative approaches that can mobilise resources for interventions that provide benefits across multiple sectors while addressing the challenge of costs. Benefits may accrue to different actors and over various time scales. Blended financing approaches that combine public and private resources, payment for ecosystem services schemes that compensate landowners for environmental benefits, and green bonds that mobilise investment for ecological projects represent examples of financing innovations that can support integrated sustainable development.

Monitoring and evaluation systems for integrated sustainable development require indicators and methods that can assess progress across multiple domains while capturing the complex relationships and interactions between environmental, Health, and social outcomes. Integrated monitoring systems that track environmental conditions, health outcomes, and social indicators simultaneously can provide a more comprehensive understanding of development progress, while enabling adaptive management approaches that adjust strategies based on monitoring results and changing conditions.

International cooperation for sustainable development requires coordination mechanisms that can address the global scale of environmental and Health challenges while respecting national sovereignty and diverse development priorities and circumstances. International agreements, technology transfer mechanisms, capacity-building programs, and financing facilities provide frameworks for cooperation, while requiring implementation mechanisms that ensure effective coordination and accountability for shared development objectives (McCoy et al., 2009).

Conclusion

Intricate relationships between ecosystem health and human well-being represent fundamental 21st-century challenges that require a comprehensive understanding and integrated responses addressing the complex interdependencies between environmental quality, biodiversity conservation, and human health, while implementing transformative development approaches that sustain both human prosperity and ecological integrity within planetary boundaries. Healthy ecosystems provide essential services that directly support human health through clean air and water, climate regulation, disease control, food security, and mental health benefits. However, ecosystem degradation compromises these services, creating conditions that increase human vulnerability to diseases, natural disasters, and other health threats, disproportionately affecting vulnerable populations.

Biodiversity loss emerges as a particularly critical driver of ecosystem degradation, affecting human health through multiple pathways, including the disruption of natural disease regulation mechanisms, the loss of genetic resources for medicine and agriculture, and the degradation of ecosystem services that support human wellbeing. The ongoing sixth mass extinction represents an unprecedented threat to biological diversity that has evolved over millions of years, while creating simplified ecosystems that are potentially less stable and resilient than diverse natural systems.

Environmental pollution poses significant threats to both ecosystems and human health through air and water contamination, soil degradation, and disruption of ecological processes. One Health and conservation medicine approaches provide essential frameworks for understanding the interconnections between ecosystem health, animal health, and human health through integrated strategies that recognise shared health determinants across human and natural systems.

Planetary health concepts emphasise the fundamental dependence of human health on Earth's natural systems, while recognising that human activities have reached scales that affect Earth system processes, determining environmental conditions suitable for human civilisation. The planetary boundaries framework provides scientific evidence that humanity has exceeded safe operating limits for several critical Earth system processes while approaching dangerous thresholds for others.

The Sustainable Development Goals provide comprehensive frameworks for integrated action, requiring implementation approaches that address complex relationships and potential trade-offs between different development objectives. Future challenges include the impacts of climate change, the continued loss of biodiversity, which threatens ecosystem services, the increasing risks of disease emergence, persistent pollution problems, and the growing global population and consumption, both of which are increasing pressure on natural systems.

COVID-19 provided stark reminders of the connections between ecosystem health and human health, while demonstrating both human vulnerability to disease emergence associated with environmental degradation and the potential for coordinated global action. Success requires a fundamental recognition that ecosystem health and human well-being are mutually dependent objectives, requiring integrated approaches that enhance both environmental sustainability and human prosperity.

Acknowledgments

The authors would like to extend our appreciation to those who offered helpful commentary during the drafting process of this manuscript. We also acknowledge the role Nova Science Publishers played in enabling the work described herein.

References

Butler, C. D., Corvalan, C. F., & Koren, H. S. (2014). Human Health, wellbeing, and global ecological scenarios. *EcoHealth*, 2(4), 316-318. https://doi.org/10.1007/s10393-005-8150-9.

Cardinale, B. J., Duffy, J. E., Gonzalez, A., Hooper, D. U., Perrings, C., Venail, P., & Naeem, S. (2012). Biodiversity loss and its impact on humanity. *Nature*, 486(7401), 59-67. https://doi.org/10.1038/nature11148.

Griggs, D., Stafford-Smith, M., Gaffney, O., Rockström, J., Öhman, M. C., Shyamsundar, P., & Noble, I. (2013). Sustainable development goals for people and planet. *Nature*, 495(7441), 305-307. https://doi.org/10.1038/495305a.

Landrigan, P. J., Fuller, R., Acosta, N. J., Adeyi, O., Arnold, R., Basu, N. N., & Zhong, M. (2018). The Lancet Commission on pollution and Health. *The Lancet*, 391(10119), 462-512. https://doi.org/10.1016/S0140-6736(17)32345-0.

McCoy, D., Chand, S., & Sridhar, D. (2009). Global health funding: how much, where it comes from and where it goes. *Health Policy and Planning*, 24(6), 407-417. https://doi.org/10.1093/heapol/czp026.

Millennium Ecosystem Assessment. (2005). *Ecosystems and human wellbeing: synthesis*. Island Press. https://www.millenniumassessment.org/documents/document.356.aspx.pdf.

Myers, S. S., Gaffikin, L., Golden, C. D., Ostfeld, R. S., Redford, K. H., Ricketts, T. H., & Osofsky, S. A. (2013). Human health impacts of ecosystem alteration. *Proceedings of the National Academy of Sciences*, 110(47), 18753-18760. https://doi.org/10.1073/pnas.1218656110.

Steffen, W., Richardson, K., Rockström, J., Cornell, S. E., Fetzer, I., Bennett, E. M., & Sörlin, S. (2015). Planetary boundaries: guiding human development on a changing planet. *Science*, 347(6223), 1259855. https://doi.org/10.1126/science.1259855.

Watts, N., Amann, M., Arnell, N., Ayeb-Karlsson, S., Beagley, J., Belesova, K., & Costello, A. (2021). The 2020 report of The Lancet Countdown on Health and climate change: responding to converging crises. *The Lancet*, 397(10269), 129-170. https://doi.org/10.1016/S0140-6736(20)32290-X.

Whitmee, S., Haines, A., Beyrer, C., Boltz, F., Capon, A. G., de Souza Dias, B. F., & Yach, D. (2015). Safeguarding human Health in the Anthropocene epoch: report of The Rockefeller Foundation–Lancet Commission on planetary Health. *The Lancet*, 386(10007), 1973-2028. https://doi.org/10.1016/S0140-6736(15)60901-1.

World Health Organization. (2018). *Ambient (outdoor) air quality and Health*. World Health Organization. https://www.who.int/news-room/fact-sheets/detail/ambient-(outdoor)-air-quality-and-health.

World Health Organization. (2019). *Ten threats to global Health in 2019*. World Health Organization. https://www.who.int/news-room/spotlight/ten-threats-to-global-health-in-2019.

World Health Organization & Convention on Biological Diversity. (2015). *Connecting global priorities: biodiversity and human Health*. World Health Organization. https://www.who.int/publications/i/item/connecting-global-priorities-biodiversity-and-human-health.

Zinsstag, J., Schelling, E., Waltner-Toews, D., & Tanner, M. (2011). From "one medicine" to "one health" and systemic approaches to Health and wellbeing. *Preventive Veterinary Medicine*, 101(3-4), 148-156. https://doi.org/10.1016/j.prevetmed.2010.07.003.

Chapter 15

Community Engagement and Participatory One Health

Pratap Bhan Kaushik[1]
and Maajid Mohi Ud Din Malik[2,*]**, PhD**

[1]Department of Community Medicine, Dr. D. Y. Patil Medical College, Hospital and Research Centre, Dr. D. Y. Patil Vidyapeeth, Pune (Deemed to be University)- Sant Tukaram Nagar, Pimpri, Pune, India
[2]Department of Radiology and Imaging Technology, Dr. D. Y. Patil School of Allied Health Sciences, Dr. D. Y. Patil Vidyapeeth, Pune (Deemed to be University), Sant Tukaram Nagar, Pimpri, Pune, India

Abstract

Community engagement and participatory approaches are essential components of effective One Health implementation, recognising communities as active partners rather than passive recipients of health interventions. This approach acknowledges that sustainable health improvements require meaningful participation from all stakeholders who are affected by or can influence health outcomes across human, animal, and environmental domains. Community-based One Health initiatives demonstrate how local knowledge, resources, and leadership can be effectively mobilised to address complex health challenges that span multiple sectors, ensuring that interventions are culturally appropriate, contextually relevant, and sustainable over time. Indigenous knowledge systems and traditional practices offer valuable insights into sustainable relationships among human Health, animal health, and environmental Health, which have been developed and refined over generations. These insights provide alternative approaches to Health and development that complement and enhance scientific knowledge, while respecting cultural values and community autonomy. Effective stakeholder engagement strategies require the systematic identification and inclusion of all relevant actors, including community members, traditional leaders, healthcare providers, veterinarians, environmental managers, government officials, and civil society organisations, while creating collaborative processes that enable meaningful participation in decision-making about health interventions and policies. Cultural competency in health programs involves understanding and respecting diverse cultural beliefs, practices, and social structures that influence health behaviours and outcomes. This understanding enables the development of interventions that are aligned with community values and preferences, rather than imposing external models that may be inappropriate or unsustainable. Participatory research methods would allow communities to be active participants in generating knowledge about their own health challenges and solutions while building local capacity for ongoing health

* Corresponding Author's Email: maajid.malik@dpu.edu.in

In: Advances in the One Health Approach
Editors: Maajid Mohi Ud Din Malik, Abhay Saraf, Harshal Tukaram Pandve et al.
ISBN: 979-8-90134-202-2

improvement and problem-solving that can continue beyond specific project cycles. Building trust and sustainable partnerships requires a long-term commitment, transparent communication, shared decision-making, and mutual respect that acknowledges the expertise and contributions of all partners, while addressing power imbalances and structural inequities that may limit community participation and hinder the benefits of health interventions.

Keywords: community engagement, participatory Health, One Health, indigenous knowledge, stakeholder engagement, cultural competency, participatory research, community partnerships, Sustainable Development Goal 3, health equity

Introduction

Community engagement and participatory approaches to One Health represent fundamental shifts from top-down, expert-driven models of health intervention toward collaborative frameworks that recognise communities as essential partners in identifying health challenges, designing appropriate solutions, and implementing sustainable interventions that address the interconnected nature of human, animal, and environmental Health (Laverack, 2013). The recognition that health outcomes are determined by complex interactions among biological, environmental, social, and cultural factors necessitates approaches that engage communities as active participants in understanding and addressing these determinants, while respecting local knowledge, values, and priorities that may differ from external professional perspectives. Community engagement in One Health acknowledges that effective and sustainable health improvements cannot be achieved through technical interventions alone but require social mobilisation, behaviour change, and community ownership that can only be developed through meaningful participation in all phases of intervention design, implementation, and evaluation. The diversity of communities affected by One Health challenges, ranging from rural agricultural communities to urban settlements, indigenous populations to immigrant groups, requires flexible and adaptive engagement approaches that can respond to different cultural contexts, social structures, and community priorities while maintaining core principles of participation, empowerment, and respect for community autonomy. Participatory One Health approaches recognise that communities possess valuable knowledge about local health challenges, environmental conditions, and cultural practices that influence health outcomes, while also acknowledging that communities have the right and responsibility to make informed decisions about interventions that affect their Health and wellbeing. Success in implementing participatory One Health requires sustained commitment to building relationships, developing trust, sharing power, and creating mechanisms for community voice and influence that can transform traditional professional-community dynamics while achieving health improvements that are meaningful, sustainable, and equitable for all community members.

15.1. Community-Based One Health Initiatives

Community-based One Health initiatives represent locally driven approaches to addressing health challenges that recognise the interconnected nature of human, animal, and environmental

Health, while mobilising community resources, knowledge, and leadership to develop and implement contextually appropriate solutions that are sustainable and responsive to local priorities and conditions (Zinsstag et al., 2015). These initiatives demonstrate how communities can serve as primary agents of change in improving health outcomes across multiple domains while building local capacity for ongoing problem identification, solution development, and program implementation that continues beyond external project support.

Successful community-based One Health initiatives typically emerge from community-identified priorities rather than externally imposed agendas, beginning with participatory assessment processes that enable communities to identify and prioritise health challenges that affect human, animal, and environmental Health within their local context while considering the complex relationships and interactions between these different health domains. These assessments often reveal health challenges that span traditional sectoral boundaries and require integrated approaches that address multiple factors simultaneously, such as zoonotic disease transmission associated with livestock management practices, water quality issues that affect both human and animal health, or environmental degradation that increases disease transmission risks while reducing livelihood opportunities.

Community health worker programs represent one crucial model for community-based One Health implementation, training community members to serve as bridges between formal health services and community needs while providing integrated services that address human Health, animal health, and environmental Health within a unified framework. These programs recognise that health challenges in many communities cannot be addressed effectively through separate human health and veterinary services but require integrated approaches that consider the relationships between human and animal Health while addressing environmental factors that affect both. Community health workers who are trained in One Health approaches can provide more comprehensive and effective services while building community capacity for ongoing health improvement.

Livestock vaccination campaigns that integrate human health education and services demonstrate how community-based initiatives can address multiple health objectives simultaneously while maximising efficiency and community engagement. These campaigns can provide animal vaccinations that prevent the transmission of zoonotic diseases while also delivering human health services, including immunisations, health screenings, and health education, that address related health issues. The integration of human and animal health services can improve coverage and reduce costs while demonstrating the practical benefits of One Health approaches to community members.

Water and sanitation projects that address human Health, animal health, and environmental Health simultaneously illustrate how community-based initiatives can tackle complex challenges that require integrated solutions involving multiple stakeholders and technical approaches. Community-managed water systems that provide safe water for human consumption while also addressing livestock watering needs and promoting environmental protection can achieve numerous objectives, thereby building community capacity for ongoing system management and maintenance. Table 15.1 presents community-based One Health initiative models and implementation approaches.

Zoonotic disease surveillance and response initiatives that engage communities as active participants in disease detection and reporting can improve early warning systems while building community capacity for disease prevention and control. Community members who are trained to recognise signs of zoonotic diseases in animals and humans can provide early detection, enabling a rapid response while also implementing prevention measures that reduce transmission risks. These initiatives require trust between communities and health authorities, along with feedback systems that demonstrate how community reporting contributes to disease prevention and control efforts.

Environmental conservation initiatives that explicitly address human Health and animal health benefits can mobilise community support for conservation while demonstrating the practical benefits of ecosystem protection for community wellbeing. Community-managed protected areas, reforestation projects, and sustainable resource management programs that emphasise health benefits can achieve conservation objectives while providing economic and Health benefits that sustain community engagement and support.

School-based One Health education programs can foster an understanding of the connections between human, animal, and environmental Health among young people, while also creating opportunities for community engagement through students' families and broader social networks. These programs can combine formal education with practical activities, including school gardens, animal care, and environmental monitoring that demonstrate One Health principles while building knowledge and skills that students can apply in their families and communities.

Community-based research initiatives that engage community members as co-researchers can generate knowledge about local One Health challenges while building community capacity for ongoing problem identification and solution development. These initiatives recognise that community members possess valuable knowledge about local conditions and can contribute meaningfully to research design, data collection, and interpretation, while building local capacity for evidence-based decision-making.

Challenges in implementing community-based One Health initiatives include coordinating across multiple sectors and stakeholder groups with different priorities and operating procedures, securing sustainable funding for long-term community engagement and capacity building activities, addressing technical capacity limitations that may require ongoing professional support, and balancing community autonomy with technical requirements for effective health interventions. Successful initiatives typically require flexible implementation approaches that can adapt to changing community needs and contexts while maintaining core commitments to community participation and empowerment.

Evaluation of community-based One Health initiatives requires indicators that capture both health outcomes and process outcomes, including community participation, capacity building, and sustainability of community-led activities (Conrad et al., 2013). Process evaluation is particularly important for understanding how community engagement contributes to health outcomes while identifying lessons learned that can inform replication and scaling of successful approaches.

15.2. Indigenous Knowledge and Traditional Practices

Indigenous knowledge systems and traditional practices represent sophisticated frameworks for understanding and managing relationships between human Health, animal health, and environmental Health that have been developed and refined over generations through direct experience and observation of local ecosystems and their effects on community wellbeing

(Berkes, 2012). These knowledge systems offer valuable insights into sustainable approaches to Health and development that are often more holistic and integrated than conventional sectoral approaches, while providing culturally appropriate and contextually relevant solutions that have been tested and adapted over long periods of time.

Traditional ecological knowledge encompasses a detailed understanding of local ecosystems, including plant and animal species, ecological relationships, seasonal patterns, and environmental changes that affect the availability and quality of natural resources used for food, medicine, and other purposes essential for community health and wellbeing. This knowledge often includes a sophisticated understanding of ecological indicators that signal environmental changes affecting human and animal Health, traditional management practices that maintain ecosystem health while providing sustainable resource use, and integrated approaches to resource management that consider multiple objectives simultaneously.

Traditional medicine systems represent comprehensive approaches to Health that often integrate understanding of human Health with knowledge of medicinal plants, animal-derived medicines, and environmental factors that influence Health and disease, while providing culturally appropriate treatment approaches that may be more accessible and acceptable to community members than formal healthcare services. These systems typically include diagnostic approaches that consider environmental and social factors in addition to physical symptoms. These treatment protocols combine plant-based medicines with dietary recommendations and lifestyle modifications, as well as prevention strategies that emphasise maintaining balance and harmony between individuals and their environment.

Traditional livestock management practices often demonstrate integrated approaches to animal health, human Health, and environmental Health that maintain productive and sustainable agricultural systems while preventing disease transmission and ecological degradation. These practices may include rotational grazing systems that maintain pasture health while preventing overgrazing, traditional breeding practices that maintain genetic diversity and disease resistance, and integrated pest and disease management approaches that combine multiple prevention and treatment strategies.

Traditional food systems that combine crop production, livestock management, wild resource harvesting, and food processing typically provide diverse and nutritious diets while maintaining ecological sustainability and cultural identity. These systems often incorporate a sophisticated understanding of the seasonal availability and nutritional properties of different foods, traditional food preservation and preparation techniques that maintain food safety and nutritional value, as well as social institutions that ensure food security and equitable distribution within communities.

Indigenous governance systems and social institutions that manage natural resources and community health often provide models for participatory and sustainable management approaches that integrate multiple stakeholder perspectives while maintaining accountability and transparency in decision-making processes. These systems typically include traditional authorities and decision-making processes that consider long-term sustainability and community wellbeing, conflict resolution mechanisms that address disputes over resource use and management, and institutions that maintain and transmit knowledge across generations. Table 15.2 illustrates indigenous knowledge domains and their contributions to One Health.

Table 15.1. Community-based one health initiative models and implementation approaches

Initiative Type	Primary Activities	Target Health Domains	Community Roles	Professional Roles	Sustainability Factors	Success Indicators
Community Health Worker Programs	Training, service delivery, and health education	Human, animal, environmental	Service provision, peer education, community mobilisation	Training, supervision, technical support	Community ownership, continued training, integration with health systems	Coverage rates, health outcomes, and community satisfaction
Integrated Vaccination Campaigns	Animal vaccination, human immunisation, health promotion	Human, animal	Community mobilisation, logistical support, follow-up	Technical delivery, training, and planning	Regular campaigns, supply systems, and community demand	Vaccination coverage, disease reduction, and community participation
Water and Sanitation Projects	Infrastructure development, hygiene promotion, and environmental protection	Human, animal, environmental	Construction, maintenance, behaviour change	Technical design, training, quality assurance	Community management, financial sustainability, and technical support	Water quality, health outcomes, system functionality
Zoonotic Disease Surveillance	Community reporting, case identification, and response coordination	Human, animal	Surveillance activities, reporting, and community education	Training, laboratory support, and investigation	Community engagement, reporting systems, and response capacity	Detection timeliness, response effectiveness, and community participation
Environmental Conservation	Habitat protection, restoration, and sustainable use	Environmental, human, animal	Conservation activities, monitoring, and enforcement	Technical guidance, policy support, and financing	Community benefits, governance systems, and economic incentives	Ecological indicators, community livelihoods, conservation outcomes

Table 15.2. Indigenous knowledge domains and contributions to One Health

Knowledge Domain	Traditional Practices	One Health Contributions	Modern Applications	Integration Challenges	Validation Approaches	Preservation Strategies
Medicinal Plants	Herbal medicine, pharmacology	Natural product drug discovery	Pharmaceutical development, traditional medicine integration	Intellectual property, standardisation	Ethnobotanical studies, clinical trials	Documentation, cultivation, and youth education
Ecosystem Management	Rotational use, conservation practices	Sustainable resource management	Conservation strategies, ecosystem restoration	Scale differences, regulatory conflicts	Ecological monitoring, impact assessment	Traditional governance, community protocols
Animal Husbandry	Breeding, healthcare, and feeding	Sustainable livestock systems	Genetic conservation, disease prevention	Technology integration, market access	Breeding records, health monitoring	Farmer training, breed conservation
Food Systems	Crop diversity, processing, preservation	Nutrition security, food safety	Crop breeding, food security	Modernisation pressures, climate change	Nutritional analysis, yield studies	Seed banking, cultural practices
Environmental Indicators	Weather prediction, ecosystem health	Early warning systems	Climate adaptation, monitoring	Scientific validation, communication	Comparative studies, indicator development	Knowledge documentation, training
Social Institutions	Governance, conflict resolution	Participatory management	Community engagement, policy development	Power structures, legal recognition	Institutional analysis, outcome assessment	Leadership development, institutional strengthening

Climate change adaptation strategies developed by indigenous communities often demonstrate innovative approaches to managing environmental variability and change, which can inform broader adaptation efforts while maintaining cultural practices and enhancing community resilience. These strategies may include diversification of livelihood activities to reduce vulnerability to environmental changes, modification of traditional practices to respond to changing environmental conditions, and development of new practices that combine traditional knowledge with new information about environmental changes.

Integration of indigenous knowledge with scientific knowledge and modern health approaches requires respectful and collaborative processes that recognise the validity and value of both knowledge systems while addressing potential conflicts or contradictions between different approaches. Successful integration typically involves dialogue between knowledge holders from various traditions, collaborative research that combines different methodologies and perspectives, and development of hybrid methods that incorporate elements from multiple knowledge systems.

Intellectual property and benefit-sharing considerations are crucial when working with indigenous knowledge, necessitating clear agreements on how knowledge will be utilised, how benefits will be shared, and how communities will maintain control over their knowledge while potentially contributing to broader health and development objectives. These considerations require an understanding of international frameworks, including the Convention on Biological Diversity and traditional knowledge protocols, while respecting community preferences regarding knowledge sharing and commercialisation.

Documentation and preservation of indigenous knowledge requires approaches that respect community preferences about what knowledge should be shared and how it should be transmitted while building capacity for ongoing knowledge development and adaptation. Community-based documentation projects that train community members to record and preserve their own knowledge can be more appropriate and sustainable than external documentation efforts, ensuring that communities maintain control over their own knowledge.

Capacity building for indigenous knowledge preservation and application may include training programs for young community members, development of community-based education systems that combine traditional and modern knowledge, and creation of institutions that can maintain and adapt traditional expertise while engaging with contemporary health and development systems. These efforts require long-term commitment and resources while respecting community autonomy and cultural values.

Challenges in incorporating indigenous knowledge into One Health approaches include addressing scepticism from professional communities about the validity and reliability of traditional knowledge, overcoming communication barriers between different knowledge traditions, addressing power imbalances that may limit indigenous community participation in health and development programs, and ensuring that integration processes do not undermine or appropriate indigenous knowledge without providing proper benefits to knowledge holders.

15.3. Stakeholder Engagement Strategies

Stakeholder engagement represents a fundamental component of successful One Health implementation that requires systematic identification, analysis, and inclusion of all actors who are affected by or can influence health outcomes across human, animal, and environmental domains while creating collaborative processes that enable meaningful participation in decision-making about health interventions and policies (Reed, 2008). Effective stakeholder engagement recognises that One Health challenges involve multiple sectors, disciplines, and communities with different perspectives, priorities, and resources while requiring coordination and collaboration that can bridge these differences to achieve shared health objectives.

Stakeholder identification and mapping processes provide systematic approaches to identifying all relevant actors and understanding their roles, interests, influence, and relationships within One Health systems while ensuring that engagement processes include all stakeholders who should participate in collaborative decision-making. These processes typically begin with the broad categorisation of stakeholder groups, including community members, traditional leaders, healthcare providers, veterinarians, environmental managers, government officials, civil society organisations, private sector actors, and academic institutions, while recognising that stakeholder configurations may vary significantly between different contexts and health challenges.

Primary stakeholders typically include those who are directly affected by One Health challenges and interventions, such as community members who experience health risks, livestock owners whose animals may be affected by disease control measures, healthcare workers who must implement new protocols, and environmental managers who must integrate health considerations into natural resource management activities. These stakeholders often have the strongest interest in One Health outcomes, while also possessing valuable knowledge about local conditions and constraints that affect the feasibility and effectiveness of interventions.

Secondary stakeholders may include those who are indirectly affected by One Health challenges and interventions or who can influence outcomes through their professional roles, resources, or decision-making authority, such as government officials who control policy and funding decisions. These civil society organisations advocate for specific constituencies, private sector actors who provide goods and services, and academic institutions that generate knowledge and train professionals. While secondary stakeholders may have less direct interest in specific One Health outcomes, their support and cooperation are often crucial for the successful implementation of interventions.

Stakeholder analysis processes examine the interests, influence, and relationships of different stakeholders, identifying potential areas of collaboration and conflict that may impact the implementation of One Health. This analysis typically considers each stakeholder's primary interests and priorities related to One Health challenges, their level of influence or decision-making authority that can affect intervention outcomes, their resources and capacities that can contribute to intervention success, and their relationships with other stakeholders that may facilitate or hinder collaboration.

Engagement strategy development requires tailored approaches that respond to the diverse characteristics, interests, and preferences of different stakeholders, while ensuring that all stakeholders have appropriate opportunities for meaningful participation in One Health activities. These strategies typically consider various levels of engagement, ranging from information sharing to consultation, to collaboration, and community control. In contrast, matching engagement approaches to stakeholder preferences and the nature of the decisions being made.

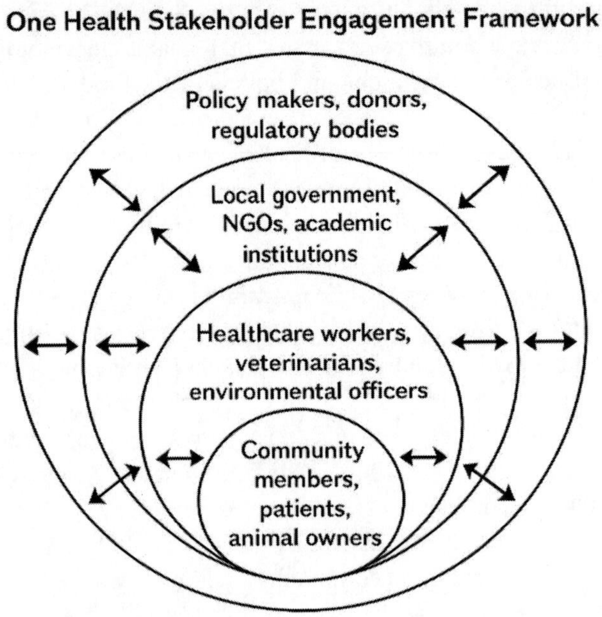

Figure 19. Comprehensive stakeholder engagement framework for One Health.

Figure 19 illustrates a multi-layered stakeholder engagement model, depicting the complex network of actors involved in One Health initiatives. The diagram shows concentric circles representing different levels of engagement, with the core containing primary beneficiaries (community members, patients, animal owners). The next ring shows direct implementers (healthcare workers, veterinarians, environmental officers, community health workers). The middle ring contains supporting institutions (local government, NGOs, academic institutions, private sector partners). The outer ring shows enabling stakeholders (policy makers, international donors, regulatory bodies, professional associations). Bidirectional arrows indicate the flow of information, resource sharing, and collaborative relationships among all levels of the organisation. The diagram emphasises different engagement mechanisms, including community meetings, technical working groups, policy consultations, multi-stakeholder platforms, and knowledge-sharing networks. Specific examples are provided for each stakeholder category, showing their unique contributions and interests. The framework demonstrates how engagement strategies must be tailored to different stakeholder groups while maintaining coordination and communication across all levels to achieve integrated One Health outcomes.

Multi-stakeholder platforms represent essential mechanisms for bringing together diverse stakeholders to address One Health challenges through collaborative planning, implementation, and evaluation processes that can coordinate activities across sectors while building shared understanding and commitment to One Health objectives. These platforms may operate at different scales, ranging from local community committees to national One Health networks, while providing forums for dialogue, joint problem-solving, and coordinated action that can address complex health challenges requiring multisectoral responses.

Community engagement strategies within broader stakeholder engagement frameworks require particular attention to ensuring that community voices are heard and respected within multi-stakeholder processes while avoiding tokenism or superficial consultation that does not provide communities with meaningful influence over decisions that affect their Health and wellbeing. Effective community engagement may require separate community processes that build community capacity and consensus before engaging in broader multi-stakeholder forums, while ensuring that community representatives have adequate support and resources to participate effectively.

Government engagement strategies must address the complex institutional arrangements and political considerations that influence government participation in One Health initiatives, while building support from various government sectors and levels that may have different priorities and operating procedures. Government engagement may require separate discussions with multiple ministries and agencies to identify champions and build coalitions that support One Health approaches within government systems.

Private sector engagement strategies must address the business interests and constraints that affect private sector participation while identifying opportunities for mutual benefit that can sustain private sector involvement in One Health initiatives. Private sector engagement may involve pharmaceutical companies, food producers, agricultural input suppliers, technology companies, and other businesses that can contribute resources, expertise, or market access to support One Health objectives while achieving their own business objectives.

Conflict resolution and negotiation processes may be necessary when stakeholders have competing interests or disagreements about One Health priorities and approaches, requiring facilitation processes that can help stakeholders identify common ground while addressing legitimate differences in perspectives and priorities. These processes may involve neutral facilitators who can help stakeholders communicate effectively while developing agreements that balance different interests and priorities.

Communication and feedback systems are crucial for sustaining stakeholder engagement over time, ensuring that stakeholders receive information about One Health activities and outcomes that demonstrate the value of their participation and contributions. These systems must be adaptable to different stakeholder preferences and communication channels, while providing regular opportunities for stakeholder input and feedback that can enhance the implementation of One Health.

Monitoring and evaluation of stakeholder engagement processes should assess both the quality of engagement processes and their contribution to One Health outcomes while identifying lessons learned that can improve future engagement efforts. This evaluation may include indicators of stakeholder participation, satisfaction with engagement processes, changes in stakeholder knowledge and attitudes, and contributions of stakeholder engagement to improved health outcomes (Doherty & Clayton, 2011).

15.4. Cultural Competency in Health Programs

Cultural competency in health programs encompasses the knowledge, skills, and attitudes that enable health professionals and organisations to work effectively with people from diverse cultural backgrounds, while respecting the cultural beliefs, practices, and social structures that influence health behaviours and outcomes (Beach et al., 2006). In One Health contexts, cultural competency requires understanding how different cultures conceptualise relationships between human Health, animal health, and environmental Health while developing interventions that are aligned with cultural values and practices rather than imposing external models that may be inappropriate or unsustainable within specific cultural contexts.

Cultural assessment processes provide systematic approaches to understanding the cultural factors that may influence One Health program implementation and outcomes while identifying opportunities for cultural adaptation that can improve program relevance and effectiveness. These assessments typically examine cultural beliefs about Health and illness causation, traditional practices related to human and animal healthcare, social structures and decision-making processes that affect health-related behaviours, communication patterns and preferences that influence health education and promotion activities, and cultural values and priorities that may affect the acceptance of health interventions.

Health beliefs and explanatory models vary significantly across cultures, encompassing a range of concepts that include biomedical perspectives, traditional healing theories, spiritual and religious frameworks, and integrated approaches that combine multiple perspectives on health and illness causation. Understanding these belief systems is crucial for developing health interventions that align with cultural understanding while addressing potential conflicts between traditional and biomedical approaches, which can impact the acceptance and effectiveness of interventions.

Traditional healing systems and practices represent critical cultural resources that can complement or conflict with formal health services, providing culturally appropriate treatment options that may be more accessible and acceptable to community members than conventional medical care. Cultural competency requires understanding these traditional systems and identifying opportunities for collaboration and integration that can improve overall health outcomes while respecting traditional healing practices and the practitioners who employ them.

Social structures and relationships, including family systems, community leadership, gender roles, and authority patterns, significantly influence health-related decision-making and behaviour change, while affecting who can participate in health programs and how health interventions should be designed and implemented. Cultural competency requires understanding these social dynamics and adapting program approaches to work effectively within existing social structures while addressing potential barriers to participation that may affect specific population groups.

Language and communication considerations are crucial for culturally competent health programs, necessitating not only the literal translation of health information but also its cultural adaptation to ensure that messages are appropriate and meaningful within specific cultural contexts. Effective cross-cultural communication may require an understanding of nonverbal communication patterns, cultural norms for discussing sensitive health topics, and proper channels and messengers for health information within specific cultural groups. Table 15.3 illustrates the cultural competency components and their application in one health program.

Religious and spiritual considerations can significantly influence health beliefs and practices, affecting the acceptance of specific health interventions that may conflict with religious teachings or spiritual practices. Cultural competency requires understanding these religious and spiritual dimensions while identifying approaches that respect religious beliefs while achieving health objectives through culturally appropriate methods.

Gender and age considerations reflect cultural variations in gender roles, age-based authority, and access to resources and decision-making, which can significantly impact who can participate in health programs and how interventions should be designed to effectively reach different population groups. Cultural competency requires understanding these demographic factors while developing targeted approaches that can address the specific needs and constraints of various groups within communities.

Economic and livelihood considerations reflect cultural values and practices related to resource use, financial activities, and household decision-making, which can impact the feasibility and sustainability of health interventions, as well as influence community priorities and resource allocation decisions. Cultural competency requires understanding these economic dimensions while designing interventions that are compatible with local livelihood systems and financial constraints.

Adaptation strategies for cultural competency may include modification of intervention content to align with cultural beliefs and practices, adjustment of implementation approaches to work within existing social structures and communication patterns, training of program staff in cultural competency skills and knowledge, partnership with cultural leaders and organisations that can provide cultural guidance and community access, and development of culturally appropriate evaluation methods that capture meaningful outcomes within specific cultural contexts.

Training and capacity building for cultural competency should address both individual competency development for health professionals and organisational competency development for health programs and institutions that can create supportive environments for culturally competent practice. Personal training may include cultural awareness education, cross-cultural communication skills, and specific knowledge about the cultural groups served by health programs. Organisational development, on the other hand, may encompass policy development, staff recruitment and retention, and program design processes that incorporate cultural considerations.

Quality assurance for culturally competent health programs requires monitoring and evaluation approaches that assess both the cultural appropriateness of program processes and their effectiveness in achieving health outcomes within specific cultural contexts. This may include community feedback processes, cultural competency assessments for program staff, and outcome evaluation that considers cultural factors that may influence program effectiveness and sustainability.

15.5. Participatory Research Methods

Participatory research methods in One Health represent collaborative approaches to knowledge generation that engage communities, practitioners, and other stakeholders as active participants in research design, implementation, and interpretation while building local capacity for ongoing problem identification, solution development, and evidence-based decision making that can continue beyond specific research projects (Cargo & Mercer, 2008). These methods recognise that communities and practitioners possess valuable knowledge and expertise that can contribute to research, while also acknowledging that research should address questions and priorities relevant and beneficial to the people affected by the research findings.

Community-based participatory research (CBPR) approaches in One Health contexts involve partnerships between researchers and communities, engaging community members as co-researchers who participate in all phases of the research process, from problem identification and research question development through data collection, analysis, and dissemination of findings. These partnerships recognise that communities possess detailed knowledge of local health challenges, environmental conditions, and social factors that affect health outcomes, while also having the capacity to contribute meaningfully to research activities when provided with appropriate training and support.

Participatory action research (PAR) combines research activities with action for social change, engaging participants in investigating their own conditions while developing and implementing interventions to address identified problems. In One Health contexts, PAR approaches may involve communities in researching local zoonotic disease risks while simultaneously implementing prevention measures, investigating environmental health hazards to develop community-based solutions, or studying traditional health practices to strengthen their integration with formal health services.

Participatory epidemiology represents a specific application of participatory research methods that engages communities and animal owners in collecting and analysing health data about human and animal populations while building local capacity for disease surveillance and response. These approaches may involve training community members to recognise and report disease symptoms, collect biological samples, and participate in outbreak investigations while contributing to broader surveillance systems that can detect and respond to health threats more effectively than conventional surveillance approaches.

Photovoice and visual methods enable participants to document their experiences and perspectives on health challenges through photography, video, and other visual media, providing powerful tools for community education and advocacy that can raise awareness about health issues and mobilise support for interventions. In One Health contexts, these methods may be used to document environmental health hazards, human-animal interactions that affect Health, or community assets and resources that can contribute to health improvement.

Digital storytelling approaches enable communities to create multimedia narratives about their health experiences and perspectives, providing accessible methods for sharing knowledge and advocating for change that can reach diverse audiences, including policymakers, funders, and other communities facing similar challenges. These approaches may be particularly valuable for documenting indigenous knowledge and traditional practices while building support for community-based health interventions. Table 15.4 illustrates participatory research methods and their applications in One Health.

Participatory mapping and geographic information systems (GIS) approaches enable communities to create maps of health risks, resources, and interventions, while building local capacity for spatial analysis and planning that informs the design and implementation of health programs. These methods may involve community members in mapping disease outbreaks, environmental hazards, healthcare resources, or traditional resource management areas while providing tools for community-based planning and advocacy.

Focus group discussions and key informant interviews conducted within participatory research frameworks emphasise the expertise and perspectives of community participants while creating opportunities for dialogue and learning that benefits both researchers and community members. These methods can be used to explore community understanding of health challenges, evaluate the acceptability of interventions, or identify barriers and facilitators for health behaviour change while building relationships and trust between researchers and communities.

Table 15.3. Cultural competency components and application in One Health programs

Competency Component	Assessment Methods	Program Adaptations	Implementation Strategies	Common Challenges	Success Indicators	Sustainability Factors
Health Beliefs and Practices	Ethnographic studies, key informant interviews	Integration of traditional and biomedical approaches	Collaboration with traditional healers, respectful dialogue	Conflicting belief systems, professional scepticism	Community acceptance, treatment compliance	Traditional healer engagement, community education
Social Structures and Relationships	Social network analysis, community mapping	Gender-appropriate programming, leadership engagement	Work with traditional authorities, respect family dynamics	Power imbalances, exclusion of marginalised groups	Inclusive participation, community ownership	Leadership development, social mobilisation
Communication Patterns	Focus groups, communication preferences surveys	Culturally appropriate messaging, trusted messengers	Use of local languages, community health workers	Language barriers, sensitive topics	Message comprehension, behaviour change	Communication infrastructure, ongoing training
Values and Priorities	Participatory assessments, community consultations	Program alignment with cultural values	Community-driven priority setting, flexible implementation	Competing priorities, external pressures	Community buy-in, program sustainability	Value alignment, community autonomy
Economic and Livelihood Systems	Household surveys, economic assessments	Cost considerations, livelihood integration	Income-generating components, affordability measures	Economic constraints, opportunity costs	Program affordability, economic benefits	Economic sustainability, market development

Table 15.4. Participatory research methods and applications in One Health

Method	Primary Purposes	Participant Roles	Capacity Building Components	Data Collection Approaches	Analysis Methods	Knowledge Translation
Community-Based Participatory Research	Community problem-solving, capacity building	Co-researchers, decision-makers	Research skills, critical thinking	Surveys, interviews, observations	Collaborative analysis, community interpretation	Community presentations, policy briefs
Participatory Action Research	Social change, empowerment	Change agents, investigators	Leadership, organising, research	Action research cycles, reflection	Participatory analysis, action planning	Community organising, advocacy
Participatory Epidemiology	Disease surveillance, outbreak response	Data collectors, analysts	Epidemiology basics, surveillance	Community reporting, sample collection	Participatory analysis, mapping	Surveillance reports, community feedback
Photovoice	Documentation, advocacy	Photographers, storytellers	Photography, narrative skills	Photography, discussion groups	Thematic analysis, exhibit development	Photo exhibits, community forums
Digital Storytelling	Narrative sharing, awareness	Storytellers, media creators	Digital media, communication	Video/audio recording, editing	Story analysis, audience feedback	Online sharing, community screenings
Participatory Mapping	Spatial analysis, planning	Mappers, spatial analysts	GIS basics, spatial thinking	GPS data, sketching, and interviews	Spatial analysis, map interpretation	Community maps, planning documents

Table 15.5. Trust and partnership building strategies and implementation approaches

Strategy	Core Activities	Timeline	Partner Responsibilities	Success Indicators	Common Obstacles	Mitigation Approaches
Relationship Building	Social activities, dialogue, shared experiences	Ongoing, intensive early phase	Mutual participation, openness	Quality of interactions, partner satisfaction	Time constraints, cultural barriers	Dedicated time, cultural facilitators
Transparent Communication	Information sharing, regular updates	Continuous	Honest communication, accessible formats	Information flow, understanding	Language barriers, technical complexity	Translation, plain language
Shared Decision-Making	Joint planning, consensus building	Major decisions	Active participation, compromise	Decision influence, implementation commitment	Power imbalances, competing interests	Facilitation, conflict resolution
Capacity Building	Training, resource sharing, mentoring	Long-term investment	Skill development, resource provision	Enhanced capabilities, sustainability	Resource limitations, uneven capacity	Graduated support, peer learning
Accountability Systems	Monitoring, reporting, feedback	Regular cycles	Progress tracking, responsiveness	Commitment fulfilment, problem resolution	Weak systems, poor follow-through	Clear agreements, regular review
Conflict Resolution	Mediation, negotiation, problem-solving	As needed	Good faith engagement, flexibility	Conflict resolution, relationship maintenance	Entrenched positions, mistrust	Neutral facilitation, relationship focus

Participatory evaluation approaches engage stakeholders in assessing the processes and outcomes of health interventions, while building capacity for ongoing monitoring and evaluation that supports adaptive management and continuous improvement of health programs. These approaches recognise that community members and other stakeholders are the ultimate judges of intervention success while possessing important insights about program implementation and effectiveness that may not be captured through conventional evaluation methods.

Ethical considerations in participatory research include ensuring that community participants have meaningful control over research processes and outcomes, protecting participant confidentiality and privacy, addressing power imbalances between researchers and communities, and ensuring that research benefits are shared appropriately with participating communities. These considerations require ongoing attention and negotiation throughout research partnerships while respecting community preferences and cultural values about knowledge sharing and use.

Capacity building for participatory research may include training programs for community members in research methods and skills, institutional development for community-based organisations that can support ongoing research activities, and professional development for researchers in participatory processes and community engagement approaches. This capacity building requires long-term commitment and resources while recognising that research partnerships should build sustainable capacity that continues beyond specific projects.

Quality and rigour in participatory research require attention to both conventional research standards and participatory criteria, including community ownership, empowerment, and social change outcomes that reflect the values and objectives of participatory approaches. This may involve mixed-methods approaches that combine quantitative and qualitative methods, using participatory processes to ensure that research addresses community priorities and produces actionable findings.

Dissemination and knowledge translation in participatory research emphasise community-driven approaches to sharing research findings and implementing recommendations while building capacity for ongoing advocacy and policy engagement that can promote broader adoption of research-based interventions (Wallerstein et al., 2017). These approaches may include community presentations, policy briefs, media engagement, and peer education activities that enable community participants to share their knowledge and experiences with broader audiences.

15.6. Building Trust and Partnerships

Building trust and sustainable partnerships represents a fundamental prerequisite for effective community engagement in One Health initiatives, requiring long-term commitment, transparent communication, shared decision-making, and mutual respect that acknowledges the expertise and contributions of all partners while addressing power imbalances and structural inequities that may limit community participation and benefit from health interventions (Jagosh et al., 2012). Trust-building is particularly important in One Health contexts because these initiatives often involve complex technical concepts, multiple stakeholder groups with different priorities, and interventions that may require significant behaviour changes or resource commitments from community members.

Trust development processes typically begin with relationship-building activities that enable different partners to get to know each other personally, while establishing common ground and shared values that provide a foundation for ongoing collaboration. These processes often require a significant time investment in informal interactions, social activities, and dialogue opportunities that allow partners to develop a mutual understanding and respect, while identifying shared interests and complementary strengths that can contribute to partnership success.

Transparency and communication represent essential elements of trust building that require the open and honest sharing of information about program objectives, resources, constraints, and decision-making processes, while ensuring that all partners have access to the information and they need to participate meaningfully in partnership activities. Transparency also requires acknowledging the uncertainties, limitations, and potential risks associated with health interventions, while providing realistic expectations about what partnerships can achieve and the challenges they may face.

Shared decision-making processes ensure that all partners have meaningful opportunities to influence decisions that affect their participation and benefit from partnership activities while respecting different forms of expertise and knowledge that partners bring to collaborative efforts. These processes may require developing new governance structures and decision-making procedures that can accommodate different partner preferences and constraints while maintaining efficient and effective partnership operations.

Power sharing and equity considerations address structural inequalities and power imbalances that may limit community participation in health partnerships while ensuring that benefits and burdens of partnership activities are distributed fairly across different partner groups. This may require explicit attention to issues such as resource allocation, capacity-building support, decision-making authority, and recognition of partner contributions, while developing mechanisms to address conflicts and grievances that may arise in partnership relationships.

Cultural humility and respect for community autonomy require external partners to approach communities with genuine respect for local knowledge, values, and decision-making authority while avoiding paternalistic attitudes or approaches that assume external expertise is superior to community knowledge and experience. Cultural humility involves ongoing learning about community perspectives and preferences while adapting partnership approaches to align with community values and priorities rather than imposing external models.

Accountability mechanisms ensure that partners fulfil their commitments and responsibilities outlined in partnership agreements, while providing processes for addressing problems or conflicts that may arise during the implementation of the partnership. These mechanisms may include regular partner meetings, progress reporting systems, feedback processes, and conflict resolution procedures that enable partners to address issues constructively while maintaining partnership relationships and momentum.

Reciprocity and mutual benefit ensure that all partners receive meaningful benefits from participation in health partnerships while contributing their unique resources and expertise to shared objectives. This may require careful attention to balancing giving and receiving across partners, while ensuring that community partners receive adequate compensation, recognition, and capacity-building support for their contributions to partnership activities. Table 15.5 shows trust and partnership-building strategies and implementation approaches.

Sustainability planning ensures that partnerships can continue to function effectively over time, adapting to changing conditions while maintaining partner engagement and commitment beyond the initial project period. This requires developing partnership structures, funding mechanisms, and capacity that can support ongoing collaboration while building institutional memory and leadership that can guide the evolution and development of partnerships.

Leadership development within partnerships involves building capacity among all partners to take leadership roles in partnership activities while rotating leadership responsibilities and supporting emerging leaders who can guide partnership activities over time. This may include formal leadership training programs, mentoring relationships, and opportunities for partners to take on increasing responsibility and authority within partnership activities.

Learning and adaptation processes enable partnerships to enhance their effectiveness over time, responding to changing conditions and emerging opportunities that may necessitate modifications to partnership approaches and activities. These processes may include regular reflection and evaluation activities, peer learning opportunities, and structured processes for incorporating lessons learned into partnership planning and implementation.

Documentation and knowledge sharing enable partnerships to capture and share their experiences with broader audiences, contributing to the evidence base on practical partnership approaches and strategies. This may include case study development, best practice documentation, and participation in professional networks and conferences where partnership experiences can be shared with other practitioners and researchers.

Evaluating trust and partnership quality requires indicators and methods that assess the strength and effectiveness of partnership relationships, identifying areas for improvement and strategies to enhance partnership performance. This evaluation may include partner satisfaction surveys, relationship quality assessments, and an analysis of partnership outcomes and impacts that can demonstrate the value of investing in trust and partnership-building activities.

Challenges in building trust and partnerships may include historical experiences of exploitation or broken promises that foster scepticism about external partnerships, competing demands and priorities that limit partner availability and engagement, resource constraints that restrict capacity for partnership activities, and cultural differences that lead to misunderstandings or conflicts between partners. Addressing these challenges requires a sustained commitment, cultural competency, and flexible approaches that can adapt to the needs and preferences of partners.

Success factors for trust and partnership building include genuine commitment to shared decision-making and mutual benefit, adequate resources and time for relationship-building activities, cultural competency and respect for community values and preferences, transparency and accountability in partnership operations, and leadership that can model collaborative approaches while building capacity for ongoing partnership development and sustainability (Israel et al., 2010).

Conclusion

Community engagement and participatory approaches to One Health represent fundamental shifts in how health interventions are conceptualised, designed, and implemented, moving from expert-driven models toward collaborative frameworks recognising communities as essential partners in identifying health challenges, developing appropriate solutions, and implementing sustainable interventions addressing interconnected human, animal, and environmental health. Meaningful community participation is not merely desirable but essential for achieving health outcomes that are relevant, acceptable, sustainable, and equitable for the communities they serve.

Community-based One Health initiatives demonstrate how local knowledge, resources, and leadership can be leveraged to address complex health challenges while building community capacity for ongoing problem identification, solution development, and program implementation that continues beyond external project support. Indigenous knowledge systems and traditional practices offer sophisticated frameworks for understanding and managing relationships among human health, animal health, and environmental health, providing valuable insights into sustainable approaches that complement and enhance scientific knowledge while respecting cultural values and community autonomy.

Stakeholder engagement strategies that systematically identify and include all relevant actors while creating collaborative processes for meaningful participation in decision-making represent essential components of successful One Health implementation. Cultural competency in health programs requires an understanding and respect for diverse cultural beliefs, practices, and social structures that influence health behaviours and outcomes. This involves developing interventions aligned with cultural values rather than imposing external models.

Participatory research methods enable communities to be active participants in generating knowledge about their own health challenges and solutions while building local capacity for ongoing problem identification and evidence-based decision-making. Building trust and sustainable partnerships requires a long-term commitment, transparent communication, shared decision-making, and mutual respect, acknowledging the expertise and contributions of all partners while addressing power imbalances and structural inequities.

The integration of community engagement into One Health implementation necessitates fundamental changes in how health professionals perceive their roles and relationships with communities, as well as the development of new competencies for collaboration, cultural humility, and shared decision-making. Future directions must address ongoing challenges, including power imbalances that limit meaningful participation, resource constraints that limit sustained engagement capacity, institutional barriers that prevent effective cross-sectoral collaboration, and evaluation systems that inadequately capture the benefits of participatory approaches.

COVID-19 highlighted both the importance of community engagement for effective health responses and the challenges of maintaining meaningful participation during health emergencies. Success requires sustained commitment from all stakeholders to fundamental changes in power relationships, resource allocation, and accountability systems, creating genuine partnerships between communities and professionals while achieving health outcomes that are meaningful and beneficial for all participants.

Acknowledgments

The authors would like to extend our appreciation to those who offered helpful commentary during the drafting process of this manuscript. We also acknowledge the role Nova Science Publishers played in enabling the work described herein.

References

Beach, M. C., Price, E. G., Gary, T. L., Robinson, K. A., Gozu, A., Palacio, A., & Cooper, L. A. (2006). Cultural competence: a systematic review of health care provider educational interventions. *Medical Care*, 44(4), 356-373. https://doi.org/10.1097/01.mlr.0000204405.99746.c2.

Berkes, F. (2012). *Sacred ecology*. Routledge. https://doi.org/10.4324/9780203123843

Cargo, M., & Mercer, S. L. (2008). The value and challenges of participatory research: strengthening its practice. *Annual Review of Public Health*, 29, 325-350. https://doi.org/10.1146/annurev.publhealth.29.091307.083824.

Conrad, P., Malouin, R., Neale, A., Kusano, C., Meurice, C., Lynch, M., & Coimbra Jr, C. E. A. (2013). Community-based participatory research in One Health. *Comparative Immunology, Microbiology and Infectious Diseases*, 36(3), 259-265. https://doi.org/10.1016/j.cimid.2013.02.001.

Doherty, I. A., & Clayton, S. (2011). The psychological impacts of global climate change. *American Psychologist*, 66(4), 265-276. https://doi.org/10.1037/a0023141.

EcoHealth, 9(2), 107-110. https://doi.org/10.1007/s10393-012-0772-8.

Israel, B. A., Coombe, C. M., Cheezum, R. R., Schulz, A. J., McGranaghan, R. J., Lichtenstein, R., & Burris, A. (2010). Community-based participatory research: a capacity-building approach for policy advocacy aimed at eliminating health disparities. *American Journal of Public Health*, 100(11), 2094-2102. https://doi.org/10.2105/AJPH.2009.170506.

Jagosh, J., Macaulay, A. C., Pluye, P., Salsberg, J., Bush, P. L., Henderson, J., & Greenhalgh, T. (2012). Uncovering the benefits of participatory research: implications of a realist review for health research and practice. *The Milbank Quarterly*, 90(2), 311-346. https://doi.org/10.1111/j.1468-0009.2012.00665.x.

Laverack, G. (2013). *Health activism: foundations and strategies*. Sage Publications. https://doi.org/10.4135/9781446269626.

Reed, M. S. (2008). Stakeholder participation for environmental management: a literature review. *Biological Conservation*, 141(10), 2417-2431. https://doi.org/10.1016/j.biocon.2008.07.014.

Wallerstein, N., Duran, B., Oetzel, J. G., & Minkler, M. (Eds.). (2017). *Community-based participatory research for Health: advancing social and Health equity*. John Wiley & Sons. https://doi.org/10.1002/9781119239631.

World Health Organization & UNICEF. (2020). *Community engagement considerations for COVID-19: community feedback and rumor tracking*. World Health Organization. https://www.who.int/publications/i/item/community-engagement-considerations-for-covid-19-community-feedback-and-rumor-tracking.

World Health Organization. (2017). *Community engagement: a health promotion guide for universal health coverage driven by primary health care*. World Health Organization. https://www.who.int/publications/i/item/community-engagement-a-health-promotion-guide-for-universal-health-coverage-driven-by-primary-health-care.

World Health Organization. (2018). *Taking a multisectoral one health approach: a tripartite guide to addressing zoonotic diseases in countries*. World Health Organization. https://www.who.int/publications/i/item/taking-a-multisectoral-one-health-approach-a-tripartite-guide-to-addressing-zoonotic-diseases-in-countries.

Chapter 16

Epidemiological Methods in One Health Research

Maajid Mohi Ud Din Malik[1,*], PhD
and Rajesh S. Kuber[2]
[1]Department of Radiology and Imaging Technology, Dr. D. Y. Patil School of Allied Health Sciences, Dr. D. Y. Patil Vidyapeeth· Pune (Deemed to be University), Sant Tukaram Nagar, Pimpri, Pune, India
[2]Department of Radio-Diagnosis, Dr. D. Y. Patil Medical College, Hospital and Research Centre, Dr. D. Y. Patil Vidyapeeth, Pune (Deemed to be University), Sant Tukaram Nagar, Pimpri, Pune, India

Abstract

Epidemiological methods form the cornerstone of One Health research, providing essential frameworks for understanding the complex interconnections between human, animal, and environmental Health. This chapter examines the application of epidemiological study designs specifically within One Health contexts, addressing the unique challenges and opportunities presented by multidisciplinary investigations. Traditional epidemiological approaches, including cross-sectional, cohort, and case-control studies, require adaptation when applied to One Health scenarios due to the need for simultaneous consideration of multiple hosts, environmental factors, and transmission pathways. Outbreak investigation methodologies in One Health settings demand coordinated responses across human Health, veterinary medicine, and environmental science sectors. Environmental and ecological epidemiology have emerged as critical components for understanding disease patterns at the human-animal-environment interface. Key challenges include managing data quality across diverse disciplines, addressing methodological bias, and ensuring effective multidisciplinary collaboration. This chapter provides comprehensive guidance for researchers conducting One Health epidemiological investigations, with emphasis on study design selection, data integration strategies, and addressing the inherent complexities of transdisciplinary research. The connection to Sustainable Development Goal 3 (Good Health and Well-being) underscores the global significance of practical One Health epidemiological approaches.

Keywords: One Health, epidemiological methods, outbreak investigation, environmental Health, multidisciplinary research, zoonotic diseases, ecological epidemiology, study design, data integration, Sustainable Development Goal 3

---

* Corresponding Author's Email: maajid.malik@dpu.edu.in

In: Advances in the One Health Approach
Editors: Maajid Mohi Ud Din Malik, Abhay Saraf, Harshal Tukaram Pandve et al.
ISBN: 979-8-90134-202-2

Introduction

Epidemiological methods form the scientific foundation for understanding disease patterns and health outcomes at the complex intersection of human, animal, and environmental health domains. The application of traditional epidemiological approaches to One Health research presents unique methodological challenges that require innovative adaptations and novel analytical frameworks. As global health challenges increasingly transcend species boundaries and environmental contexts, the need for rigorous epidemiological methods that can accommodate multi-species populations, diverse data sources, and complex transmission pathways has become critically important for advancing both scientific understanding and evidence-based policy development.

The evolution of epidemiological methods within One Health contexts reflects the growing recognition that many contemporary health threats cannot be adequately understood or addressed through single-discipline approaches. Zoonotic disease outbreaks, antimicrobial resistance, food safety challenges, and environmental health hazards require integrated investigation methods that can simultaneously examine human, animal, and environmental factors while accounting for their complex interactions. This methodological integration demands careful attention to study design considerations, data quality standards, and analytical approaches that maintain scientific rigour while accommodating the inherent complexity and interdisciplinary nature of One Health research questions.

16.1. Study Designs for One Health Investigations

One Health investigations require sophisticated epidemiological approaches that can simultaneously address health outcomes across human, animal, and environmental domains. The integration of traditional epidemiological methods with transdisciplinary perspectives represents a paradigm shift from conventional single-sector health research. The Competencies for One Health Field Epidemiology (COHFE) Framework, developed by the FAO, WHO, and WOAH, establishes standardised approaches for training frontline responders in interconnected health fields, emphasising the critical importance of methodological rigour in One Health epidemiology (WHO, 2024).

The selection of appropriate study designs in One Health research depends on multiple factors, including the nature of the health threat, available resources, temporal considerations, and the specific research questions being addressed (Munnangi & Boktor, 2023). Cross-sectional studies in One Health contexts provide snapshots of health status across multiple species and environmental conditions simultaneously, offering valuable insights into prevalence patterns and potential risk factors at the human-animal-environment interface. These studies are beneficial for baseline assessments and surveillance activities, though they face unique challenges in standardising case definitions and exposure measures across different populations and species.

Cohort studies represent the gold standard for establishing temporal relationships between exposures and health outcomes in One Health research. Prospective cohort designs enable investigators to follow populations of humans and animals, as well as monitor environmental conditions over time, providing robust evidence for causal inferences. However, the complexity of maintaining long-term follow-up across multiple sectors presents significant logistical challenges. Retrospective cohort studies offer cost-effective alternatives, but they require high-quality historical data from diverse sources, which may not always be available or compatible across different disciplines.

Case-control studies provide efficient approaches for investigating rare diseases or outcomes with long latency periods in One Health contexts. These studies are particularly valuable when investigating zoonotic disease outbreaks or environmental health incidents where rapid identification of risk factors is essential. The challenge in One Health case-control studies lies in selecting appropriate control groups that represent the same underlying populations across human, animal, and environmental domains while avoiding selection bias.

Hybrid study designs have emerged as innovative approaches tailored explicitly for One Health investigations. Case-crossover studies allow individuals to serve as their own controls, which is particularly useful when investigating transient exposures or trigger events at the human-animal-environment interface. Nested case-control studies within established cohorts offer a cost-effective means of conducting detailed exposure assessments using expensive laboratory methods or specialised environmental measurements. The Generalizable One Health Framework (GOHF) provides a five-step structure for implementing One Health approaches in disease control programs, emphasising the importance of systematic study design selection based on specific programmatic needs (Ribeiro et al., 2022).

The integration of spatial epidemiological methods has become increasingly crucial in One Health research, particularly for understanding disease transmission patterns and environmental determinants of Health. Geographic Information Systems (GIS) and remote sensing technologies enable researchers to examine spatial distributions of health outcomes across multiple species while simultaneously assessing environmental factors such as land use patterns, climate variables, and ecosystem characteristics. Spatial analytical approaches provide valuable insights into disease clustering, transmission pathways, and environmental risk factors that would not be apparent through traditional epidemiological methods (Zhang et al., 2024). Advanced spatial epidemiological frameworks integrate traditional epidemiology with geography, statistics, environmental science, and ecology, offering comprehensive approaches for analysing spatial dimensions of Health and disease across multiple species. Table 16.1 shows a comparison of epidemiological study designs in health research.

Table 16.1. Comparison of epidemiological study designs in One Health research

Study Design	Strengths in One Health Context	Limitations	Best Applications
Cross-sectional	Rapid assessment across sectors; Cost-effective; Baseline establishment	Cannot establish causality; Temporal bias risk	Surveillance; Prevalence studies
Cohort (Prospective)	Strong causal inference; Multiple outcome assessment	Expensive; Long follow-up periods	Disease emergence studies
Cohort (Retrospective)	Cost-effective; Utilises existing data	Data quality issues; Limited exposure assessment	Historical outbreak analysis
Case-control	Efficient for rare diseases; Rapid results	Recall bias; Control selection challenges	Outbreak investigations
Ecological	Population-level insights; Utilises routine data	Ecological fallacy; Limited individual-level data	Policy evaluation
Nested case-control	Cost-effective biomarker studies	Limited to a single cohort	Mechanistic studies

16.2. Outbreak Investigation Methodologies

Outbreak investigation in One Health contexts requires coordinated, multisectoral approaches that can rapidly identify sources, modes of transmission, and appropriate control measures across human, animal, and environmental domains. The traditional steps for outbreak investigation must be adapted to address the complexity of investigations that span multiple disciplines and jurisdictions. Emergency preparedness and response protocols increasingly recognise that effective outbreak control requires simultaneous investigation and intervention across all relevant sectors.

The initial phase of a One Health outbreak investigation involves confirming the outbreak through analysis of surveillance data from human Health, animal health, and environmental monitoring systems. This process requires standardised case definitions that can be applied consistently across different sectors while maintaining sensitivity for early detection. The European Centre for Disease Prevention and Control and European Food Safety Authority have developed coordinated approaches for zoonotic avian influenza investigations, emphasising the critical importance of establishing clear communication protocols and joint response mechanisms before outbreaks occur (ECDC & EFSA, 2025).

Descriptive epidemiology in One Health outbreak investigations encompasses the systematic characterisation of cases by person, place, and time across all affected sectors. This includes a detailed analysis of human cases, affected animal populations, and relevant environmental conditions. The challenge lies in developing comparable analytical frameworks that can accommodate the different biological and social characteristics of affected populations while maintaining epidemiological rigour. Geographic information systems play crucial roles in visualising outbreak patterns and identifying potential foci of transmission or transmission pathways.

Analytical epidemiology in outbreak investigations requires rapid deployment of case-control or cohort study methods to test specific hypotheses about outbreak sources and transmission mechanisms. These analytical studies must be designed to capture exposures relevant to all potentially affected populations, including direct animal contact, environmental exposures, and consumption of contaminated food or water. The Johns Hopkins Bloomberg School of Public Health has developed comprehensive training programs specifically focused on One Health outbreak investigation methodologies, emphasising the importance of interdisciplinary team coordination (Johns Hopkins, 2024).

Environmental investigations form integral components of One Health outbreak investigations, requiring systematic assessment of potential contamination sources, transmission pathways, and ecological factors that may have contributed to disease emergence or spread. These investigations often involve water quality testing, air sampling, soil analysis, and assessment of waste management systems. The complexity of environmental investigations increases significantly when dealing with vector-borne diseases or environmentally persistent pathogens that may affect multiple host species over extended periods. Participatory epidemiological approaches have proven valuable in One Health contexts, particularly for engaging local communities in disease surveillance and outbreak detection activities (Zhou et al., 2022).

Laboratory coordination represents a critical challenge in One Health outbreak investigations, as different sectors often utilise different diagnostic protocols, laboratory networks, and reporting systems. Establishing coordinated laboratory response protocols ensures that specimens from humans, animals, and environmental sources are processed using compatible methods, enabling a meaningful comparison of results. The development of standardised laboratory protocols for priority pathogens has been identified as a key need for improving outbreak response effectiveness.

Communication and coordination mechanisms are crucial for effective One Health outbreak investigations, necessitating established protocols for information sharing among human health authorities, veterinary services, environmental agencies, and other relevant stakeholders. The U.S. One Health Coordination Unit, launched in 2024, brings together 24 agencies to enhance collaboration and coordination for the prevention, detection, and response to zoonotic diseases (CDC, 2025). These coordination mechanisms must address both technical aspects of investigation protocols and administrative challenges related to jurisdiction, authority, and resource allocation.

Risk communication during One Health outbreak investigations requires carefully crafted messaging that addresses concerns of multiple stakeholder groups while avoiding public panic or unnecessary disruption of economic activities. Messages must be scientifically accurate while remaining accessible to diverse audiences, including healthcare providers, veterinarians, farmers, environmental health professionals, and the public. Cultural competency and community engagement are critical when investigations involve animal husbandry practices, food traditions, or environmental exposures that are deeply embedded in local communities.

16.3. Cross-Sectional, Cohort, and Case-Control Studies

Cross-sectional studies in One Health research provide valuable snapshots of health status and risk factor distributions across human, animal, and environmental domains at specific points in time. These studies are beneficial for establishing baseline conditions, monitoring trends over time, and identifying potential associations between exposures and health outcomes. The design and implementation of cross-sectional studies in One Health contexts requires careful consideration of sampling strategies that ensure representative data collection across all relevant populations and environmental conditions.

Sampling strategies for One Health cross-sectional studies must account for the different population structures and accessibility challenges associated with human communities, animal populations, and environmental monitoring sites. Human populations can be sampled using standard epidemiological approaches, such as cluster sampling or stratified random sampling. In contrast, animal populations require specialised veterinary epidemiological methods that consider herd structures, management practices, and species-specific behavioural patterns. Environmental sampling requires spatial sampling designs that capture relevant environmental gradients and potential exposure pathways.

Data collection in One Health cross-sectional studies presents unique challenges related to standardisation of measurement protocols, quality control across different types of data, and integration of diverse data sources. Survey instruments must be designed to capture comparable exposure information across different populations while respecting cultural and practical constraints. Biological specimen collection requires protocols that ensure sample integrity and comparability across different types of specimens from various species and environmental sources.

Cohort studies represent the strongest observational study design for establishing causal relationships in One Health research, as they enable the establishment of temporal relationships between exposures and health outcomes across multiple domains. Prospective cohort studies allow investigators to implement standardised data collection protocols from the beginning of follow-up, ensuring high-quality exposure and outcome data. However, the logistical challenges and costs associated with maintaining long-term follow-up across multiple sectors can be substantial.

The design of One Health cohort studies necessitates careful consideration of follow-up protocols that can accommodate the diverse life spans, mobility patterns, and accessibility characteristics of both human and animal populations. Human cohorts can be followed through routine healthcare contacts, periodic surveys, and linkage to health registries, whereas animal cohorts require coordination with veterinary services and the owners of the animals. Environmental monitoring requires sustained sampling protocols that can detect changes in environmental conditions over time while accounting for seasonal variations and long-term trends.

Outcome ascertainment in One Health cohort studies must address the challenge of identifying comparable health outcomes across different populations and species. Case definitions must be developed that can be applied consistently while accounting for species-specific disease manifestations and diagnostic capabilities. The integration of electronic health records, veterinary databases, and environmental monitoring systems can provide efficient mechanisms for outcome ascertainment but requires careful attention to data quality and completeness.

Case-control studies offer efficient approaches for investigating rare diseases or outbreaks in One Health contexts, providing the ability to rapidly identify risk factors and generate hypotheses about disease causation. The selection of appropriate cases and controls represents a critical challenge in One Health case-control studies, requiring careful consideration of population definitions and potential sources of bias. Cases must be defined using consistent criteria across different populations, while controls must be selected from the same underlying populations that gave rise to the cases.

Control selection in One Health case-control studies requires innovative approaches that ensure representativeness across human, animal, and environmental domains. Human controls can be selected using standard epidemiological methods, such as random digit dialling or registry sampling. In contrast, animal controls require coordination with veterinary services and consideration of herd or flock structures. Environmental controls may be selected based on spatial or temporal matching criteria that ensure comparable ecological conditions.

Exposure assessment in One Health case-control studies must capture the full range of potential exposures at the human-animal-environment interface, including direct animal contact, consumption of animal products, environmental exposures, and indirect exposures through shared ecological contamination. Retrospective exposure assessment presents challenges related to recall bias and the availability of historical exposure data. The use of biological markers and environmental sampling can provide objective measures of exposure but requires specialised laboratory capabilities and may not capture historical exposures. Table 16.2 presents key considerations for implementing a one-health study.

Table 16.2. Key considerations for One Health study implementation

Study Component	Human Health Considerations	Animal Health Considerations	Environmental Health Considerations
Sampling	Population registries; Healthcare utilisation	Herd/flock structures; Owner cooperation	Spatial distribution; Seasonal variation
Case Definition	Clinical criteria; Laboratory confirmation	Species-specific manifestations; Diagnostic availability	Contamination thresholds; Measurement methods
Exposure Assessment	Occupational history; Lifestyle factors	Husbandry practices; Feed sources	Land use; Climate factors
Follow-up	Healthcare contacts; Vital statistics	Veterinary records; Owner reports	Monitoring networks; Remote sensing
Quality Control	Medical record validation; Laboratory QC	Veterinary oversight; Species expertise	Environmental standards; Laboratory accreditation

16.4. Ecological and Environmental Epidemiology

Ecological epidemiology represents a fundamental component of One Health research, focusing on the study of health outcomes at the population level while examining relationships between environmental exposures and disease patterns across human, animal, and environmental domains. Unlike individual-level studies, ecological studies use aggregate data to investigate associations between exposures and health outcomes at the group or population level, making them particularly suitable for examining large-scale environmental influences on health outcomes.

Geographic boundaries, temporal periods, or other grouping characteristics relevant to the research question can define the unit of analysis in ecological studies. Geographic ecological studies compare health outcomes between different regions, countries, or administrative units while examining corresponding differences in environmental exposures or risk factors. Temporal ecological studies investigate changes in health outcomes over time in relation to changes in environmental conditions or policy interventions. Mixed ecological studies combine both geographic and temporal dimensions to provide more comprehensive assessments of exposure-outcome relationships.

Environmental exposures in ecological studies encompass a broad range of factors, including air pollution, water quality, climate variables, land-use patterns, and ecosystem characteristics. These exposures are typically measured as area-level aggregates such as mean pollution concentrations, percentage of land under different uses, or average meteorological conditions. The availability of environmental monitoring data and satellite-based measurements has dramatically enhanced the capacity to conduct ecological studies examining environmental determinants of health outcomes across large geographic areas and extended time periods.

The ecological fallacy represents a fundamental limitation of environmental studies, occurring when associations observed at the group level are incorrectly assumed to apply to individuals within those groups (Morgenstern, 1995). This limitation is significant in One Health contexts where individual-level variation in exposure and susceptibility may be substantial. Researchers must carefully interpret ecological study results and avoid making inappropriate inferences about individual-level relationships based on aggregate-level findings.

Spatial epidemiological methods have emerged as powerful tools for examining environmental determinants of health outcomes in One Health research. Geographic Information Systems (GIS) enable researchers to integrate health outcome data with detailed ecological data at multiple spatial scales, from local microenvironments to regional ecosystems. Remote sensing data provide consistent measurements of environmental conditions across large areas and over extended time periods, enabling studies that would not be feasible using ground-based measurements alone.

Temporal ecological studies are particularly valuable for evaluating the health impacts of environmental policy interventions or changes in environmental conditions over time. These studies can examine how changes in air quality regulations, water treatment practices, or land use policies affect health outcomes across different populations. Time-series analyses can identify both short-term and long-term relationships between environmental exposures and health outcomes while controlling for seasonal patterns and long-term trends.

Multi-level ecological studies attempt to address some limitations of traditional ecological studies by incorporating data at multiple levels of aggregation. These studies may combine individual-level data with area-level environmental exposures, allowing for more sophisticated analyses that can distinguish between individual-level and contextual effects on health outcomes. However, multi-level studies require more complex analytical approaches and may still be subject to certain forms of ecological bias.

Environmental epidemiology in One Health contexts requires integration of environmental health assessment methods with traditional epidemiological approaches. Environmental health risk assessment provides frameworks for evaluating potential health impacts of environmental exposures based on toxicological data and exposure modelling. These approaches complement epidemiological studies by providing mechanistic insights into how environmental exposures may affect health outcomes across different species.

Climate change epidemiology has emerged as a critical area of environmental epidemiology research, examining how changing climate conditions affect disease patterns and health outcomes. Climate variables such as temperature, precipitation, and extreme weather events can directly affect human and animal Health while also influencing vector ecology, pathogen survival, and food security. Climate change epidemiology necessitates the collection of long-term data and the application of sophisticated modelling approaches to distinguish climate effects from other temporal trends.

16.5. Challenges in Multidisciplinary Research

Multidisciplinary research in One Health settings presents unique methodological and practical challenges that require innovative solutions and adaptive management approaches. The integration of knowledge, methods, and perspectives from human medicine, veterinary medicine, environmental science, and other relevant disciplines creates both opportunities and obstacles for conducting rigorous epidemiological research. Effective multidisciplinary collaboration requires careful attention to communication, coordination, and harmonisation of research methods across different scientific traditions and professional cultures.

Communication challenges in multidisciplinary One Health research stem from differences in professional vocabularies, conceptual frameworks, and analytical traditions across different disciplines. Medical professionals, veterinarians, environmental scientists, and public health practitioners may use different terminology to describe similar concepts or may have different interpretations of standard terms. Establishing shared vocabularies and conceptual frameworks early in research projects is essential for effective collaboration and meaningful integration of findings across disciplines.

Methodological harmonisation represents a significant challenge in multidisciplinary One Health research, as different disciplines may have different standards for study design, data collection, laboratory methods, and statistical analysis. Human health research typically follows clinical and epidemiological standards established by medical research communities, while veterinary research follows standards developed by veterinary and agricultural research communities. Environmental research adheres to standards established by the environmental science and public health communities. Reconciling these different methodological traditions requires careful negotiation and may involve compromises that are acceptable to all participating disciplines.

Data integration challenges arise from differences in data collection protocols, measurement units, quality control procedures, and data management systems across different disciplines. Human health data are typically collected using standardised clinical and epidemiological protocols with established quality control procedures. In contrast, animal health data may be collected using different protocols that reflect species-specific considerations and veterinary practices. Environmental data are collected using various protocols that adhere to ecological monitoring standards and regulatory requirements.

Institutional coordination presents practical challenges for multidisciplinary One Health research, as different sectors may have different institutional structures, administrative procedures, and regulatory requirements. Human health research typically requires approval from institutional review boards, which focus on the protection of human subjects, while animal research requires approval from institutional animal care and use committees. Environmental research may require permits from environmental regulatory agencies and coordination with land management authorities.

Resource allocation and funding represent ongoing challenges for multidisciplinary One Health research, as traditional funding mechanisms are often organised around single-discipline research programs. Multidisciplinary projects may fall between traditional funding categories or may require coordination between multiple funding agencies with different priorities and procedures. The National Institutes of Health, National Science Foundation, and other funding agencies have increasingly recognised the need for multidisciplinary funding mechanisms. Still, challenges remain in securing adequate support for complex One Health research projects.

Quality control and assurance across multiple disciplines require comprehensive protocols that address the diverse standards and procedures employed by various research communities. Laboratory quality control must address differences in analytical methods, reference standards, and proficiency testing programs used by human Health, veterinary, and environmental laboratories. Field data collection quality control must address differences in training requirements, certification procedures, and supervision protocols used by different professional communities.

Ethical considerations in multidisciplinary One Health research require attention to the different moral frameworks and regulatory requirements applicable to human subject's research, animal research, and environmental research. Human subjects research must comply with informed consent requirements and institutional review board oversight. In contrast, animal research must comply with oversight from an animal care and use committee and adhere to animal welfare standards. Environmental research may involve considerations related to environmental justice, community engagement, and potential impacts on natural resources.

Professional training and capacity building represent long-term challenges for developing effective multidisciplinary One Health research capabilities. Traditional educational programs in medicine, veterinary medicine, environmental science, and public Health provide discipline-specific training but may not adequately prepare professionals for effective multidisciplinary collaboration. The Competencies for One Health Field Epidemiology (COHFE) Framework represents a significant step toward addressing these training needs; however, comprehensive capacity-building efforts are necessary across all relevant disciplines. Health inequalities and disparities in health outcomes across different populations and regions further complicate the challenges of implementing practical One Health approaches (Lübker & Murtin, 2023).

Figure 20 shows A circular diagram illustrating the interconnected nature of the One Health research collaboration. At the center is "Integrated One Health Research Team" with six spoke-like connections radiating outward to different disciplinary domains: Human Health (showing medical doctors, epidemiologists, and public health professionals), Animal Health (showing veterinarians and animal scientists), Environmental Health (showing environmental scientists and ecologists), Laboratory Sciences (showing diagnostic laboratories and research facilities), Data Sciences (showing biostatisticians and data managers), and Policy/Regulatory (showing health officials and regulators). Double-headed arrows between adjacent domains indicate the need for collaboration between every pair of disciplines. Surrounding the entire framework are boxes showing key challenges: "Communication Barriers," "Methodological Differences," "Institutional Coordination," "Resource Allocation," "Quality Control," and "Training Needs."

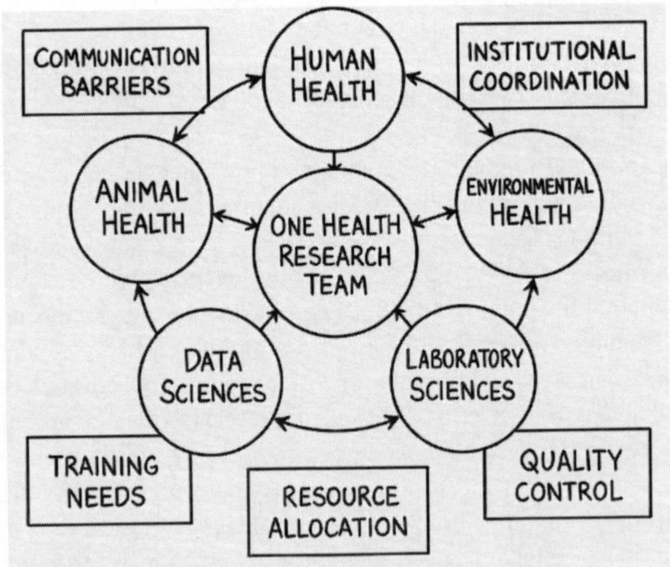

Figure 20. One Health research collaboration framework.

16.6. Data Quality and Bias Considerations

Data quality represents a fundamental concern in One Health epidemiological research, as the validity and reliability of study findings depend critically on the accuracy, completeness, and comparability of data collected across human, animal, and environmental domains. The complexity of managing data quality across multiple disciplines, measurement systems, and data sources requires comprehensive quality assurance programs and systematic attention to potential sources of bias and error. Global health measurement initiatives, such as the Global Burden of Disease Study, provide essential frameworks for standardising health outcome measurement across different populations and regions. However, adaptation for One Health contexts requires additional considerations (Wang et al., 2016).

Measurement error represents a pervasive challenge in One Health research, as different measurement systems, instruments, and protocols may have various levels of precision, accuracy, and reliability. Human health measurements typically follow established clinical and laboratory standards with well-characterised performance characteristics. In contrast, animal health measurements may use different standards that reflect species-specific considerations and veterinary practice requirements. Environmental measurements follow yet different standards that reflect environmental monitoring objectives and regulatory requirements.

Laboratory quality control necessitates coordination among human diagnostic laboratories, veterinary diagnostic laboratories, and environmental testing laboratories, each of which may have distinct quality assurance programs, proficiency testing requirements, and accreditation standards. The Checklist for One Health Epidemiological Reporting of Evidence (COHERE) provides guidelines for ensuring adequate reporting of laboratory quality control measures in One Health studies (Davis et al., 2017). Standardisation of laboratory methods across different types of laboratories may not always be feasible, but documenting differences and assessing their impact on study findings is essential.

Missing data present particular challenges in One Health research, as different data collection systems may exhibit distinct patterns of missing data that reflect systematic differences in data collection procedures, accessibility of study populations, or resource limitations. Human health data may be missing due to healthcare utilisation patterns, privacy concerns, or administrative limitations, while animal health data may be missing due to access limitations, owner cooperation, or veterinary service availability. Environmental data may be missing due to equipment failures, maintenance requirements, or budget constraints.

Selection bias can occur in One Health studies when study participants or sampling units are not representative of the target populations or when different selection mechanisms operate across various domains of the survey. Human participants may be selected based on healthcare utilisation patterns that are not representative of the general population. In contrast, animal populations may be selected based on ownership patterns, management practices, or geographic accessibility. Environmental sampling sites may be chosen based on accessibility, regulatory requirements, or historical monitoring patterns.

Information bias encompasses various forms of bias related to the collection, classification, or interpretation of exposure and outcome data in One Health studies. Recall bias may affect the retrospective assessment of exposures in human populations. In contrast, information about animal exposures may be subject to limitations in owner recall or the completeness of veterinary records. Environmental exposure assessment may be subject to measurement error related to spatial or temporal variability in environmental conditions.

Confounding represents a significant concern in One Health epidemiological studies, as the complex relationships between human, animal, and environmental factors create numerous opportunities for spurious associations. Traditional approaches to confounding control may be inadequate in One Health contexts, where confounders may operate at multiple levels and across different domains of the study. Unmeasured confounding may be particularly problematic when available data collection systems do not capture important risk factors.

Temporal bias can occur in One Health studies when exposure and outcome measurements are not aligned correctly in time or when relevant temporal relationships are not adequately captured. Disease incubation periods may vary between species, making it challenging to establish appropriate time windows for exposure assessment. Environmental exposures may have complex temporal patterns that require sophisticated modelling approaches to characterise adequately.

Spatial bias may occur in One Health studies when geographic patterns in data collection, exposure assessment, or outcome measurement create systematic differences that are not related to the underlying relationships of interest. Spatial clustering of cases or exposures may reflect surveillance artefacts, reporting patterns, or accessibility factors rather than authentic epidemiological relationships. Geographic information systems and spatial analytical methods can help identify and address some forms of spatial bias.

Verification and validation procedures are crucial for ensuring data quality in One Health studies, necessitating systematic approaches to verifying data accuracy, identifying outliers, and resolving discrepancies. Data verification involves checking data for internal consistency, completeness, and adherence to established protocols, whereas data validation entails comparing the collected data with external standards or alternative data sources. These procedures must be adapted to accommodate the diverse types of data and data sources utilised in One Health research.

Conclusion

Epidemiological methods provide essential frameworks for conducting rigorous One Health research; however, their application in multidisciplinary contexts requires careful adaptation and innovative approaches to address the unique challenges presented by investigations that span human, animal, and environmental health domains. The evolution of One Health epidemiological methods reflects growing recognition that many contemporary health challenges cannot be adequately addressed through single-discipline approaches and require integrated, transdisciplinary research strategies.

The selection of appropriate study designs for One Health investigations depends on multiple factors, including research objectives, available resources, temporal considerations, and the specific characteristics of the health outcomes and exposures being investigated. Cross-sectional studies provide valuable snapshots of health status across multiple domains, while cohort studies offer the most substantial evidence for causal relationships, albeit at a greater cost and complexity. Case-control studies provide efficient approaches for investigating rare diseases and outbreaks, though they require careful attention to control selection and exposure assessment challenges.

Outbreak investigation methodologies must be adapted to address the coordination and communication challenges inherent in multisectoral response efforts. Effective outbreak investigation requires established protocols for information sharing, coordinated case definitions, integrated analytical approaches, and joint control measures across all relevant sectors. The development of standardised outbreak investigation protocols and training programs designed explicitly for One Health contexts represents an essential priority for improving outbreak response capabilities.

Ecological and environmental epidemiological approaches provide valuable tools for examining population-level relationships between environmental exposures and health outcomes across multiple species and domains. However, these approaches require careful attention to the ecological fallacy and other limitations associated with aggregate-level analyses. The integration of spatial analytical methods and environmental monitoring data has greatly enhanced the capacity to conduct sophisticated environmental epidemiological studies relevant to One Health questions.

The challenges associated with multidisciplinary One Health research require sustained attention to communication, coordination, and methodological harmonisation across different professional communities and scientific traditions. Effective interdisciplinary collaboration entails establishing shared vocabularies, compatible research protocols, and integrated data management systems. Professional training and capacity-building efforts must be enhanced to prepare researchers for effective participation in multidisciplinary One Health research teams.

Data quality and bias considerations necessitate comprehensive quality assurance programs that address the diverse standards, procedures, and potential sources of error associated with various types of data and measurement systems. The development of standardised quality control protocols and reporting guidelines designed explicitly for One Health research represents an essential priority for enhancing the reliability and comparability of research findings across different studies and settings.

The connection between One Health epidemiological research and Sustainable Development Goal 3 (Good Health and Well-being) underscores the global significance of developing effective methods for investigating health outcomes at the human-animal-environment interface. The 2030 Agenda for Sustainable Development recognises Health as both a driver and outcome of sustainable development, emphasising the need for integrated approaches that address the complex determinants of Health across multiple domains (United Nations Development Programme, 2023). However, monitoring progress towards environment and health-related SDGs remains challenging, with persistent inequalities and concerning trends in key environmental indicators that are vital to human survival (Racioppi et al., 2020). The sustainable development framework provides essential context for One Health epidemiological research by emphasising the interconnected nature of health, environmental, and social determinants (Marmot & Bell, 2018).

Future developments in One Health epidemiological methods will likely include the enhanced integration of digital health technologies, artificial intelligence applications, and real-time surveillance systems, which can provide more timely and comprehensive data for investigating health outcomes across multiple domains. The development of standardised data sharing platforms and interoperable data systems will be essential for facilitating more effective multidisciplinary collaboration and enabling larger-scale One Health research initiatives.

The success of One Health epidemiological research ultimately depends on the development of a sustainable research infrastructure that can support long-term, multidisciplinary investigations addressing priority health challenges. This infrastructure must include not only technical capabilities for data collection and analysis but also institutional mechanisms for coordination, funding, and professional development across multiple sectors and disciplines.

Acknowledgments

The authors would like to extend our appreciation to those who offered helpful commentary during the drafting process of this manuscript. We also acknowledge the role Nova Science Publishers played in enabling the work described herein.

References

Davis, M. F., Rankin, S. C., Schurer, J. M., Cole, S., Conti, L., Rabinowitz, P., ... & Toribio, J. A. (2017). Checklist for One Health Epidemiological Reporting of Evidence (COHERE). *One Health*, 4, 14-21. https://doi.org/10.1016/j.onehlt.2017.07.001.

European Centre for Disease Prevention and Control & European Food Safety Authority. (2025). Coordinated One Health investigation and management of outbreaks in humans and animals caused by zoonotic avian influenza viruses. *EFSA Journal*, 23(1), e9183.

Johns Hopkins Bloomberg School of Public Health. (2024). The One Health approach to outbreaks and spillover events. *Public Health On Call*. https://publichealth.jhu.edu/2025/the-one-health-approach-to-outbreaks-and-spillover-events.

Lübker, C., & Murtin, F. (2023). Changes in longevity inequality by education among OECD countries before the COVID-19 pandemic. *BMC Public Health*, 23(1), 1646. https://doi.org/10.1186/s12889-023-16492-z.

Marmot, M., & Bell, R. (2018). The sustainable development goals and health equity. *Epidemiology*, 29(1), 5-7. https://doi.org/10.1097/EDE.0000000000000773.

Morgenstern, H. (1995). Ecologic studies in epidemiology: concepts, principles, and methods. *Annual Review of Public Health*, 16(1), 61-81. https://doi.org/10.1146/annurev.pu.16.050195.000425.

Munnangi, S., & Boktor, S. W. (2023). Epidemiology of study design. In *StatPearls*. StatPearls Publishing. https://www.ncbi.nlm.nih.gov/books/NBK470342/.

Racioppi, F., Dasgupta, S., Sturts, R., & Kolbenstetter, T. (2020). Reaching the sustainable development goals through healthy environments: are we on track? *European Journal of Public Health*, 30(Supplement_1), i14-i18. https://doi.org/10.1093/eurpub/ckz218.

Ribeiro, C. S., van de Burgwal, L. H., & Regeer, B. J. (2022). A generalisable one health framework for the control of zoonotic diseases. *Scientific Reports*, 12(1), 8588. https://doi.org/10.1038/s41598-022-12619-1.

United Nations Development Programme. (2023). Sustainable Development Goals. https://www.undp.org/sustainable-development-goals.

Wang, H., Naghavi, M., Allen, C., Barber, R. M., Bhutta, Z. A., Carter, A., ... & Murray, C. J. (2016). Global, regional, and national life expectancy, all-cause mortality, and cause-specific mortality for 249 causes of death, 1980–2015: a systematic analysis for the Global Burden of Disease Study 2015. *The Lancet*, 388(10053), 1459-1544.

Zhang, L., Wilson, D. P., & Zhang, W. (2024). Spatial epidemiology and its role in prevention and control of swine viral disease. *Animals*, 14(19), 2814. https://doi.org/10.3390/ani14192814.

Zhou, T., Li, M., & Chen, R. (2022). A participatory epidemiological and One Health approach to explore the community's capacity to detect emerging zoonoses and surveillance network opportunities in the forest region of Guinea. *PLOS Neglected Tropical Diseases*, 16(7), e0010462. https://doi.org/10.1371/journal.pntd.0010462.

Chapter 17

Rapid Response Systems and Outbreak Investigation

Maajid Mohi Ud Din Malik[1,*], PhD
and Shaista Mohuiddin[2]

[1]Department of Radiology and Imaging Technology, Dr. D. Y. Patil School of Allied Health Sciences, Dr. D. Y. Patil Vidyapeeth· Pune (Deemed to be University), Sant Tukaram Nagar, Pimpri, Pune, India
[2]Indira Gandhi National Open University, Regional Centre Srinagar Saida Kadal, Rainawari, Srinagar, UT of Jammu and Kashmir, India

Abstract

Rapid response systems and outbreak investigation form the backbone of global health security, providing essential frameworks for detecting, verifying, and responding to public health emergencies that threaten populations worldwide. This chapter examines the comprehensive approaches required for effective outbreak detection and verification, from surveillance systems to international reporting mechanisms under the International Health Regulations (2005). The deployment of rapid response teams involves coordinated, multisectoral efforts that integrate epidemiological, laboratory, clinical, and logistical expertise to ensure timely and effective control of outbreaks. Field investigation protocols have evolved to incorporate standardised approaches while maintaining flexibility to address diverse pathogens and settings. Laboratory support and specimen management require robust networks that can provide accurate, timely diagnostic services while maintaining quality assurance across different jurisdictions and laboratory capabilities. Contact tracing and case management represent critical components of outbreak response that require systematic approaches adapted to disease characteristics and local contexts. International collaboration mechanisms, anchored by the International Health Regulations and supported by networks such as the Global Outbreak Alert and Response Network, enable coordinated global responses to health emergencies. The 7-1-7 strategy, emphasising detection within 7 days, reporting within 1 day, and response within 7 days, provides a framework for measuring and improving outbreak response effectiveness. This chapter provides comprehensive guidance for public health practitioners, policymakers, and international organisations involved in outbreak preparedness and response, with particular emphasis on the connections to Sustainable Development Goal 3 (Good Health and Well-being) and global health security objectives.

---

[*] Corresponding Author's Email: maajid.malik@dpu.edu.in

In: Advances in the One Health Approach
Editors: Maajid Mohi Ud Din Malik, Abhay Saraf, Harshal Tukaram Pandve et al.
ISBN: 979-8-90134-202-2

Keywords: rapid response systems, outbreak investigation, global health security, International Health Regulations, contact tracing, laboratory networks, field epidemiology, emergency response, pandemic preparedness, Sustainable Development Goals

Introduction

Rapid response systems and outbreak investigation represent the critical frontline defence mechanisms in global health security, serving as the essential bridge between disease detection and effective public health action. In an increasingly interconnected world where infectious diseases can spread from remote villages to major cities within 36 hours, the capacity to rapidly detect, verify, and respond to public health emergencies has become fundamental to protecting both local communities and global populations. The COVID-19 pandemic, mpox outbreaks, and other recent health emergencies have demonstrated both the vital importance of robust rapid response capabilities and the persistent gaps in global preparedness and response infrastructure.

The evolution of outbreak investigation from descriptive field epidemiology to sophisticated, technology-enabled rapid response systems reflects advances in surveillance technologies, laboratory networks, data analytics, and international coordination mechanisms. Modern outbreak response integrates traditional epidemiological methods with digital technologies, artificial intelligence, and real-time data sharing platforms to enable faster detection, more accurate characterisation, and more effective control measures. However, the success of these systems depends critically on sustained investment in public health infrastructure, a trained workforce, and effective international collaboration frameworks that can function effectively during crisis periods when resources are strained and coordination challenges are magnified.

17.1. Outbreak Detection and Verification

Outbreak detection and verification constitute the critical first steps in effective public health emergency response, requiring sophisticated surveillance systems capable of identifying unusual patterns of disease occurrence while distinguishing actual outbreaks from standard variations in disease incidence. The Global Public Health Intelligence Network (GPHIN), maintained by the World Health Organisation, continuously monitors over 30,000 sources in nine languages, analysing more than 20,000 online news reports daily to identify potential public health events of international concern (Health Knowledge, 2024). This comprehensive approach recognises that more than 60% of initial outbreak reports originate from informal sources, including social media and electronic discussion groups, highlighting the importance of multi-source surveillance systems.

The verification process involves systematic assessment of reported events through multiple channels, including formal reports from ministries of health, WHO regional and country offices, national public health organisations, military and civilian laboratories, academic institutions, and non-governmental organisations. The WHO outbreak toolkit provides standardised tools and protocols for field investigators and epidemiologists operating in complex emergencies and resource-limited settings, addressing the critical need for data consistency and practical information sharing across teams, locations, and timeframes (WHO, 2024c). The toolkit includes disease-specific and generic investigation protocols that can be rapidly deployed when outbreaks are suspected or confirmed.

Modern outbreak detection systems increasingly rely on integrated approaches that combine traditional surveillance methods with digital technologies and artificial intelligence. The 7-1-7 strategy, implemented by CDC in collaboration with international partners, aims to detect outbreaks within 7 days, report them within 1 day, and mount an effective response within 7 days (CDC, 2025b). This approach includes bottleneck analysis to help countries identify barriers to meeting these targets and direct resources where they are most needed. As of 2024, the CDC is working to expand the use of the 7-1-7 approach in 26 countries worldwide, with evidence showing significant improvements in outbreak detection and response times where it has been implemented.

Laboratory-based surveillance plays an increasingly important role in outbreak detection, particularly for pathogens that may not present with distinctive clinical syndromes in early stages. The Laboratory Response Checklist for Infectious Disease Outbreaks provides public health laboratories with standardised frameworks for rapidly identifying important outbreak response considerations, particularly when investigating previously unknown infectious disease threats (Graham et al., 2020). This checklist encompasses five central themes: laboratory investigation, laboratory response capacity and training, laboratory surveillance and data management, interjurisdictional engagement and communication, and research and ethics considerations.

Environmental surveillance systems have emerged as valuable tools for outbreak detection, particularly for pathogens that can be detected in wastewater, air samples, or other ecological media before widespread clinical recognition occurs. The COVID-19 pandemic demonstrated the utility of wastewater surveillance for early detection of community transmission, leading to expanded implementation of environmental surveillance programs for various pathogens. These systems provide complementary information to clinical surveillance and can offer early warning of emerging outbreaks or resurgence of known pathogens.

The verification process must address challenges related to diagnostic capacity, reporting systems, and information quality across diverse health system contexts. Verification protocols require coordination between clinical providers, laboratory services, public health authorities, and international organisations to ensure that reported events are accurately characterised and appropriate response measures are initiated. The International Health Regulations (2005) provide the legal framework for event verification and reporting, requiring countries to notify WHO of events that may constitute a public health emergency of international concern through designated National IHR Focal Points (CDC, 2024d).

Quality assurance in outbreak detection requires systematic attention to the performance of surveillance systems, including their sensitivity, specificity, timeliness, and representativeness of surveillance data. Performance indicators should be regularly monitored and evaluated to identify areas for improvement and ensure that surveillance systems can effectively detect and verify outbreaks across different disease types and epidemiological contexts. Training programs for surveillance personnel, laboratory workers, and healthcare providers are essential components of maintaining effective outbreak detection capabilities. Table 17.1 shows components of an effective outbreak detection and verification system.

Table 17.1. Components of effective outbreak detection and verification systems

Component	Key Functions	Quality Indicators	Challenges
Surveillance Systems	Case detection; Data collection; Pattern recognition	Sensitivity; Timeliness; Coverage	Resource limitations; Data quality
Laboratory Networks	Diagnostic confirmation; Pathogen characterisation	Accuracy; Turnaround time; Capacity	Quality control; Connectivity
Reporting Mechanisms	Information flow; Alert generation; Communication	Completeness; Speed; Reliability	Coordination; Standardization
Verification Protocols	Event assessment; Information validation	Accuracy; Consistency; Objectivity	Expertise; Access; Coordination
Digital Technologies	Data integration; Pattern detection; Early warning	Performance; User adoption; Scalability	Technical capacity; Maintenance

17.2. Rapid Response Team Deployment

Rapid response team deployment represents a critical component of outbreak control, requiring pre-established systems for mobilising multidisciplinary expertise and resources to affected areas within timeframes that can effectively interrupt disease transmission and minimise health impacts. The CDC Global Rapid Response Team (GRRT), established following lessons learned from the 2014-2016 Ebola epidemic in West Africa, provides a model for a systematic approach to deploying rapid response teams (Koon et al., 2017). The GRRT maintains a roster of trained responders searchable by technical and language skills, facilitating rapid identification of appropriate personnel to fill specific response needs across diverse outbreak scenarios.

The composition of rapid response teams must be tailored to the specific characteristics of the outbreak, including the pathogen involved, transmission patterns, affected populations, and local response capacity. Core team members typically include epidemiologists for outbreak investigation and surveillance, clinicians for case management and clinical characterisation, laboratory specialists for diagnostic support and specimen management, infection prevention and control experts for healthcare facility preparedness, risk communication specialists for community engagement, and logistical coordinators for operational support. Additional expertise may be required, depending on the outbreak characteristics, such as vector control specialists for vector-borne diseases, environmental health experts for environmentally mediated outbreaks, or anthropologists for outbreaks that require intensive community engagement.

The Global Outbreak Alert and Response Network (GOARN), established by WHO in 2000, provides a formal mechanism for coordinating international outbreak response through a collaboration of institutions and networks ready to respond rapidly to outbreaks (CDC, 2024a). Key GOARN partners include academic and scientific institutions, medical and surveillance initiatives, laboratory networks, United Nations organisations, Red Cross organisations, and international humanitarian non-governmental organisations. Since its creation, GOARN has provided support during numerous public health emergencies, including deploying more than 1,100 experts during the West Africa Ebola epidemic with expertise in surveillance, epidemiology, case finding, contact tracing, and information management.

Pre-deployment preparations are essential for effective rapid response team deployment, including training programs that prepare responders for work in diverse cultural and environmental conditions, development of standardised protocols and tools that can be rapidly implemented across different settings, establishment of logistical support systems for transportation, accommodation, and supplies, and coordination mechanisms with local health authorities and international partners. The WHO Unity Studies provide examples of standardised protocols that can be rapidly implemented for early investigation of emerging pathogens, including protocols for investigating the first few cases and their contacts (FFX), household transmission studies, and healthcare worker infection studies (WHO, 2024b).

Deployment logistics require careful coordination across multiple organisations and jurisdictions, including visa and travel arrangements for international responders, coordination with local authorities for access and permissions, establishment of command-and-control structures that integrate with existing response systems, and provision of appropriate personal protective equipment, communications systems, and other essential supplies. The complexity of deployment logistics increases significantly for outbreaks in areas affected by conflict, natural disasters, or other humanitarian emergencies that may limit access or compromise security.

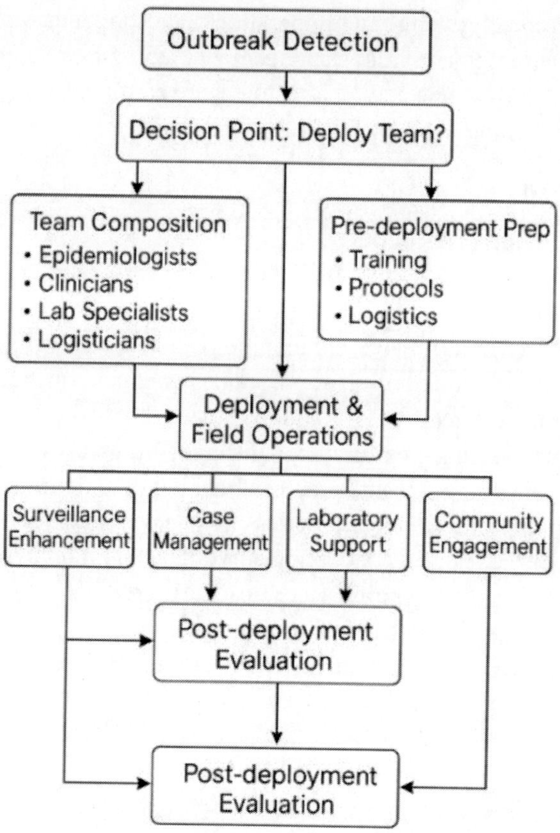

Figure 21. Rapid response team deployment framework.

Team integration with local response structures is crucial for effective outbreak response, necessitating a clear definition of roles and responsibilities, the establishment of communication protocols and information-sharing mechanisms, respect for local authority and decision-making processes, and the provision of technical assistance that builds rather than replaces local capacity. Successful integration requires cultural competency and understanding of local health systems, legal frameworks, and community contexts that may affect outbreak response activities.

Performance monitoring and evaluation of rapid response team deployment should include assessment of deployment times, team composition and competencies, integration with local response systems, achievement of response objectives, and identification of lessons learned for future improvement. A systematic evaluation of response team performance provides valuable insights for enhancing deployment procedures, training programs, and coordination mechanisms. After-action reviews should be conducted following each deployment to capture lessons learned and identify areas for improvement.

Figure 21 illustrates a comprehensive flowchart of the rapid response team deployment process. The framework begins with outbreak detection and verification, which feed into a decision point for team deployment. Once deployment is authorised, parallel processes commence, including team composition (epidemiologists, clinicians, laboratory specialists, logisticians), pre-deployment preparations (training, protocols, logistics), and coordination mechanisms (local authorities, international partners, GOARN). The central deployment phase shows integration with local systems, field operations, and ongoing support. Output streams include surveillance enhancement, case management, laboratory support, and community engagement. Feedback loops connect all phases to ensure continuous improvement, with post-deployment evaluation feeding back to enhance future response capabilities.

17.3. Field Investigation Protocols

Field investigation protocols provide systematic frameworks for conducting outbreak investigations that can generate reliable epidemiological evidence while adapting to diverse pathogen characteristics, population contexts, and resource constraints. The WHO has developed standardised outbreak investigation stages that provide structure for field investigations while maintaining flexibility for different outbreak scenarios (WHO, 2024a). These stages include confirming the outbreak, establishing case definitions, conducting active case finding, performing descriptive epidemiology, developing and testing hypotheses, implementing control measures, and conducting surveillance to monitor effectiveness.

Case definition development represents a critical early step in field investigation, requiring a balance between sensitivity for case detection and specificity for accurate case classification. Case definitions must account for clinical manifestations, epidemiological criteria, and laboratory confirmation requirements while recognising that these may evolve as more information becomes available about the outbreak. The WHO outbreak toolkit guides the development of case definitions that can be applied consistently across different investigation teams and timeframes, while allowing for refinement as outbreak characteristics become better understood. Case definitions should typically include categories for suspected, probable, and confirmed cases based on available diagnostic capabilities and clinical presentation patterns.

Active case finding represents a cornerstone of field investigation that requires systematic approaches to identifying cases beyond those that present for medical care. Active case-finding methods include reviewing medical records, conducting interviews with healthcare providers and community members, conducting household-to-household surveys in affected areas, and conducting contact tracing of known cases. The intensity and scope of active case finding should be proportional to the characteristics of the outbreak, its transmission patterns, and the available resources. Standardised data collection forms should be used to ensure consistency in information gathering and facilitate data analysis and interpretation.

Descriptive epidemiology analysis provides the foundation for understanding outbreak patterns and generating hypotheses about sources, modes of transmission, and risk factors. The classical epidemiological approach of analysing cases by person, place, and time remains fundamental to field investigations. However, modern investigations increasingly incorporate additional dimensions such as molecular epidemiology, environmental factors, and social network analysis. Epidemic curves offer visual representations of outbreak patterns over time, providing insight into transmission dynamics, incubation periods, and the effectiveness of control measures.

Analytical epidemiology studies may be conducted during field investigations to test specific hypotheses about outbreak sources and transmission mechanisms. Case-control studies are commonly used during outbreak investigations due to their efficiency and ability to generate rapid results; however, cohort studies may be more suitable for specific outbreak scenarios. Study design must account for the urgent nature of outbreak response while maintaining epidemiological rigour sufficient to generate reliable evidence for control measures. The International Severe Acute Respiratory and Emerging Infection Consortium (ISARIC) has developed standardised protocols for clinical characterisation that can be rapidly implemented during outbreaks of emerging infections (Dunning et al., 2020).

Environmental investigations form integral components of many field investigations, particularly for outbreaks involving foodborne, waterborne, or vector-borne transmission. Environmental investigations may include assessments of food preparation and distribution systems, water quality testing, sanitation system evaluation, vector surveillance and control measures, and evaluations of healthcare facility infection prevention and control practices. Environmental sampling should be coordinated with epidemiological investigations to test specific hypotheses and guide the implementation of control measures.

Laboratory coordination requires integration of field investigation activities with diagnostic testing, pathogen characterisation, and quality assurance procedures. Field investigators must understand laboratory capabilities and limitations, as well as specimen collection and transport requirements, and the turnaround times for various types of testing. The GOARN Emerging and Dangerous Pathogens Laboratory Network provides support for field investigations through deployment of mobile laboratories and diagnostic expertise, particularly for outbreaks involving high-consequence pathogens or areas with limited laboratory capacity.

Data management and analysis systems must be capable of handling the volume and complexity of data generated during field investigations while providing real-time analysis capabilities that can guide ongoing response activities. Digital data collection platforms have increasingly replaced paper-based systems, offering advantages including reduced data entry errors, real-time data access, and automated analysis capabilities. However, digital systems require technical expertise and a reliable communication infrastructure that may not be available in all outbreak settings.

Quality control procedures should be implemented throughout field investigations to ensure the accuracy, completeness, and reliability of the data. Quality control measures include training investigation teams on standardised protocols, supervising and mentoring junior investigators, conducting regular data reviews, and cleaning procedures, and validating findings through multiple data sources. Inter-rater reliability assessments should be performed when multiple investigators are involved in data collection to ensure consistency in data collection procedures.

17.4. Laboratory Support and Specimen Management

Laboratory support and specimen management represent critical components of outbreak response that require coordinated networks capable of providing accurate, timely diagnostic services while maintaining quality assurance standards across diverse jurisdictions and technical capabilities. The WHO emphasises that laboratory information is critical for disease surveillance and control programs, providing support before outbreaks through early case detection and during outbreaks through confirmation of cases and characterisation of etiological agents (WHO EMRO, 1996). Laboratory networks operate at multiple levels, from field laboratories that provide basic diagnostic capabilities in resource-limited settings to international reference laboratories that can identify rare or dangerous pathogens and provide specialised diagnostic reagents.

Specimen collection and transport systems must be designed to maintain specimen integrity while ensuring safe handling procedures that protect healthcare workers, laboratory personnel, and the general public. Standardised protocols for specimen collection, packaging, and transport are essential for maintaining diagnostic accuracy and preventing laboratory-acquired infections. The Laboratory Response Checklist for Infectious Disease Outbreaks identifies specimen management as a critical early response consideration, emphasising the need for standardised protocols that can be rapidly implemented across different outbreak scenarios (Graham et al., 2020). Specimen transport networks must account for varying geographic distances, transportation infrastructure limitations, and regulatory requirements for shipping infectious materials.

Laboratory capacity requirements vary significantly depending on the characteristics of the outbreak, including the type of pathogen, diagnostic complexity, specimen volumes, and turnaround time requirements. Field laboratories can be deployed to provide basic diagnostic capabilities in areas where laboratory services are limited or nonexistent, offering advantages such as reduced specimen transport requirements, faster turnaround times, and increased testing capacity during surge periods. Regional laboratories typically offer more comprehensive diagnostic services and often serve as referral centres for field laboratories. International reference laboratories, including WHO collaborating centres, provide specialised services, such as the identification of rarely encountered organisms, characterisation of pathogenic microorganisms, and the provision of diagnostic reagents that may not be commercially available.

Quality assurance programs are essential for maintaining laboratory reliability and ensuring that diagnostic results can be trusted for clinical and public health decision-making. Quality assurance encompasses internal quality control procedures within individual laboratories, external quality assessment programs that provide proficiency testing across laboratory networks, and accreditation processes that verify compliance with international standards. The Strengthening Laboratory Management Toward Accreditation (SLMTA) program, supported by the CDC through PEPFAR, has assisted over 400 laboratories in low- and middle-income countries in achieving accreditation to international quality standards since 2013 (CDC, 2025c).

The selection and validation of diagnostic tests require careful consideration of test performance characteristics, available resources, and public health objectives. Rapid diagnostic tests may be prioritised during outbreak response due to their ability to provide results at the point of care. However, they may have reduced sensitivity or specificity compared to reference laboratory methods. Molecular diagnostic methods offer high sensitivity and specificity but require specialised equipment and technical expertise that may not be available in all settings. Serological testing may be valuable for outbreak investigation and surveillance, but it requires careful interpretation, considering the timing of specimen collection relative to disease onset.

Data management systems must integrate laboratory results with epidemiological investigation data while maintaining appropriate confidentiality and security protections. Laboratory information management systems (LIMS) can facilitate specimen tracking, result reporting, and quality control monitoring, though implementation requires technical infrastructure and training that may be challenging in resource-limited settings. Standardised data formats and communication protocols are essential for effective information sharing between laboratories and public health authorities.

Surge capacity planning addresses the need to rapidly scale up laboratory services during outbreak situations when testing demands may exceed routine capacity. Surge capacity strategies include pre-positioning of diagnostic supplies and reagents, training additional laboratory personnel, establishing agreements with reference laboratories for overflow testing, and deploying mobile laboratory units to affected areas. The GOARN Emerging and Dangerous Pathogens Laboratory Network deployed more than 25 mobile laboratories, with over 200 experts, during the West Africa Ebola epidemic, demonstrating the potential for a coordinated laboratory surge response (CDC, 2024a).

Biosafety and biosecurity considerations are critical during outbreak response when laboratories may be handling unfamiliar or high-consequence pathogens. Biosafety protocols must be tailored to the risk level associated with the pathogen, while allowing for efficient diagnostic operations. The European Network of Biosafety Level 4 Laboratories (Euronet-P4) provides a model for international collaboration in high-containment laboratory operations, including the standardisation of biosafety procedures, the sharing of protocols and reagents, and the coordination of training programs (Nisii et al., 2009). Biosecurity measures must protect against both accidental exposure and intentional misuse of dangerous pathogens while maintaining the collaborative relationships essential for effective outbreak response. Table 17.2 presents the laboratory network's capabilities and requirements.

17.5. Contact Tracing and Case Management

Contact tracing and case management represent fundamental strategies for controlling infectious disease outbreaks through systematic identification, assessment, management, and support of individuals who may have been exposed to infectious pathogens. The World Health Organisation's 2024 guidelines on contact tracing define contact tracing as "the systematic process of identifying, assessing, managing, and supporting contact persons of infectious individuals" and emphasise its role in breaking chains of transmission through the early identification and management of cases (WHO, 2024d). Contact tracing has been effectively used for various diseases, including tuberculosis and Ebola virus disease, and most recently during the COVID-19 pandemic. However, implementation approaches must be adapted to disease characteristics, transmission patterns, and local contexts.

Case investigation forms the foundation of contact tracing efforts and must be conducted systematically to identify potential sources of infection and mechanisms of transmission. The WHO's interim guidance for mpox surveillance emphasises that case investigation should consist of clinical examination in a well-ventilated room using appropriate personal protective equipment, questioning about possible sources of exposure, and safe collection and dispatch of specimens for laboratory examination (WHO, 2024e). Case investigation interviews should use standardised forms to ensure consistent data collection while allowing flexibility to explore unique aspects of individual cases that may provide critical epidemiological insights.

Contact identification requires systematic approaches to determine who may have been exposed to infected individuals based on the pathogen's known or expected modes of transmission. Contact definitions must be established early in outbreak response and should specify the types of interactions, time periods, and settings that constitute potential exposure. The WHO guideline on contact tracing notes that contact definitions may evolve as understanding of outbreak characteristics improves, emphasising the importance of evidence-based revisions that are thoroughly communicated and documented (WHO, 2024d). Contact identification methods include interviews with cases or their proxies, review of medical records, household visits, and increasingly, digital proximity tracing applications.

Risk stratification enables the prioritisation of contact management activities based on the likelihood of infection and the potential for onward transmission. High-risk contacts may require more intensive monitoring, testing, or quarantine measures, while lower-risk contacts may be managed through self-monitoring or periodic check-ins. Risk stratification criteria should consider factors such as the type and duration of exposure, timing relative to the infectious period, use of personal protective equipment, and individual susceptibility factors, including immunocompromised status or underlying health conditions.

Contact monitoring involves systematic follow-up of identified contacts to detect early signs of infection and facilitate prompt diagnosis and treatment. The WHO's mpox guidance recommends that contacts of probable and confirmed cases monitor themselves daily for signs or symptoms for 21 days from the last contact with an infectious case (WHO, 2024e). Monitoring methods may include daily telephone calls, text message systems, mobile applications, or in-person visits, depending on available resources, technology, and individual circumstances. Monitoring protocols should specify what symptoms to watch for, when and how to report these symptoms, and procedures for evaluating symptomatic contacts.

Case management encompasses the clinical care and support services provided to individuals diagnosed with infectious diseases, including isolation measures to prevent the transmission of the disease to others. Clinical management protocols should be developed based on available evidence about treatment options, supportive care requirements, and infection prevention and control measures. Healthcare facilities must be prepared to provide appropriate isolation accommodations and clinical care while protecting healthcare workers and other patients from exposure. Community-based case management may be applicable for mild cases of certain diseases, provided adequate isolation and monitoring can be maintained.

Table 17.2. Laboratory network capabilities and requirements

Laboratory Level	Primary Functions	Diagnostic Capabilities	Quality Requirements	Resource Needs
Field Laboratories	Point-of-care testing; Basic confirmation	Rapid tests; Basic microscopy; Antigen detection	Internal QC; Standard protocols	Minimal infrastructure; Portable equipment
Regional Laboratories	Comprehensive testing; Confirmatory testing	Culture; Molecular testing; Serology	External QA; Accreditation	Moderate infrastructure; Skilled staff
National Reference Labs	Advanced characterisation; Rare pathogens	Specialised testing; Antimicrobial resistance; Typing	International standards; Proficiency testing	Advanced equipment; Expert staff
International Reference Labs	Global expertise; Novel pathogens	Research-level capabilities; Experimental methods	WHO collaboration; Research standards	Maximum containment; International expertise

Support services for contacts and cases are essential components of effective contact tracing programs that address the social, economic, and psychological impacts of outbreak control measures. Support services may include the provision of necessities during quarantine periods, mental health services, assistance with employment or housing issues, and compensation for lost wages. The WHO guideline on contact tracing emphasises the importance of financial transfers and other support mechanisms to enable adherence to public health and social measures (WHO, 2024d). Failure to provide adequate support can undermine the effectiveness of contact tracing and create hardships that disproportionately affect vulnerable populations.

Digital technologies are increasingly being integrated into contact tracing programs to improve efficiency, reduce resource requirements, and enhance data management capabilities. Digital proximity tracing applications can supplement manual contact tracing by identifying potential exposures that may not be recalled during interviews. However, digital tools have limitations, including variable adoption rates, privacy concerns, and technical requirements that may limit their effectiveness in specific populations or settings. The WHO emphasises that digital tools should complement, rather than replace, human-centred contact tracing approaches.

Performance monitoring and evaluation of contact tracing programs should assess both process indicators, such as the timeliness and completeness of contact identification, and outcome indicators, such as the reduction in transmission. Key performance indicators may include the percentage of cases interviewed within a specified timeframe, the rate of contacts identified and successfully monitored, the time from case identification to contact notification, and the proportion of secondary cases identified through contact tracing versus other means. Regular evaluation enables the identification of bottlenecks and the implementation of improvements to enhance program effectiveness.

17.6. International Collaboration Mechanisms

International collaboration mechanisms provide essential frameworks for coordinating global responses to public health emergencies that transcend national boundaries and require shared expertise, resources, and coordinated action. The International Health Regulations (2005) represent the primary legal framework governing international collaboration for health emergency response, providing legally binding rules that apply to 196 countries, including all 194 WHO Member States (CDC, 2024d). The IHR establish obligations for countries to develop core capacities for disease surveillance and response, report events of international public health importance, and collaborate in global health security efforts through the sharing of information, technical assistance, and coordinated response measures.

The 2024 amendments to the International Health Regulations, adopted by the World Health Assembly, introduce significant changes that emphasise equity and solidarity in pandemic preparedness and response (Habibi et al., 2025). These amendments reflect lessons learned from the COVID-19 pandemic and shift the IHR from a primarily technical instrument to one that addresses inherently political issues, including financing, access to countermeasures, and technology transfer. The amendments establish new obligations for international cooperation, including mechanisms for sharing pathogen samples and genetic sequences, procedures for equitable access to pandemic-related health products, and frameworks for providing technical and financial assistance to countries with limited capacity.

The Global Outbreak Alert and Response Network (GOARN) represents WHO's primary mechanism for coordinating technical expertise and operational support during international health emergencies. GOARN partnerships include academic and scientific institutions, medical and surveillance initiatives, laboratory networks, United Nations organisations, Red Cross organisations, and global humanitarian non-governmental organisations that maintain constant alert status and readiness to respond rapidly to outbreaks (CDC, 2024a). The network's effectiveness has been demonstrated through its responses to multiple international health emergencies, including SARS, MERS, Ebola, Zika, and COVID-19, by providing coordinated deployments of experts and resources based on specific technical needs and country requests.

Laboratory networks play critical roles in international collaboration by providing diagnostic support, pathogen characterisation, and quality assurance across national boundaries. Multiple global laboratory networks support early detection and response to infectious disease outbreaks, including PulseNet International for foodborne disease surveillance, the WHO Global Influenza Surveillance and Response System, and the GOARN Emerging and Dangerous Pathogens Laboratory Network (CDC, 2024a). These networks facilitate the sharing of diagnostic protocols, reference materials, and expertise while maintaining quality standards through proficiency testing and accreditation programs.

Regional collaboration mechanisms complement global frameworks by addressing specific geographic, cultural, and epidemiological contexts that affect disease transmission and response capacity. The European Centre for Disease Prevention and Control maintains multinational surveillance networks for various diseases, including Legionnaires' disease, tuberculosis, antimicrobial resistance, and vaccine-preventable diseases, which facilitate a coordinated response to cross-border health threats (CDC, 2024a). Regional networks can provide a more rapid response than global mechanisms while maintaining a connection to international coordination structures for events with broader implications.

Information sharing represents a fundamental component of international collaboration that requires balancing transparency and rapid communication with protection of sensitive information and respect for national sovereignty. The WHO's Disease Outbreak News serves as a platform for sharing information about international health events. At the same time, the Global Public Health Intelligence Network monitors informal information sources to identify potential health threats. Real-time information sharing platforms enable coordinated surveillance and response activities while maintaining appropriate confidentiality protections for sensitive epidemiological and laboratory data.

Financing mechanisms for international collaboration include both standing capacity-building programs and emergency response funding that can be rapidly deployed during health emergencies. The World Bank's Pandemic Emergency Financing Facility, established following the West Africa Ebola epidemic, provides insurance-based financing for outbreak response. At the same time, the WHO Contingency Fund for Emergencies enables immediate funding for response activities (CDC, 2024a). However, sustainable financing for international collaboration remains a significant challenge, with many countries unable to maintain adequate preparedness capacities and international support mechanisms that are chronically underfunded relative to their needs.

The diplomatic and political dimensions of international collaboration necessitate careful navigation of sovereignty concerns, resource allocation disputes, and competing national interests that can impact the effectiveness of coordinated responses. The designation of Public Health Emergencies of International Concern through the IHR provides a mechanism for elevating international attention and mobilising resources. However, the political aspects of these determinations can affect their perceived legitimacy and effectiveness. WHO's role as a technical agency operating within a politically complex international system requires a careful balance between technical objectivity and diplomatic effectiveness.

Performance evaluation of international collaboration mechanisms should assess both preparedness and capacity-building, as well as emergency response effectiveness, across multiple dimensions, including timeliness, coordination, resource mobilisation, and health outcomes. The WHO's IHR Monitoring and Evaluation Framework offers systematic approaches for assessing country capacity and identifying areas for improvement through State Party Self-Assessment Annual Reporting, Joint External Evaluations, After-Action Reviews, and simulation exercises (CDC, 2024d). However, evaluating the effectiveness of international collaboration remains challenging due to the complex, multi-actor nature of global health emergency responses and the difficulty of attributing outcomes to specific intervention components.

Conclusion

Rapid response systems and outbreak investigation represent fundamental components of global health security that require coordinated, multisectoral approaches spanning detection, verification, response, and recovery phases of health emergency management. The evolution of outbreak response capabilities over the past decades reflects growing recognition that infectious disease threats can emerge anywhere and spread rapidly across international boundaries, requiring robust preparedness systems and effective international cooperation mechanisms. The COVID-19 pandemic, mpox outbreaks, and other recent health emergencies have demonstrated both the critical importance of rapid response systems and the persistent gaps in global preparedness and response capacity.

The detection and verification of outbreaks requires sophisticated surveillance systems that can identify unusual disease patterns while distinguishing true emergencies from normal epidemiological variation. The integration of traditional surveillance methods with digital technologies, artificial intelligence, and environmental monitoring systems offers promising approaches for improving the speed and accuracy of outbreak detection. However, effective detection systems require sustained investment in surveillance infrastructure, laboratory capacity, and workforce development that remains inadequate in many countries and regions.

Rapid response team deployment has evolved from ad hoc arrangements to systematic approaches that maintain trained personnel, standardised protocols, and pre-positioned resources that can be rapidly mobilised when emergencies occur. The CDC Global Rapid Response Team and WHO's Global Outbreak Alert and Response Network provide models for coordinated response that balance international technical expertise with respect for national sovereignty and local capacity. However, the effectiveness of rapid response teams depends critically on integration with local health systems and response structures, requiring ongoing attention to capacity building and coordination mechanisms.

Field investigation protocols have benefited from standardisation efforts that promote consistency and quality while maintaining flexibility to address diverse pathogen characteristics and local contexts. The WHO outbreak toolkit and other standardised investigation protocols provide valuable resources for field investigators, though their effectiveness depends on adequate training, supervision, and quality control systems. The integration of digital data collection platforms and real-time analysis capabilities offers opportunities for improving investigation efficiency and timeliness. Still, it requires technical infrastructure and expertise that may be limited in outbreak-affected areas.

Laboratory support and specimen management systems require coordinated networks that can provide accurate and timely diagnostic services while maintaining quality assurance standards across various technical capabilities and resource levels. The development of field laboratory capacity, the strengthening of national reference laboratories, and coordination with international reference centres provide a multi-tiered approach to diagnostic support that can be scaled based on outbreak characteristics and local needs. However, laboratory network sustainability requires ongoing investment in equipment, reagents, training, and quality assurance programs.

Contact tracing and case management represent critical but resource-intensive activities that require systematic approaches adapted to disease characteristics, transmission patterns, and local contexts. The WHO's disease-agnostic guideline on contact tracing provides valuable frameworks for implementation while recognising the need for disease-specific adaptations (WHO, 2024d). Digital technologies offer opportunities for enhancing contact tracing efficiency; however, human-centred approaches remain essential for building trust, providing support, and addressing the social determinants that affect program effectiveness.

International collaboration mechanisms, anchored in the International Health Regulations, provide a legal framework and operational structures for a coordinated global response to health emergencies. The 2024 amendments to the IHR reflect efforts to address equity and solidarity concerns highlighted during the COVID-19 pandemic while strengthening global health security (Habibi et al., 2025). However, effective international collaboration requires sustained political commitment, adequate financing, and resolution of sovereignty concerns that can impede coordinated response efforts.

The connection between outbreak response and Sustainable Development Goal 3 (Good Health and Well-being) underscores the broader development implications of health security investments. Effective outbreak response systems contribute to health system strengthening, reduce the economic impacts of health emergencies, and protect vulnerable populations who are disproportionately affected by infectious disease outbreaks. The estimated $13.8 trillion economic cost of the COVID-19 pandemic through 2024 demonstrates the enormous potential return on investment in outbreak preparedness and response capacity (CDC, 2024d).

Future developments in rapid response systems will likely include the enhanced integration of artificial intelligence and machine learning technologies for outbreak detection and response optimisation, the expanded use of digital platforms for coordination and information sharing, the development of more flexible and scalable laboratory networks, and strengthened community engagement approaches that build local capacity and trust. The success of these developments will depend on sustained investment in health system infrastructure, workforce development, and international cooperation mechanisms that can effectively address the complex challenges of 21st-century global health security.

The fundamental challenge facing global health security is the persistent gap between the resources required for adequate preparedness and the political will to sustain necessary investments during inter-pandemic periods. Building effective rapid response systems requires long-term commitment to capacity building, infrastructure development, and international cooperation that extends beyond crisis periods. Only through such sustained efforts can the global community develop the resilience necessary to detect, respond to, and recover from future health emergencies while advancing broader global health and development objectives.

Acknowledgments

The authors would like to extend our appreciation to those who offered helpful commentary during the drafting process of this manuscript. We also acknowledge the role Nova Science Publishers played in enabling the work described herein.

References

Dunning, J., Baillie, J. K., Cao, B., Hayden, F. G., International Severe Acute Respiratory and Emerging Infections Consortium (ISARIC). (2020). Global outbreak research: harmony not hegemony. *The Lancet*, 395(10230), 1143-1145. https://doi.org/10.1016/S0140-6736(20)30777-6.

Graham, H., Burkholder, B. T., Featherstone, J., Grein, T. W., Lowe, R., McMahon, S. A., ... & Restrepo-Méndez, M. C. (2020). Laboratory response checklist for infectious disease outbreaks—preparedness and response considerations for emerging threats. *Health Security*, 18(6), 429-438. https://doi.org/10.1089/hs.2020.0067.

Habibi, R., Eckert, S., Brassard, C., Burci, G. L., Eccleston-Turner, M., Forman, L., ... & Yamin, A. E. (2025). The 2024 amendments to the International Health Regulations: A new era for global health law in pandemic preparedness and response? *Journal of Law, Medicine & Ethics*, 53(S1), 28-39. https://doi.org/10.1017/jme.2025.15.

Health Knowledge. (2024). The steps in outbreak investigation including the use of relevant epidemiological methods. https://www.healthknowledge.org.uk/public-health-textbook/disease-causation-diagnostic/2g-communicable-disease/outbreak-investigation.

Koon, A. D., Nsoesie, E. O., Rees, C. A., Hawkins, J. B., Juma, P. A., Haskew, C., ... & Brownstein, J. S. (2017). Establishment of CDC Global Rapid Response Team to ensure global health security. *Emerging Infectious Diseases*, 23(13), S184-S189. https://doi.org/10.3201/eid2313.170711.

Nisii, C., Vincenti, D., Fusco, F. M., Gagliardini, R., Lauria, F. N., Magnavita, N., ... & Ippolito, G. (2009). European lab network prepares for high-risk pathogen threat. *The Lancet Infectious Diseases*, 9(2), 72-73. https://doi.org/10.1016/S1473-3099(09)70019-8.

Chapter 18

Statistical Methods and Data Analysis for One Health

Shaista Mohuiddin[1]
and Maajid Mohi Ud Din Malik[2,*], PhD

[1]Indira Gandhi National Open University, Regional Centre Srinagar Saida Kadal, Rainawari, Srinagar, UT of Jammu and Kashmir, India

[2]Department of Radiology and Imaging Technology, Dr. D. Y. Patil School of Allied Health Sciences, Dr. D. Y. Patil Vidyapeeth, Pune (Deemed to be University), Sant Tukaram Nagar, Pimpri, Pune, India

Abstract

Statistical methods and data analysis form the analytical foundation of One Health research, providing essential tools for understanding complex interactions between human, animal, and environmental health factors. This chapter examines the application of descriptive and analytical statistical approaches designed explicitly for One Health investigations, addressing the unique challenges of integrating diverse data types and sources across multiple disciplines. Spatial and temporal analysis methods have emerged as critical components for examining disease patterns and environmental determinants at the human-animal-environment interface, utilising geographic information systems and advanced modelling techniques to reveal spatiotemporal relationships. Disease transmission modelling provides a mechanistic framework for understanding pathogen dynamics across different hosts and environments, supporting evidence-based decision-making for outbreak control and prevention strategies. Risk factor analysis in One Health contexts requires sophisticated approaches that can identify and quantify exposures operating at multiple scales and across different populations. Meta-analysis and systematic review methodologies adapted for One Health research enable synthesis of evidence from diverse study designs and data sources while addressing methodological heterogeneity. Big data approaches and machine learning technologies offer transformative potential for One Health research through the integration of high-dimensional datasets, automated pattern recognition, and predictive modelling capabilities. The connections to Sustainable Development Goal 3 (Good Health and Well-being) and related targets emphasise the global significance of robust statistical approaches for addressing complex health challenges that require transdisciplinary solutions. This chapter provides practical guidance for researchers, analysts, and public health practitioners working at the intersection of human, animal, and environmental health domains.

* Corresponding Author's Email: maajid.malik@dpu.edu.in

In: Advances in the One Health Approach
Editors: Maajid Mohi Ud Din Malik, Abhay Saraf, Harshal Tukaram Pandve et al.
ISBN: 979-8-90134-202-2

Keywords: statistical methods, One Health, spatial analysis, temporal analysis, disease transmission modelling, risk factor analysis, meta-analysis, machine learning, big data, artificial intelligence, Sustainable Development Goal 3

Introduction

Statistical methods and data analysis form the quantitative backbone of One Health research, providing the analytical frameworks necessary to understand the complex relationships between human, animal, and environmental health factors. The interdisciplinary nature of One Health research presents unique statistical challenges that extend far beyond traditional epidemiological approaches, requiring innovative methods that can integrate diverse data types, account for multiple levels of organisation, and address the inherent complexity of multi-species, multi-environment health systems. As One Health research increasingly relies on big data, machine learning, and artificial intelligence technologies, the need for sophisticated statistical approaches that maintain scientific rigour while accommodating methodological diversity has become paramount.

The emergence of One Health as a dominant paradigm for addressing complex health challenges has coincided with rapid advances in statistical methodology, computational power, and data availability. These technological developments have enabled researchers to tackle questions that were previously intractable, including real-time disease forecasting, multi-scale risk assessment, and integrated surveillance across human, animal, and environmental domains. However, the application of advanced statistical methods to One Health research requires careful attention to assumptions, limitations, and interpretation challenges that may not be apparent in single-discipline studies. The successful implementation of statistical approaches in One Health contexts depends on close collaboration between quantitative methodologists and domain experts from human medicine, veterinary medicine, environmental science, and related fields.

18.1. Descriptive and Analytical Statistics

Descriptive and analytical statistics in One Health research require specialised approaches that can accommodate the complexity and diversity of data generated across human, animal, and environmental health domains. Traditional epidemiological methods must be adapted to address the unique characteristics of One Health investigations, including different study populations, varying data quality standards, and diverse measurement scales across disciplines. The integration of descriptive statistics from multiple domains requires careful attention to data harmonisation, standardisation procedures, and appropriate visualisation techniques that can effectively communicate findings across different professional audiences and stakeholder groups. Descriptive statistical approaches in One Health contexts encompass measures of central tendency, variability, and distribution characteristics that must be interpreted within the specific context of each health domain. Human health data typically adhere to established clinical and epidemiological standards, whereas animal health data may reflect species-specific considerations, husbandry practices, and veterinary diagnostic protocols. Environmental health data introduce additional complexity through spatial and temporal variability, measurement uncertainty, and the need to integrate multiple environmental parameters. Practical descriptive analysis requires understanding these domain-specific characteristics while developing integrated approaches that can reveal patterns and relationships across the human-animal-environment interface.

Data visualisation techniques play a critical role in One Health research by enabling researchers to explore complex, multidimensional datasets and communicate their findings to diverse audiences. Traditional epidemiological visualisation methods, including epidemic curves, scatter plots, and forest plots, must be supplemented with specialised techniques such as geographic information system (GIS) mapping, network diagrams, and interactive dashboards that can effectively display relationships across multiple domains. The choice of visualisation methods should consider the intended audience, the complexity of the data, and the specific research questions being addressed.

Analytical statistics in One Health research must address challenges related to data integration, confounding control, and causal inference across different types of studies and data sources. Regression modelling approaches require careful consideration of hierarchical data structures, spatial and temporal dependencies, and measurement errors that may affect different variables in varying ways. The Global Health Data Institute emphasises that spatial and temporal modelling requires specialised techniques that account for spatial relationships and spatiotemporal correlation in both fixed effects and random effects components (Global Health Data Institute, 2020). These approaches enable researchers to separate individual-level effects from contextual effects while accounting for dependencies that arise from shared environmental exposures or social clustering.

Hypothesis testing in One Health contexts requires multiple comparison adjustments and careful interpretation of statistical significance considering practical significance and policy relevance. The integration of evidence from numerous studies or data sources may require meta-analytical approaches that can account for heterogeneity in study designs, populations, and measurement methods. Power analysis and sample size calculations must consider the complexity of One Health study designs, including cluster sampling, multilevel data structures, and multiple outcome measures.

Quality control and data validation procedures are essential components of statistical analysis in One Health research, requiring systematic approaches to identify and address data quality issues that may arise from different collection methods, measurement protocols, and reporting standards across disciplines. Missing data patterns may be informative about underlying processes and require specialised imputation techniques that account for the reasons for missingness and the relationships between different types of variables. Outlier detection and influential observation analysis must consider the various distributions and measurement scales associated with varying types of health data.

Statistical software selection and analysis workflows must accommodate the diverse data types and analytical requirements associated with One Health research. Traditional statistical packages may need to be supplemented with specialised software for spatial analysis, network analysis, or machine learning applications. Reproducible research practices are crucial in One Health contexts, given the complexity of data integration and analysis procedures, which necessitate meticulous documentation of data processing steps, statistical methods, and sensitivity analyses. Table 18.1 shows statistical approaches for different types of one health data.

Table 18.1. Statistical approaches for different types of one health data

Data Type	Descriptive Methods	Analytical Methods	Visualisation Techniques	Special Considerations
Human Health	Prevalence rates; Incidence rates; Clinical measures	Regression models; Survival analysis; Case-control studies	Epidemic curves; Forest plots; Risk plots	Clinical validation; Ethical considerations
Animal Health	Population parameters; Disease prevalence; Production measures	Mixed models; Spatial models; Time series	Herd maps; Population pyramids; Temporal trends	Species differences; Management systems
Environmental Health	Concentration measures; Spatial distribution; Temporal patterns	Spatial statistics; Time series; Exposure models	GIS maps; Contour plots; Temporal surfaces	Measurement uncertainty; Scale effects
Integrated Data	Cross-domain indicators; Composite indices; Network measures	Multilevel models; Network analysis; Machine learning	Network diagrams: Dashboard displays; Interactive maps	Data harmonisation; Scale integration

18.2. Spatial and Temporal Analysis

Spatial and temporal analysis methods represent fundamental components of One Health research, providing essential tools for understanding how health outcomes vary across geographic locations and time periods while revealing patterns that may not be apparent through traditional analytical approaches. The Columbia University Mailman School of Public Health emphasises that spatiotemporal analysis has emerged as a crucial research area due to the development and application of novel computational techniques that enable analysis of large spatiotemporal databases (Columbia University, 2023). These approaches are particularly valuable for One Health investigations because they can reveal relationships between environmental factors, pathogen ecology, and disease outcomes that operate at multiple spatial and temporal scales.

Spatial statistical methods encompass a range of techniques designed to account for spatial relationships and dependencies in health data, including point pattern analysis, area-level analysis, and geostatistical approaches. Point pattern analysis is particularly useful for investigating disease clusters, environmental exposure sources, and animal population distributions. Area-level analysis, on the other hand, enables the examination of health outcomes aggregated at the administrative unit or ecological zone level. Geostatistical methods provide frameworks for interpolating and predicting health outcomes at unsampled locations, while quantifying the uncertainty associated with these predictions. This is particularly valuable for assessing environmental exposure and mapping disease risk.

Temporal analysis methods in One Health research must accommodate different time scales and temporal patterns that characterise different types of health data. Human disease surveillance typically operates on daily to weekly reporting cycles. At the same time, animal population dynamics may follow seasonal or annual cycles, and environmental conditions may exhibit both short-term fluctuations and long-term trends. Time series analysis techniques enable the identification of temporal trends, seasonal patterns, and cyclical behaviours while accounting for autocorrelation and other forms of temporal dependence. Advanced methods, such as state-space models and dynamic linear models, can accommodate time-varying parameters and missing observations that are commonly encountered in One Health datasets.

Spatiotemporal modelling approaches integrate spatial and temporal dimensions to provide comprehensive frameworks for understanding disease dynamics and environmental determinants of Health. The analysis of spatiotemporal data necessitates considering both temporal and spatial correlations, which adds significant complexity to the analytical process due to the continuous and discrete changes in spatial and non-spatial properties of spatiotemporal objects, as well as the influence of neighbouring objects on one another (Columbia University, 2023). Key challenges include the two-dimensional nature of space, with unlimited directionality, compared to the unidimensional, forward-only direction of time, which affects the interpretation of spatiotemporal analytical results.

Geographic Information Systems (GIS) provide essential platforms for spatial and spatiotemporal analysis in One Health research, enabling integration of health data with environmental, demographic, and infrastructure data at multiple spatial scales. GIS capabilities include spatial data management, cartographic visualisation, spatial analysis functions, and integration with statistical software packages for advanced analytical procedures. Modern GIS platforms are increasingly incorporating temporal functionality, enabling the analysis of spatiotemporal data through animated displays, temporal queries, and integrated statistical modelling capabilities.

Spatial autocorrelation represents a fundamental consideration in spatial and spatiotemporal analysis, arising when observations that are closer together in space are more similar than would be expected under spatial independence. Positive spatial autocorrelation is a common feature in health data, resulting from shared environmental exposures, social clustering, and administrative boundaries that influence healthcare access and reporting practices. Failure to account for spatial autocorrelation can lead to underestimation of standard errors, inflated significance tests, and biased parameter estimates in regression analyses.

Scale effects and the modifiable areal unit problem represent essential challenges in spatial analysis that require careful consideration in One Health research. The choice of spatial units for analysis can influence the patterns observed and the relationships detected, as different analytical units may lead to different conclusions about the same underlying phenomena. Multi-scale analysis approaches can help assess the sensitivity of findings to spatial scale choices while providing insights into the mechanisms operating at different spatial scales.

Kernel density estimation and spatial smoothing techniques provide valuable approaches for visualising and analysing spatial patterns in One Health data, enabling conversion of point data into continuous surfaces that can reveal spatial clustering and risk gradients. Bandwidth selection remains a significant methodological challenge in kernel-based methods, as inappropriate bandwidth choices can potentially obscure important spatial patterns or create artificial clustering (Stevens & Pfeiffer, 2015). Adaptive bandwidth methods and data-driven bandwidth selection procedures can help address these challenges while maintaining appropriate smoothing characteristics.

Spatial scan statistics and cluster detection methods offer formal statistical approaches for identifying unusual aggregations of health outcomes, while controlling for multiple testing issues that arise when examining numerous potential cluster locations simultaneously. These methods have been widely applied in outbreak detection, environmental health assessment, and surveillance applications; however, they require careful interpretation, considering the specific characteristics of the data and the spatial processes under investigation.

18.3. Modelling Disease Transmission

Disease transmission modelling represents a cornerstone of quantitative One Health research, providing mechanistic frameworks for understanding how pathogens spread between and within human, animal, and environmental reservoirs, while supporting evidence-based decision-making for prevention and control strategies. Mathematical models of infectious disease transmission enable researchers to integrate knowledge from diverse sources, including biologic characteristics of pathogens, patterns of contact between individuals and populations, healthcare utilisation patterns, and responses to public health interventions (Grassly & Fraser, 2008). The CDC Centre for Forecasting and Analytics emphasises that transmission models are mechanistic, using equations to represent the processes underlying disease transmission, while enabling the evaluation of different scenarios through parameter modification (CDC, 2025).

Compartmental models represent the most used framework for disease transmission modelling, dividing populations into epidemiologically relevant compartments based on infection status and disease progression stages. The basic SIR (Susceptible-Infected-Recovered) model provides a foundation for understanding the dynamics of transmission. However, One Health applications often require more complex compartmental structures that can accommodate multiple host species, environmental reservoirs, vector populations, and cross-species transmission pathways. Model complexity must be balanced against available data and analytical objectives, with simpler models often preferred when data are limited or when general insights are more important than detailed predictions (Kumar et al., 2021).

Parameter estimation and model calibration represent critical challenges in disease transmission modelling, particularly in One Health contexts where parameters may vary across species, environments, and transmission pathways. The basic reproduction number (R_0) represents a fundamental parameter that quantifies the average number of secondary infections generated by a typical infected individual in a completely susceptible population. However, One Health models often require species-specific or environment-specific reproduction numbers that reflect different transmission efficiencies, contact patterns, and susceptibility characteristics across various components of the system.

Agent-based models provide alternative approaches to compartmental models by explicitly representing individual agents (humans, animals, or environmental units) and their interactions over time and space. These models can accommodate heterogeneity in personal characteristics, complex contact patterns, and spatial structure that may be difficult to capture in compartmental models. However, agent-based models typically require more detailed data for parameterisation and greater computational resources for simulation. At the same time, their complexity can make it more challenging to understand the key drivers of model behaviour.

Network models focus explicitly on the contact structures that enable disease transmission, representing individuals or populations as nodes connected by edges that represent potential transmission pathways. Network approaches are particularly valuable for One Health applications because they can represent complex multi-species contact patterns, environmental contamination pathways, and trade or movement networks that facilitate the spread of pathogens. Network metrics such as centrality, clustering, and path length can provide insights into key vulnerabilities and optimal intervention targets within complex transmission systems.

Stochastic models incorporate random variation in transmission processes, demographic events, and environmental conditions that can affect disease dynamics. Stochasticity is particularly important for understanding extinction and invasion dynamics, outbreak probability distributions, and the effects of small population sizes or rare events. One Health applications often require stochastic approaches because environmental variability, climate fluctuations, and demographic stochasticity can have an essential impact on multi-species transmission systems.

Environmental transmission models explicitly incorporate environmental reservoirs, contamination dynamics, and environmental factors that affect pathogen survival and transmission efficiency. These models are essential for understanding waterborne diseases, foodborne pathogens, vector-borne diseases, and other environmentally-mediated transmission pathways that are central to many One Health challenges. Environmental models must account for physical processes, such as dispersion, dilution, and decay, while incorporating biological processes, including pathogen replication and host-pathogen interactions.

Model validation and uncertainty quantification are essential components of disease transmission modelling that require systematic approaches to assess model performance and characterise prediction uncertainty. Validation approaches include comparison with historical data, out-of-sample prediction assessment, and cross-validation procedures that evaluate model performance under different conditions. The COVID-19 pandemic highlighted both the utility and limitations of disease transmission models, emphasising the importance of clearly communicating model assumptions, uncertainties, and appropriate interpretation of model predictions (Grant et al., 2024).

Sensitivity analysis provides essential tools for understanding how model predictions depend on parameter values and structural assumptions, enabling identification of key uncertainties and priorities for additional data collection. Global sensitivity analysis methods can systematically explore the effects of simultaneous variation in multiple parameters while identifying parameter interactions that may not be apparent through local sensitivity analysis approaches.

Figure 22 illustrates a comprehensive diagram of multi-species disease transmission modelling in One Health contexts. The framework displays three interconnected transmission cycles: Human-to-Human (showing susceptible, exposed, infected, and recovered compartments with healthcare interventions), Animal-to-Animal (depicting domestic and wild animal populations with management and ecological factors), and Environmental Reservoir (representing pathogen persistence in water, soil, or vector populations). Bidirectional arrows connect all three cycles, illustrating zoonotic transmission (from animals to humans), reverse zoonosis (from humans to animals), and environmental contamination/exposure pathways. Control measures are outlined for each cycle, including vaccination, treatment, vector control, environmental remediation, and behavioural interventions. Parameter flows indicate how transmission rates, contact patterns, and intervention effectiveness vary between and within each cycle.

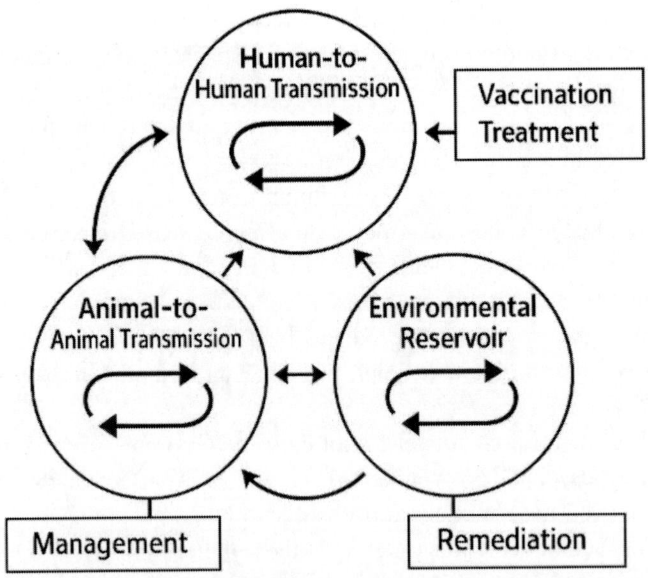

Figure 22. Integrated One Health disease transmission modelling framework.

18.4. Risk Factor Analysis

Risk factor analysis in One Health contexts requires sophisticated statistical approaches that can identify, quantify, and interpret exposures operating at multiple scales while accounting for complex interactions between human, animal, and environmental factors. Traditional epidemiological approaches to risk factor analysis must be expanded to accommodate the multilevel nature of One Health data, where individual-level risks may be influenced by factors operating at multiple levels, including household, community, regional, and global levels, across different temporal scales. The International Journal of Epidemiology emphasises that mathematical modelling approaches are increasingly being used to address health disparities and understand how social determinants and environmental factors interact to influence disease risk across different populations (Richard & Lipsitch, 2024).

Exposure assessment represents a fundamental challenge in One Health risk factor analysis, requiring integration of direct and indirect exposure pathways that may operate through different environmental media, contact patterns, and temporal windows. Human exposures may occur through occupational contact with animals, consumption of animal products, recreational activities in natural environments, or residence in areas with specific environmental characteristics. Animal exposures may involve feed contamination, water sources, air quality, and contact with other animals or humans. Environmental exposures encompass a broad range of factors, including climate variables, land-use patterns, pollution sources, and ecosystem characteristics, that affect pathogen survival and transmission.

Hierarchical modelling approaches provide essential tools for risk factor analysis in One Health contexts by explicitly accounting for the multilevel structure of exposure and outcome data. Mixed-effects models enable separation of individual-level and contextual effects while accounting for clustering within households, herds, geographic areas, or time periods. These approaches can accommodate random effects that capture unobserved heterogeneity while enabling estimation of both fixed effects for specific risk factors and variance components that quantify the importance of different levels of organisation.

Confounding control in One Health risk factor analysis requires careful consideration of factors that may affect multiple components of the system while potentially creating spurious associations or masking authentic relationships. Traditional confounding control methods, such as stratification, matching, and multivariable adjustment, must be supplemented with approaches that can address confounding by indication, selection bias, and measurement error, which may affect different types of variables in varying ways. Causal inference methods, including directed acyclic graphs, instrumental variables, and quasi-experimental designs, provide frameworks for identifying and addressing sources of bias in observational studies.

Time-varying exposures and dynamic risk factors require specialised analytical approaches that can accommodate changes in exposure status, cumulative effects, and lagged relationships between exposures and outcomes. Time-to-event analysis methods, including Cox regression and parametric survival models, enable the investigation of how risk factors affect the timing of disease occurrence while accounting for censoring and competing risks. Joint modelling approaches can simultaneously analyse longitudinal exposure data and time-to-event outcomes while accounting for measurement error and missing data in exposure assessments.

Interaction analysis in One Health contexts must consider biological, statistical, and public health dimensions of interaction while addressing the increased complexity that arises from multiple exposure types and outcome measures. Biological interactions may reflect mechanistic relationships between different pathogens, host factors, or environmental conditions that affect disease susceptibility or severity. Statistical interactions can be assessed through product terms in regression models, though interpretation requires careful attention to the scale of measurement and the specific research questions being addressed.

Machine learning approaches are increasingly complementing traditional statistical methods for risk factor analysis by enabling the investigation of high-dimensional exposure data, nonlinear relationships, and complex interaction patterns that may be difficult to specify a priori. Random forests, gradient boosting, and neural network methods can identify significant predictors from large numbers of candidate variables while providing measures of variable importance and prediction accuracy. However, machine learning approaches require careful attention to interpretability, generalizability, and validation to ensure that findings are robust and relevant for public health decision-making (Chen et al., 2024).

Environmental risk factor analysis requires specialised approaches that can account for spatial and temporal variability in exposure while addressing measurement error and spatial confounding that may affect environmental exposure assessments. Geospatial exposure modelling approaches combine ecological monitoring data, satellite imagery, dispersion models, and geographic information systems to provide spatially and temporally resolved exposure estimates that can be linked to health outcome data. Hybrid modelling approaches that combine mechanistic environmental models with statistical calibration methods can improve exposure prediction accuracy while quantifying prediction uncertainty (Lash et al., 2024).

Causal mediation analysis provides valuable tools for understanding the pathways through which risk factors influence health outcomes, enabling the investigation of both direct effects and indirect effects that operate through intermediate variables. Mediation analysis is particularly relevant for One Health applications because environmental factors may affect human Health both directly and indirectly through impact on animal populations, pathogen ecology, or food systems. Modern mediation analysis methods can accommodate nonlinear relationships, multiple mediators, and time-varying mediators while providing measures of the proportion of effects mediated through different pathways.

18.5. Meta-Analysis and Systematic Reviews

Meta-analysis and systematic review methodologies provide essential tools for synthesising evidence from diverse studies and data sources in One Health research. However, traditional approaches require adaptation to address the methodological heterogeneity and interdisciplinary nature characteristic of One Health investigations. The complexity of integrating evidence across human medicine, veterinary medicine, environmental science, and other disciplines creates unique challenges for evidence synthesis that require specialised approaches and careful attention to study quality assessment, data extraction procedures, and heterogeneity analysis (Mengist et al., 2023). Systematic reviews in One Health contexts must accommodate different study designs, outcome measures, and analytical approaches while maintaining rigorous standards for evidence evaluation and synthesis.

Study identification and selection procedures for One Health systematic reviews require comprehensive search strategies that span multiple databases, disciplines, and publication types while addressing the challenge of inconsistent terminology across different fields. Search terms must capture concepts from human Health, animal health, environmental Health, and their intersections, while database selection should include medical, veterinary, environmental, and multidisciplinary sources. Grey literature searches are significant for One Health topics because relevant evidence may be published in government reports, conference proceedings, and technical documents that are not indexed in traditional academic databases.

The quality assessment of studies included in One Health systematic reviews necessitates consideration of study design quality, reporting standards, and methodological rigour across various disciplines that may employ different established practices and quality criteria. The Newcastle-Ottawa Scale, Cochrane Risk of Bias tools, and other established quality assessment instruments may need to be adapted or supplemented to address the specific characteristics of One Health studies. Quality assessment should consider both internal validity (the risk of bias within studies) and external validity (the generalizability of findings across different settings, populations, and contexts).

Data extraction procedures must accommodate diverse outcome measures, exposure definitions, and analytical approaches while maintaining consistency and completeness across included studies. Standardised data extraction forms should capture study characteristics, population characteristics, exposure and outcome definitions, analytical methods, and results while allowing for flexibility to accommodate the diversity of study types and data presentations found in One Health literature. Multiple reviewers should independently extract data, using procedures to resolve discrepancies and ensure accuracy.

Heterogeneity assessment and management represent critical challenges in One Health meta-analyses due to the diversity of study designs, populations, exposures, and outcomes that characterise this field. Statistical heterogeneity can be assessed using standard measures, such as the I^2 statistic and Cochran's Q test; however, these measures should be supplemented with clinical and methodological assessments of heterogeneity sources. Random-effects models are typically preferred over fixed-effects models when substantial heterogeneity is present. However, the choice of model should be justified based on the specific characteristics of the included studies.

Subgroup analysis and meta-regression provide essential tools for exploring sources of heterogeneity while investigating how study characteristics, population factors, or methodological differences affect effect estimates. Meta-regression should only be considered when at least 10 studies are available, and the number of covariates should be limited relative to the number of studies to avoid overfitting (Mengist et al., 2023). Pre-specified subgroup analyses based on biologically or methodologically relevant factors are preferable to post-hoc analyses, as observed patterns may influence the data.

Publication bias assessment requires systematic approaches to identify and address the selective publication of studies with statistically significant or favourable results. Funnel plots provide a visual assessment of publication bias, but should be supplemented with formal statistical tests, such as Egger's test or Begg's test, when sufficient studies are available. Asymmetrical funnel plots may indicate publication bias; however, other factors, such as study quality differences, clinical heterogeneity, or chance, may also contribute to funnel plot asymmetry.

Table 18.2. Meta-analysis considerations for One Health research

Component	Traditional Approaches	One Health Adaptations	Special Challenges	Solutions
Search Strategy	Medical databases; Clinical terms	Multidisciplinary databases; Cross-sector terminology	Inconsistent terminology; Multiple disciplines	Comprehensive search terms; Expert consultation
Study Selection	Clinical criteria; Population focus	Cross-species criteria; Environmental factors	Diverse study designs; Mixed populations	Inclusive criteria; Multiple reviewers
Quality Assessment	Medical bias tools: Clinical validity	Adapted tools; Cross-disciplinary standards	Different quality standards; Varied methodologies	Modified assessment tools; Discipline-specific criteria
Data Extraction	Clinical outcomes; Standard measures	Multi-domain outcomes; Diverse measures	Heterogeneous data types; Varied scales	Flexible extraction forms; Standardisation procedures
Synthesis Methods	Clinical homogeneity; Fixed populations	Methodological diversity; multi-species data	High heterogeneity; Complex interactions	Random effects models; Subgroup analysis

Network meta-analysis approaches enable the simultaneous comparison of multiple interventions or exposures, incorporating both direct and indirect evidence from different studies. These methods are particularly valuable for One Health applications where multiple intervention strategies may be compared across various settings, populations, or pathogen systems. Network meta-analysis requires careful attention to transitivity assumptions and consistency between direct and indirect evidence while providing rankings of intervention effectiveness and credible intervals for all pairwise comparisons.

Individual participant data (IPD) meta-analysis represents the gold standard for evidence synthesis when primary study data are available, enabling standardised analyses, investigation of individual-level factors, and more sophisticated statistical modelling approaches than are possible with aggregate data meta-analysis. IPD meta-analysis can address some limitations of traditional meta-analysis approaches, including standardisation of outcome definitions, investigation of nonlinear relationships, and assessment of effect modification by individual-level characteristics.

One Health-specific considerations for systematic reviews include the need to address interdisciplinary evidence synthesis, integrate quantitative and qualitative evidence, and consider implementation factors that affect the translation of evidence into practice across different sectors and disciplines. Mixed-methods systematic reviews may be appropriate when both quantitative and qualitative evidence are relevant to the research question, requiring specialised approaches for integrating various types of evidence while maintaining methodological rigour. Table 18.2 shows meta-analysis considerations for one health research.

18.6. Big Data Approaches and Machine Learning

Big data approaches and machine learning technologies offer transformative potential for One Health research by enabling the integration and analysis of high-dimensional datasets from diverse sources, while providing automated pattern recognition, predictive modelling, and decision support capabilities that can enhance traditional epidemiological and statistical methods. The integration of artificial intelligence with mechanistic epidemiological modelling has emerged as a rapidly advancing field, with 245 eligible studies identified in a recent scoping review, highlighting its practical value, including advances in disease forecasting, model parameterisation, and calibration (Shi et al., 2025). However, key research gaps remain, including the need for better incorporation of realistic decision-making considerations, expanded exploration of diverse datasets, and further investigation into biological and socio-behavioural mechanisms.

Machine learning applications in One Health epidemiology encompass supervised learning for prediction and classification tasks, unsupervised learning for pattern discovery and data exploration, and reinforcement learning for optimisation of intervention strategies and resource allocation. Supervised learning approaches, including random forests, support vector machines, and gradient boosting methods, can be trained on labelled datasets to predict disease outcomes, classify risk levels, or identify high-priority surveillance targets. These methods can accommodate high-dimensional predictor sets, nonlinear relationships, and complex interaction patterns while providing measures of prediction accuracy and variable importance.

Deep learning methods, including artificial neural networks, convolutional neural networks, and recurrent neural networks, offer powerful approaches for analysing complex data types such as medical images, genomic sequences, environmental sensor data, and natural language text. Deep learning models have been applied to detect outbreaks of infectious diseases, with dynamic neural network models developed to predict outbreak risk using historical epidemiological data, air travel volumes, vector distribution, and socioeconomic factors (Zeng et al., 2021). Transfer learning approaches can overcome overfitting problems due to small datasets by adapting models trained on large datasets to specific One Health applications.

Natural language processing (NLP) techniques provide essential capabilities for extracting structured information from unstructured text sources, including medical records, veterinary reports, environmental monitoring reports, and social media data. NLP applications in One Health encompass automated surveillance of disease reports, extraction of exposure information from clinical notes, sentiment analysis of public health communications, and monitoring of online discussions related to health topics. Large language models and transformer architectures have shown particular promise for biomedical text processing while requiring careful attention to bias, accuracy, and interpretability.

Artificial intelligence-enabled public health surveillance systems integrate multiple data sources and analytical techniques to provide early warning of disease outbreaks, monitor population health trends, and support real-time decision making. These systems can incorporate traditional surveillance data, environmental monitoring data, social media signals, search engine queries, and mobile phone data to provide comprehensive situational awareness capabilities. However, implementation requires careful attention to data quality, privacy protection, validation procedures, and integration with existing public health infrastructure (Rajesh et al., 2023).

Predictive modelling using machine learning approaches enables the forecasting of disease trends, the identification of high-risk populations and geographic areas, and the assessment of intervention impacts under different scenarios. Ensemble methods that combine predictions from multiple algorithms can improve prediction accuracy while providing measures of prediction uncertainty. Model interpretability techniques, including feature importance measures, partial dependence plots, and model-agnostic explanation methods, help ensure that machine learning models provide actionable insights rather than black-box predictions.

Geospatial machine learning approaches integrate machine learning methods with geographic information systems and spatial data to address location-specific prediction tasks and recognise spatial patterns. These approaches can be applied to predict disease risk maps, identify environmental exposure hotspots, optimise surveillance network placement, and support targeted intervention strategies. Spatial cross-validation procedures are essential for providing an unbiased assessment of model performance while accounting for spatial autocorrelation in the data.

Data integration and harmonisation represent fundamental challenges for big data approaches in One Health research, requiring methods that can combine datasets with different formats, measurement scales, temporal resolutions, and quality standards. Federated learning approaches enable the training of machine learning models across distributed datasets without requiring centralised data sharing, which can address privacy concerns and data governance issues while allowing analysis of larger and more diverse datasets. However, federated approaches require careful attention to data compatibility and model aggregation procedures.

Quality assurance and validation procedures are vital for machine learning applications in public Health because model complexity can make it difficult to identify errors, biases, or inappropriate generalisations. Cross-validation procedures should account for temporal dependencies, spatial clustering, and hierarchical data structures that are common in One Health datasets. External validation using independent datasets is essential for assessing generalizability, while ongoing monitoring is necessary to detect model degradation over time.

Ethical considerations and bias mitigation require systematic attention in machine learning applications for One Health research, including fairness across different populations, transparency in algorithmic decision-making, and protection of individual privacy. Algorithmic bias can arise from biased training data, inappropriate model specifications, or differential performance across population subgroups. Bias detection and mitigation techniques should be integrated into model development and deployment procedures while maintaining focus on public health objectives and equity considerations (Chen et al., 2024).

Figure 23 illustrates a comprehensive flowchart that depicts the machine learning workflow for One Health applications. The pipeline begins with diverse data sources, including human health data (such as EHRs, surveillance, and genomics), animal health data (such as veterinary records, production data, and movement data), environmental data (such as satellite imagery, sensor networks, and climate data), and additional sources (such as social media, mobile data, and economic indicators). These feed into a Data Integration Platform, which displays data cleaning, harmonisation, and quality control processes. The integrated data flows to a Machine Learning Engine containing multiple algorithm types (supervised learning for prediction/classification, unsupervised learning for pattern discovery, deep learning for complex data types, and reinforcement learning for optimisation). Outputs branch into three main applications: Disease Surveillance and Early Warning (outbreak detection, risk prediction, and monitoring dashboards), Risk Assessment and Prediction (risk factor identification, spatial risk mapping, and temporal forecasting), and Decision Support Systems (intervention optimisation, resource allocation, and policy recommendations). Feedback loops connect outputs back to data sources and the ML engine for continuous improvement.

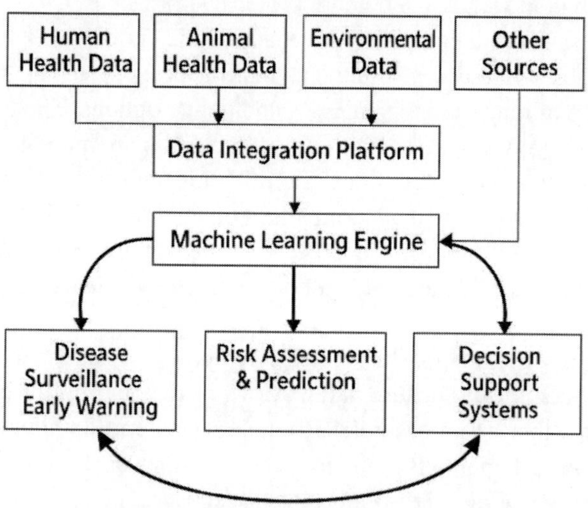

Figure 23. Machine Learning Pipeline for One Health Data Integration.

Conclusion

Statistical methods and data analysis form the analytical backbone of One Health research, providing essential tools for understanding the complex interactions between human, animal, and environmental health factors, while supporting evidence-based decision-making for prevention, control, and policy interventions. The evolution of statistical approaches in One Health contexts reflects growing recognition that traditional single-discipline analytical methods, while valuable, are insufficient for addressing the multidimensional challenges that characterise health issues at the human-animal-environment interface. The integration of diverse data types, analytical approaches, and technological innovations presents unprecedented opportunities for advancing One Health science, while also requiring careful attention to methodological rigour, validity, and practical applicability.

Descriptive and analytical statistics form the foundation of One Health research, though their application requires adaptation to accommodate the unique characteristics of multidisciplinary data integration. The challenge of harmonising data from human medicine, veterinary medicine, environmental science, and other disciplines requires sophisticated approaches to data standardisation, quality control, and visualisation that can effectively communicate findings across different professional communities. The development of integrated analytical frameworks that maintain disciplinary rigour while enabling transdisciplinary synthesis remains an ongoing challenge that requires continued methodological innovation and collaborative growth.

Spatial and temporal analysis methods have emerged as critical components of One Health research, enabling investigation of geographic and temporal patterns that reveal important insights about disease ecology, environmental determinants, and population dynamics. The increasing availability of high-resolution spatial and temporal data, combined with advances in computational methods and software tools, has dramatically expanded the potential for sophisticated spatiotemporal analyses. However, the complexity of spatiotemporal data requires careful attention to analytical assumptions, scale effects, and interpretation challenges that may not be apparent in traditional epidemiological approaches.

Disease transmission modelling provides mechanistic frameworks that are essential for understanding pathogen dynamics in complex, multi-species systems, while supporting the quantitative evaluation of intervention strategies and policy options. The COVID-19 pandemic demonstrated both the power and limitations of transmission modelling, emphasising the importance of model validation, uncertainty quantification, and clear communication of model assumptions and limitations. Future developments in transmission modelling will likely involve the better integration of environmental factors, social behaviours, and intervention dynamics, while addressing challenges related to model complexity, parameter uncertainty, and computational requirements.

Risk factor analysis in One Health contexts requires sophisticated approaches that can identify and quantify complex exposure pathways while accounting for multilevel influences and interaction effects that operate across different scales and domains. The integration of traditional epidemiological methods with machine learning approaches presents promising opportunities for investigating high-dimensional exposure data and complex interaction patterns. However, these approaches require careful attention to interpretability, validation, and bias mitigation to ensure that findings are robust and actionable.

Meta-analysis and systematic review methodologies adapted for One Health research enable the synthesis of evidence from diverse study designs and disciplines while addressing the methodological heterogeneity that characterises this field. The development of One Health-specific guidelines for systematic reviews and meta-analyses represents a crucial priority for establishing standards and best practices that can enhance the quality and utility of evidence synthesis efforts. Individual participant data meta-analyses and network meta-analyses offer particularly promising approaches for addressing some limitations of traditional meta-analytical methods in One Health contexts.

Big data approaches and machine learning technologies hold transformative potential for One Health research, enabling the integration of high-dimensional datasets, the identification of complex patterns, and the support of predictive modelling applications. The rapid advancement of artificial intelligence technologies, including deep learning, natural language processing, and computer vision, provides new opportunities for analysing diverse data types and supporting real-time surveillance and decision-making applications. However, the successful implementation of these technologies requires careful attention to data quality, algorithmic bias, validation procedures, and ethical considerations.

The connection between advanced statistical methods and Sustainable Development Goal 3 (Good Health and Well-being) underscores the global significance of methodological innovation in addressing complex health challenges that transcend traditional disciplinary boundaries. The World Health Organisation's 2024 World Health Statistics highlight the importance of robust analytical approaches for monitoring progress toward SDG targets, while identifying persistent health inequalities and emerging challenges (WHO, 2024). The Global Burden of Disease Study demonstrates how systematic analytical approaches can provide comprehensive assessments of health outcomes across countries and time periods while informing policy priorities and resource allocation decisions (GBD 2023 Cancer Collaborators, 2024).

Future developments in statistical methods for One Health research will likely include the enhanced integration of artificial intelligence with traditional epidemiological approaches, the development of real-time analytical platforms for surveillance and response, and the creation of standardised frameworks for multidisciplinary data integration and analysis. The success of these developments will depend on continued collaboration between statisticians, epidemiologists, data scientists, and domain experts across human medicine, veterinary medicine, and environmental science.

The fundamental challenge for statistical methods in One Health research is maintaining analytical rigour and validity while accommodating the complexity and interdisciplinary nature that characterise this field. This requires ongoing methodological innovation, the collaborative development of standards and best practices, and sustained investment in training and capacity building to prepare researchers to apply sophisticated analytical methods effectively in transdisciplinary contexts. Only through such efforts can the statistical sciences fully realise their potential to support One Health research and contribute to addressing the complex health challenges of the 21st century.

Acknowledgments

The authors would like to extend our appreciation to those who offered helpful commentary during the drafting process of this manuscript. We also acknowledge the role Nova Science Publishers played in enabling the work described herein.

References

Chen, S., Yu, J., Chamouni, S., Martinez-Gutierrez, M., Gozzer, E., Franco, O. H., & Muka, T. (2024). Integrating machine learning and artificial intelligence in life-course epidemiology: pathways to innovative public health solutions. *BMC Medicine*, 22(1), 354. https://doi.org/10.1186/s12916-024-03566-x.

Columbia University Mailman School of Public Health. (2023). Spatiotemporal analysis. *Population Health Methods*. https://www.publichealth.columbia.edu/research/population-health-methods/spatiotemporal-analysis.

GBD 2023 Cancer Collaborators. (2024). The global, regional, and national burden of cancer, 1990–2023, with forecasts to 2050: A systematic analysis for the Global Burden of Disease Study 2023. *Institute for Health Metrics and Evaluation*. https://www.healthdata.org/research-analysis/library/global-regional-and-national-burden-cancer-1990-2023-forecasts-2050.

Global Health Data Institute. (2020). Global health data methods: Spatial and spatio-temporal modelling. https://globalhealthdata.org/spatial-and-spatio-temporal-modelling/.

Grant, R., Rubin, M., Abbas, M., Pittet, D., Srinivasan, A., Jernigan, J. A., & Slayton, R. B. (2024). Expanding the use of mathematical modeling in healthcare epidemiology and infection prevention and control. *Infection Control & Hospital Epidemiology*, 45(8), 930-935. https://doi.org/10.1017/ice.2024.97.

Grassly, N. C., & Fraser, C. (2008). Mathematical models of infectious disease transmission. *Nature Reviews Microbiology*, 6(6), 477-487. https://doi.org/10.1038/nrmicro1845.

Kumar, A., Khatri, P., Patel, K., Rizvi, S. Z., & Kumar, S. (2021). Statistical modeling for the prediction of infectious disease dissemination with special reference to COVID-19 spread. *Frontiers in Public Health*, 9, 645405. https://doi.org/10.3389/fpubh.2021.645405.

Lash, T. L., VanderWeele, T. J., Haneuse, S., & Rothman, K. J. (2024). A review of geospatial exposure models and approaches for health data integration. *Journal of Exposure Science & Environmental Epidemiology*, 34(5), 712-728. https://doi.org/10.1038/s41370-024-00712-8.

Mengist, B., Adem, F., Tilahun, A., Tilahun, D., Degu, A., Dewana, Z., & Mohammed, A. (2023). A 7-step guideline for qualitative synthesis and meta-analysis of observational studies in health sciences. *Frontiers in Public Health Reviews*, 4, 1605454. https://doi.org/10.3389/phrs.2023.1605454.

Rajesh, A., Pai, C., Jha, R., Nair, A., Cherian, S., Abraham, S., & Ravi, V. (2023). Using artificial intelligence to improve public Health: A narrative review. *Frontiers in Public Health*, 11, 1198397. https://doi.org/10.3389/fpubh.2023.1198397.

Richard, D. M., & Lipsitch, M. (2024). What's next: using infectious disease mathematical modelling to address health disparities. *International Journal of Epidemiology*, 53(1), dyad180. https://doi.org/10.1093/ije/dyad180.

Shi, Z., Zhang, Q., Yan, K., Liu, S., Wang, J., Lee, V. J., & Chughtai, A. A. (2025). Integrating artificial intelligence with mechanistic epidemiological modeling: A scoping review of opportunities and challenges. *Nature Communications*, 16, 55461. https://doi.org/10.1038/s41467-024-55461-x.

Stevens, K. B., & Pfeiffer, D. U. (2015). Spatial and temporal epidemiological analysis in the big data era. *Preventive Veterinary Medicine*, 122(1-2), 213-220. https://doi.org/10.1016/j.prevetmed.2015.07.012.

World Health Organisation. (2024). World health statistics 2024: Monitoring health for the SDGs, sustainable development goals. https://www.who.int/publications/i/item/9789240094703.

Zeng, D., Cao, Z., & Neill, D. B. (2021). Artificial intelligence–enabled public health surveillance—From local detection to global epidemic monitoring and control. In *Artificial Intelligence in Medicine* (pp. 437-453). Academic Press. https://doi.org/10.1016/B978-0-12-821259-2.00022-3.

Chapter 19

Survey Design, Sampling, and Mixed Methods Research

Harshal Tukaram Pandve[1], MD
and Maajid Mohi Ud Din Malik[2,*], PhD
[1]Community Medicine (PSM), Pimpri Chinchwad Municipal Corporation's Postgraduate Medical Institute and Yashwantrao Chavan Memorial Hospital, Pimpri, Pune, India
[2]Department of Radiology and Imaging Technology, Dr. D. Y. Patil School of Allied Health Sciences, Dr. D. Y. Patil Vidyapeeth, Pune (Deemed to be University), Sant Tukaram Nagar, Pimpri, Pune, India

Abstract

The integration of human, animal, and environmental health domains in One Health research requires sophisticated methodological approaches that can address the inherent complexity of multisectoral, interdisciplinary investigations. This chapter examines survey design, sampling strategies, and mixed methods research approaches essential for conducting robust One Health studies across diverse populations, species, and environments. Survey methodology in One Health contexts must accommodate the unique challenges of studying interconnected health systems, requiring innovative sampling strategies that span taxonomic boundaries and environmental gradients. Mixed methods research approaches provide particularly valuable frameworks for capturing both quantitative patterns and qualitative insights necessary for understanding complex health phenomena at the human-animal-environment interface. Data collection tools and technologies have evolved to support real-time, multi-domain surveillance and monitoring. However, validity and reliability considerations become increasingly complex when research spans multiple disciplines and sectors. These methodological advances directly support Sustainable Development Goal 3 (Good Health and Well-being) by providing the evidence base necessary for the development of comprehensive health policies and interventions. The chapter synthesises current best practices and emerging innovations in One Health research methodology, providing practical guidance for researchers, policymakers, and practitioners seeking to implement scientifically rigorous, ethically sound, and practically relevant studies.

Keywords: One Health, survey design, mixed methods research, sampling strategies, multisectoral surveillance, interdisciplinary research, SDG 3

---

* Corresponding Author's Email: maajid.malik@dpu.edu.in

In: Advances in the One Health Approach
Editors: Maajid Mohi Ud Din Malik, Abhay Saraf, Harshal Tukaram Pandve et al.
ISBN: 979-8-90134-202-2

Introduction

The emergence of One Health as a unifying framework for addressing complex health challenges has fundamentally transformed approaches to health research methodology. One Health recognises that the health of humans, animals, and ecosystems are interconnected and interdependent, requiring integrated approaches that transcend traditional disciplinary boundaries (Zinsstag et al., 2017). This paradigm shift has created unprecedented demands for research methodologies that can capture the dynamic relationships between human behaviour, animal populations, and environmental processes while maintaining scientific rigour across multiple domains and scales of inquiry.

Contemporary global health challenges, from emerging infectious diseases and antimicrobial resistance to environmental degradation and climate change, increasingly demonstrate the limitations of siloed research approaches that examine human, animal, and ecological Health in isolation. The COVID-19 pandemic, zoonotic disease outbreaks, and growing recognition of the health impacts of biodiversity loss have underscored the urgent need for research methodologies that can address these complex, interconnected phenomena (Stärk et al., 2023). Survey design, sampling strategies, and mixed methods research approaches represent critical methodological foundations for generating the evidence base necessary to understand and address these challenges through comprehensive, integrated interventions that recognise the fundamental interconnectedness of Health across all domains.

19.1. Survey Methodology in Complex Populations

Survey methodology within One Health research contexts presents unique challenges that distinguish it from traditional single-domain health surveys. The fundamental complexity arises from the need to study interconnected populations across human, animal, and environmental domains simultaneously, requiring methodological approaches that can capture the dynamic relationships between these traditionally separated sectors (Lebov et al., 2017). Complex populations in One Health research often exhibit characteristics that violate assumptions underlying conventional survey designs, including non-random spatial distribution, temporal variability in accessibility, and interdependent health outcomes that cannot be adequately addressed through siloed approaches.

The conceptualisation of target populations in One Health surveys requires careful consideration of the multiple levels at which health interactions occur. At the individual level, surveys must account for the reality that human health outcomes are influenced by direct and indirect contact with animal populations and environmental exposures, necessitating sampling frameworks that can capture these multifaceted relationships (Galiè et al., 2024). Community-level surveys face the additional challenge of defining meaningful boundaries when ecological, social, and economic systems transcend traditional geographic and administrative divisions. Population heterogeneity becomes particularly complex when considering that different domains may exhibit distinct demographic patterns, seasonal variations, and response rates to survey instruments.

Methodological frameworks for One Health surveys must integrate knowledge from epidemiology, veterinary medicine, environmental science, and social research to develop appropriate study designs. The multimedia, multi-pathway, multi-receptor methodology exemplified in environmental health assessments provides one model for structuring complex survey approaches, allowing researchers to trace exposures and outcomes across multiple domains and pathways (Lebov et al., 2017). This approach requires careful mapping of conceptual frameworks that visualise how health hazards move between ecological compartments and affect different populations, informing both sampling strategies and questionnaire design.

Survey instrument development for complex One Health populations requires attention to domain-specific knowledge systems, cultural contexts, and communication patterns. Questionnaires must be designed to capture information that may be familiar to professionals in one domain but require translation or explanation for participants from other sectors. For example, surveys examining zoonotic disease risk may need to elicit information about animal husbandry practices from human participants while also collecting data on human health behaviours that may impact animal populations. This necessitates collaborative instrument development processes that engage expertise from multiple disciplines during the design phase. The development of adjusted indicators for measuring disease burden across species boundaries, such as zoonotic disability-adjusted life years (zDALY), demonstrates the importance of methodological innovations that can capture health impacts across traditional domain boundaries (Torgerson et al., 2018).

The integration of different temporal scales presents another methodological challenge in One Health survey design. Human health surveys typically focus on relatively short-term exposures and outcomes. In contrast, environmental health assessments often require data collection over multiple seasons or years to capture meaningful variations in ecological conditions. Animal health surveys may need to account for breeding cycles, migration patterns, or management practices that create periodic accessibility constraints. Survey methodologies must accommodate these varying temporal requirements while maintaining coherence in the overall research design.

Response rate optimisation in complex One Health populations requires an understanding of the different incentives, constraints, and communication preferences that characterise each domain. Human participants may be motivated by individual health benefits or community improvement goals. In contrast, animal health data collection often depends on cooperation from veterinarians, farmers, or wildlife managers, whose participation is influenced by different professional and economic considerations. Environmental monitoring may rely on partnerships with regulatory agencies, research institutions, or community organisations that operate according to distinct organisational cultures and priorities. Recent surveys across European countries have demonstrated significant variation in One Health awareness and implementation across different professional sectors, highlighting the importance of tailored engagement strategies for various stakeholder groups (Chiesa et al., 2021). Table 19.1 shows survey design considerations for one Health complex populations.

Table 19.1. Survey design considerations for One Health complex populations

Domain	Population Characteristics	Key Challenges	Methodological Adaptations
Human	Diverse socioeconomic, cultural, and geographic contexts	Variable health literacy, privacy concerns, and temporal constraints	Multi-language instruments, culturally adapted protocols, flexible scheduling
Animal	Domestic vs. wild species, seasonal accessibility, and owner cooperation	Species-specific sampling requirements, welfare considerations, and jurisdictional issues	Collaborative protocols with veterinarians, non-invasive methods, and regulatory compliance
Environmental	Spatial and temporal heterogeneity, regulatory oversight	Technical expertise requirements, equipment constraints, and access permissions	Standardised protocols, quality assurance, and multi-agency coordination
Cross-domain	Interconnected systems, shared exposures, emergent properties	Disciplinary boundaries, communication barriers, and analytical complexity	Integrated frameworks, interdisciplinary teams, systems approaches

19.2. Sampling Strategies Across Species and Environments

Sampling strategies in One Health research must address the fundamental challenge of obtaining representative data across taxonomically diverse populations that occupy different ecological niches and respond to distinct selective pressures. The development of sampling frameworks that can accommodate both human populations and animal species requires integration of methods from social research, wildlife biology, veterinary epidemiology, and environmental science (Gortázar et al., 2024). Traditional sampling approaches developed for single-domain research often prove inadequate when applied to the complex, interconnected systems that characterise One Health investigations.

Probability sampling methods face challenges when applied across species and environments due to the fundamental differences in population structures, spatial distributions, and accessibility patterns. Human populations may be sampled using established demographic and geographic frameworks, but animal populations often exhibit markedly different distribution patterns that do not align with human administrative boundaries. Wild animal populations may be clustered around resource patches, exhibit seasonal migration patterns, or demonstrate social structures that create dependencies between sampling units. Domestic animal populations are constrained by human management systems that create artificial clustering and may introduce systematic biases related to socioeconomic factors or management practices.

Stratified sampling approaches provide valuable frameworks for One Health research when strata are defined based on ecological, epidemiological, or management criteria that are relevant across multiple domains. Ecosystem-based stratification enables researchers to define sampling units based on habitat characteristics, environmental gradients, or land-use patterns that influence the health of all constituent populations. For example, agricultural systems may be stratified by farming intensity, crop types, or water management practices that create distinct risk profiles for human, animal, and environmental health outcomes. Urban environments can be stratified by population density, infrastructure characteristics, or the availability of green spaces, which influence disease transmission dynamics across species.

Cluster sampling methods offer practical advantages for One Health research when natural clustering occurs at scales that encompass multiple domains. Geographic clusters based on watersheds, administrative units, or ecological boundaries may provide sampling frameworks that capture relevant variation while maintaining logistical feasibility. However, cluster sampling in One Health contexts requires careful consideration of the different clustering patterns that may characterise each domain, as clusters that are meaningful for human health outcomes may not align with those most relevant for animal or environmental health assessment.

Adaptive and sequential sampling strategies have emerged as particularly valuable approaches for One Health research, allowing sampling protocols to be modified based on initial findings or changing conditions in the study system. Sequential sampling may involve initial broad-scale surveys to identify areas of interest, followed by more intensive sampling in targeted locations where cross-domain interactions are most evident. Adaptive sampling protocols can respond to disease outbreaks, environmental changes, or management interventions that alter the risk profile of study populations during the research period.

Non-invasive sampling methods have become increasingly crucial for One Health research, particularly when studying wildlife populations where traditional capture methods may be impractical, ethically problematic, or likely to introduce bias (Cantu-Salinas et al., 2022). Environmental sampling approaches that detect genetic material, antibodies, or pathogens in water, soil, or other ecological matrices can provide information about the presence and health status of multiple species without the need for direct sampling of individual animals. These approaches are particularly valuable for surveillance of emerging diseases or assessment of population health in areas where direct access is limited.

Integrated sampling designs that collect data from multiple domains simultaneously offer opportunities to maximise information content while minimising research costs and environmental impact. For example, sampling protocols that collect human biological specimens, domestic animal samples, and ecological specimens from the same households or geographic areas can provide insights into shared exposures and transmission pathways that would not be apparent from single-domain studies. However, integrated sampling requires careful coordination of protocols, equipment, and personnel to ensure that sampling procedures for one domain do not compromise the quality or feasibility of sampling in other domains.

19.3. Mixed Methods Research Approaches

Mixed methods research approaches have gained recognition as particularly well-suited to One Health investigations due to their capacity to integrate quantitative and qualitative data collection and analysis methods across multiple domains and scales of inquiry (Gupta et al., 2016). The inherent complexity of One Health systems, characterised by dynamic interactions between human behaviour, animal populations, and environmental processes, often requires research designs that can capture both measurable patterns and the contextual factors that shape these patterns. The mixed methods approach offers frameworks for integrating the breadth of quantitative surveys with the depth of qualitative investigations, allowing researchers to develop a more comprehensive understanding of complex health phenomena.

Sequential explanatory designs represent one of the most widely applied mixed-methods approaches in One Health research, involving initial quantitative data collection followed by qualitative investigations designed to explain or expand upon the quantitative findings. This approach may begin with cross-sectional surveys of human populations to identify patterns of zoonotic disease risk, followed by ethnographic investigations to understand the cultural, economic, and social factors that shape human-animal interactions in high-risk areas. The qualitative phase can provide insights into the mechanisms underlying quantitative associations, identify intervention opportunities that may not be apparent from survey data alone, and generate hypotheses for future research.

Sequential exploratory designs reverse this process, beginning with qualitative investigations to understand the dimensions of a One Health problem before developing quantitative instruments to measure these dimensions across broader populations. This approach is particularly valuable when studying emerging health issues where existing survey instruments may not capture relevant domains or when working in cultural contexts where the meaning and significance of health concepts may differ from those underlying standardised instruments. Qualitative investigations can inform the development of culturally appropriate survey questions, identify relevant outcome measures, and ensure that quantitative research addresses priorities identified by affected communities.

Concurrent mixed methods designs collect both quantitative and qualitative data simultaneously, allowing for the triangulation of findings and the identification of convergent or divergent patterns across different types of data. In One Health contexts, concurrent designs may involve simultaneous administration of structured surveys and semi-structured interviews to varying subsets of the same population, or the collection of quantitative health data alongside qualitative assessments of community perceptions and experiences. This approach can be particularly valuable for evaluating One Health interventions, where qualitative assessments of acceptability, feasibility, and unintended consequences can complement quantitative measures of health outcomes.

Transformative mixed methods frameworks explicitly incorporate social justice and equity considerations into research design and implementation, addressing the reality that health disparities often affect the most vulnerable populations across human, animal, and environmental domains. These approaches recognise that One Health research takes place within contexts of unequal power relationships and may inadvertently reinforce existing inequities if not carefully designed to promote inclusive participation and equitable benefit distribution. Transformative frameworks require attention to community engagement, participatory research methods, and capacity building that extends beyond the immediate research objectives.

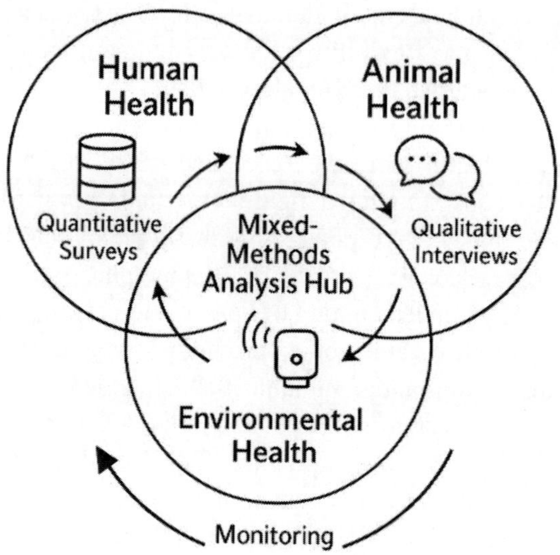

Figure 24. Integrated Mixed Methods Framework for One Health Research.

Complex mixed methods designs integrate multiple phases of data collection and analysis over extended time periods, allowing researchers to adapt their methods based on emerging findings and changing conditions within the study systems. These designs may incorporate multiple sequential and concurrent phases, intervention components, and feedback loops that enable responsive research processes. For example, a complex mixed-methods study of antimicrobial resistance might begin with quantitative surveillance to identify patterns of resistance, followed by qualitative investigations of prescribing practices and livestock management, concurrent implementation of interventions in selected sites, and ongoing mixed-methods evaluation of the impacts and adaptation processes of the interventions.

Figure 24 shows A conceptual diagram illustrating the integration of quantitative and qualitative methods across human, animal, and environmental health domains. The diagram illustrates three overlapping circles representing the traditional One Health domains, with arrows indicating data flow between concurrent quantitative surveys (represented by databases), qualitative investigations (represented by interview symbols), and environmental monitoring (represented by sensor symbols). A central coordination hub illustrates how data integration is achieved through mixed-methods analysis, resulting in integrated findings and recommendations. Feedback loops show how findings from each domain inform adaptive sampling and method selection in other domains.

19.4. Qualitative Research in One Health

Qualitative research methods provide essential tools for understanding the complex social, cultural, and behavioural dimensions of One Health systems that cannot be adequately captured through quantitative approaches alone. The interconnected nature of human, animal, and environmental Health is mediated through human knowledge systems, cultural practices, and decision-making processes that require in-depth investigation to understand their influence on health outcomes (Galiè et al., 2024). Qualitative methods offer approaches for exploring these dimensions while maintaining the flexibility necessary to adapt to the diverse contexts and unexpected findings that characterise One Health research.

Ethnographic approaches provide valuable frameworks for understanding how different communities conceptualise Health, perceive risks, and make decisions that affect human-animal-environment interactions. Extended fieldwork enables researchers to observe daily practices, seasonal patterns, and crisis responses that shape health outcomes, which may not be apparent through survey research or brief site visits. Ethnographic research can reveal how local knowledge systems integrate an understanding of human, animal, and environmental Health in ways that differ from scientific frameworks, providing insights essential for developing culturally appropriate interventions and communication strategies.

In-depth interview methods enable exploration of individual experiences, decision-making processes, and knowledge systems that influence One Health outcomes. Semi-structured interviews can explore topics such as animal care practices, environmental risk perceptions, or healthcare-seeking behaviours while maintaining sufficient flexibility to pursue emergent themes and unexpected connections. Key informant interviews with veterinarians, healthcare providers, environmental managers, and community leaders can provide expert perspectives on system dynamics, institutional barriers, and potential intervention opportunities that may not be accessible through other methods.

Focus group discussions offer opportunities to explore community-level perspectives, social norms, and collective decision-making processes that shape One Health outcomes. Focus groups can reveal how communities understand relationships between human, animal, and environmental Health, identify priorities for intervention or research, and explore the feasibility and acceptability of potential health measures. The group interaction format can stimulate discussion of topics that individuals might not raise spontaneously, while also revealing areas of consensus or disagreement within communities.

Participatory research methods engage community members as co-researchers, recognising that local knowledge and priorities are essential for understanding and addressing One Health challenges. Participatory approaches may include community mapping exercises to identify health hazards and resources, photovoice projects to document environmental conditions and health experiences, or community-based monitoring programs that engage local participants in data collection and interpretation. These methods can build research capacity within communities while ensuring that research addresses locally identified priorities and generates actionable findings.

Digital ethnographic methods have emerged as valuable approaches for understanding how One Health issues are discussed, understood, and acted upon in online spaces. Social media analysis can reveal how disease outbreaks are perceived and discussed by different stakeholders, how health information spreads through networks, and how public understanding of One Health issues evolves. Online forums and discussion groups may provide access to specialised knowledge communities, such as livestock producers, pet owners, or environmental activists, whose perspectives might be difficult to access through traditional research methods.

Narrative analysis approaches focus on how individuals and communities construct stories about Health, illness, and recovery that incorporate relationships between human, animal, and environmental factors. Illness narratives can reveal how people understand the causal relationships between environmental exposures, animal contact, and health outcomes, providing insights into the mental models that influence behaviour and healthcare-seeking. Community narratives about environmental change, animal disease outbreaks, or successful health interventions can inform the design and implementation of intervention strategies.

19.5. Data Collection Tools and Technologies

Data collection tools and technologies for One Health research have undergone rapid evolution in recent years, driven by advances in sensor technology, mobile computing, genomic sequencing, and data integration platforms that enable real-time, multi-domain surveillance and monitoring (CDC, 2025). These technological innovations have created unprecedented opportunities for conducting comprehensive One Health investigations while also introducing new challenges related to data quality, standardisation, and integration across different technical platforms and organisational systems.

Digital data collection platforms have transformed survey administration and field data collection by enabling real-time data entry, automated quality checks, and immediate feedback to research teams. Mobile applications designed for epidemiological fieldwork can accommodate complex survey instruments, support multimedia data collection, including photographs and audio recordings, and function in areas with limited internet connectivity through offline data storage and synchronisation capabilities. These platforms can integrate GPS coordinates, timestamp data, and device identifiers to enhance data quality and enable spatial-temporal analysis of health outcomes.

Biological sampling technologies have expanded the range of specimens that can be collected and analysed in One Health research, while reducing the invasiveness and cost of sample collection. Point-of-care diagnostic devices enable rapid testing for infectious diseases, biomarkers, or environmental contaminants, eliminating the need for laboratory infrastructure. This facilitates research in resource-limited settings and provides real-time feedback to study participants. Dried blood spot technology and other simplified sampling methods reduce storage and transportation requirements while maintaining sample integrity for subsequent analysis.

Environmental monitoring technologies provide continuous or frequent measurements of environmental parameters that influence Health across multiple domains. Air quality monitors, water quality sensors, and soil contamination assessment tools can provide high-resolution data on environmental exposures that affect human, animal, and ecological Health simultaneously. Remote sensing technologies, including satellite imagery and drone-based monitoring, enable assessment of environmental conditions over large spatial scales and in areas that are difficult to access through traditional sampling methods.

Genomic sequencing technologies have revolutionised pathogen surveillance and outbreak investigation by enabling rapid identification of infectious agents, characterisation of antimicrobial resistance patterns, and reconstruction of transmission pathways across species and geographic boundaries (Franco-Rocha et al., 2024). Whole genome sequencing can provide insights into pathogen evolution, identify reservoirs and transmission routes, and inform intervention strategies with unprecedented precision. Environmental DNA sequencing enables the detection of multiple species from environmental samples, providing information about biodiversity, species health, and ecosystem functioning without the need for direct animal sampling.

Geographic information systems (GIS) and spatial analysis tools enable integration of health, environmental, and demographic data across multiple scales and domains. GIS platforms can overlay human health data with animal disease surveillance information, ecological monitoring results, and land-use data to identify spatial clusters, risk factors, and opportunities for intervention. Spatial-temporal analysis tools can track disease spread across species and geographic boundaries, identify environmental factors that influence transmission, and evaluate the effectiveness of spatially targeted interventions.

Automated surveillance systems integrate multiple data sources to provide early warning of health threats that span traditional domain boundaries. Syndromic surveillance systems can detect unusual patterns of symptoms or disease in human populations that may signal environmental exposures or zoonotic disease outbreaks. Similar systems for monitoring animal health, environmental conditions, and food safety can provide complementary information, enhancing overall surveillance sensitivity and specificity. The evaluation of multisectoral collaboration in One Health surveillance systems requires systematic assessment frameworks that can capture the quality and appropriateness of cross-sector coordination throughout the surveillance process (Rüegg et al., 2019). Vector-borne disease surveillance exemplifies these integrated approaches, offering new opportunities for addressing health challenges through coordinated monitoring systems that align with broader sustainable development objectives (Vanwambeke et al., 2019).

Table 19.2. Data collection technologies for One Health research

Technology Category	Applications	Advantages	Limitations	Implementation Considerations
Mobile data collection	Field surveys, real-time entry	Immediate quality checks, GPS integration	Device limitations, connectivity issues	Training requirements, device management
Point-of-care diagnostics	Rapid pathogen detection	Real-time results, field deployment	Limited test availability, accuracy concerns	Quality control, result validation
Environmental sensors	Continuous monitoring	High-resolution temporal data	Maintenance requirements, calibration needs	Installation costs, data management
Genomic sequencing	Pathogen characterisation	High-resolution typing, transmission tracking	Cost, technical expertise	Laboratory capacity, bioinformatics support
Remote sensing	Large-scale environmental assessment	Spatial coverage, historical data	Resolution limitations, interpretation complexity	Data processing, validation methods

Data integration platforms address the challenge of combining information collected using different technologies, formats, and standards across multiple organisations and domains. Cloud-based platforms can provide secure data sharing capabilities while maintaining appropriate access controls and privacy protections. Standardised data formats and interoperability standards facilitate data sharing and analysis across different software platforms and institutional boundaries. Table 19.2 shows data collection technologies for one health research

19.6. Validity and Reliability Considerations

Validity and reliability considerations in One Health research become more complex due to the need to ensure measurement quality across multiple domains, disciplines, and methodological approaches while maintaining coherence in overall research objectives and findings (Singh & Kumar, 2016). Traditional concepts of validity and reliability must be extended and adapted to address the unique challenges of interdisciplinary research that spans different epistemological traditions, measurement scales, and analytical frameworks.

Construct validity in One Health research requires careful consideration of how key concepts are defined and operationalised across different domains and disciplinary perspectives. Health concepts that have precise meanings within human medicine may need adaptation or redefinition when applied to animal populations or environmental systems. For example, concepts such as wellness, disease burden, or quality of life may be operationalised differently across domains, requiring explicit attention to construct equivalence and comparability. Multi-domain construct validation may require evidence from multiple sources and methods to establish that measurement instruments capture the intended concepts across all relevant populations and contexts.

Content validity assessment must evaluate whether measurement instruments adequately capture the full range of relevant dimensions within each domain while maintaining coherence across domains. Expert panels for One Health research may need to include representatives from multiple disciplines to ensure that survey instruments, interview guides, or observational protocols address all relevant aspects of the phenomena under study. Content validity assessment may also require community validation to ensure that instruments capture locally relevant dimensions of Health and include culturally appropriate language and concepts.

Criterion validity presents challenges in One Health research due to the frequent absence of established gold standard measures that span multiple domains. Concurrent validity assessment may require comparison with domain-specific measures that are not directly comparable across domains. In contrast, predictive validity assessment must account for the complex temporal relationships that characterise One Health systems. Cross-domain criterion validation may require novel approaches that establish validity through convergent patterns across multiple types of evidence rather than comparison to single reference standards.

Reliability assessment must address both the consistency of measurements within domains and the coherence of measurements across domains over time and contexts. Test-retest reliability assessment may be complicated by the dynamic nature of One Health systems, where actual changes in conditions may be challenging to distinguish from measurement error. Inter-rater reliability assessment in interdisciplinary research teams requires attention to differences in professional training, conceptual frameworks, and measurement traditions that may influence consistency across different data collectors.

Internal validity considerations must address the complex causal relationships and confounding factors that characterise One Health systems. Threats to internal validity may arise from unmeasured confounders that operate across domains, temporal relationships that differ between domains, or feedback loops that violate assumptions underlying traditional analytical approaches. Selection bias may operate differently across domains if different factors influence participation or accessibility in human, animal, and environmental sampling.

External validity and generalizability assessment must consider the multiple dimensions along which One Health research findings might be generalised, including taxonomic groups, environmental conditions, cultural contexts, and management systems. Generalizability across species requires attention to phylogenetic relationships, ecological similarities, and biological constraints that may limit the transferability of findings. Generalizability across environmental contexts requires consideration of climate, habitat, land use, and other factors that may modify relationships between variables.

Measurement invariance testing provides approaches for evaluating whether measurement instruments function equivalently across different groups, contexts, or time periods. In One Health research, measurement invariance testing can be applied to assess whether survey instruments function equivalently across different cultural groups, whether biological assays yield comparable results across various species, or whether environmental monitoring protocols produce consistent results across different ecosystems.

Conclusion

The methodological approaches examined in this chapter represent essential components for conducting rigorous and meaningful One Health research that can inform the development of evidence-based policies and interventions. Survey design methodology for complex populations necessitates careful consideration of the unique challenges associated with studying interconnected systems, while maintaining scientific rigour and ethical standards. Sampling strategies must strike a balance between the competing demands of representativeness, feasibility, and comparability across diverse populations and environments. A mixed-methods approach provides valuable frameworks for capturing both the breadth and depth necessary for understanding complex One Health phenomena. At the same time, qualitative methods offer essential insights into the social, cultural, and behavioural dimensions that mediate human-animal-environment interactions.

The rapid evolution of data collection tools and technologies creates unprecedented opportunities for conducting comprehensive, real-time One Health surveillance and research. However, technological advances also introduce new challenges related to data quality, integration, and interpretation that require ongoing attention to validity and reliability considerations. The complexity of ensuring measurement quality across multiple domains, disciplines, and methodological approaches demands innovative approaches to validation and reliability assessment that extend beyond traditional single-domain frameworks.

Future directions in One Health research methodology should prioritise the development of integrated analytical frameworks that can accommodate the complex and dynamic relationships characterising One Health systems. This includes continued development of statistical methods that can handle multi-level, multi-domain data structures, as well as computational approaches that can integrate diverse data types and sources. Participatory and community-engaged research methods will become increasingly crucial as One Health initiatives seek to address health equity and ensure that research benefits extend to all affected communities.

The methodological innovations described in this chapter directly support the achievement of Sustainable Development Goal 3 by providing the evidence base necessary for comprehensive health policy development that addresses the interconnected nature of human, animal, and environmental Health. As global health challenges become increasingly complex and interconnected, the methodological approaches outlined here will be essential for developing effective, equitable, and sustainable health interventions that recognise and leverage the relationships between different health domains.

Acknowledgments

The authors would like to extend our appreciation to those who offered helpful commentary during the drafting process of this manuscript. We also acknowledge the role Nova Science Publishers played in enabling the work described herein.

References

Cantu-Salinas, L., Garcia-Espinosa, G., Hernandez-Escareño, J. J., Rodriguez-Diego, J., & Scott, M. E. (2022). A review of non-invasive sampling in wildlife disease and health research: What's new? *Animals*, *12*(13), 1719. https://doi.org/10.3390/ani12131719.

CDC. (2025). Using technologies for data collection and management. *Field Epidemiology Manual*. https://www.cdc.gov/field-epi-manual/php/chapters/data-collection-management.html.

Franco-Rocha, O. Y., Mendoza-Torres, E., Villalobos-Delgado, L., Rivera-Dominguez, A. J., Martinez-Hernandez, S. L., Gaytan-Garcia, M. J., Rincon-Orozco, B., & Wheldon, C. W. (2024). Pathogen genomics and One Health: A scoping review of current practices in zoonotic disease research. *medRxiv*. https://doi.org/10.1101/2024.02.05.24302264.

Galiè, A., McLeod, A., Campbell, Z. A., Ngwili, N., Terfa, Z. G., & Thomas, L. F. (2024). Gender considerations in One Health: A framework for researchers. *Frontiers in Public Health*, *12*, 1345273. https://doi.org/10.3389/fpubh.2024.1345273.

Gortázar, C., Diez-Delgado, I., Barasona, J. A., Vicente, J., De la Fuente, J., & Boadella, M. (2024). Overcoming the limitations of wildlife disease monitoring. *Research Directions: One Health*, *2*, e5. https://doi.org/10.1017/one.2024.2.

Gupta, M., Prasad, S., & Singh, D. (2016). Application of mixed method approach in public health research. *Indian Journal of Community Medicine*, *41*(2), 93-97. https://doi.org/10.4103/0970-0218.173495.

Chiesa, F., Tomassone, L., Savic, S., Bellato, A., Mihalca, A. D., Modry, D., Häsler, B., & De Meneghi, D. (2021). A survey on One Health perception and experiences in Europe and neighboring areas. *Frontiers in Public Health*, *9*, 609949. https://doi.org/10.3389/fpubh.2021.609949.

Lebov, J., Grieger, K., Womack, D., Zaccaro, D., Whitehead, N., Kowalcyk, B., & MacDonald, P. D. M. (2017). A framework for One Health research. *One Health*, *3*, 44-50. https://doi.org/10.1016/j.onehlt.2017.03.004.

Rüegg, S. R., McMahon, B. J., Häsler, B., Esposito, R., Nielsen, L. R., Ifejika Speranza, C., Ehlinger, T., Peyre, M., Aragrande, M., Zinsstag, J., Davies, P., Mihalca, A. D., Roe, E. J., Christley, R. M., Urban, P., Pilot,

E., Ma, L., van Nistelrooij, A., Limon, G., ... Buttigieg, S. C. (2019). One Health surveillance: A matrix to evaluate multisectoral collaboration. *Frontiers in Veterinary Science*, *6*, 109. https://doi.org/10.3389/fvets.2019.00109.

Singh, A. S., & Kumar, M. (2016). Validity and reliability of the experience-sampling method. *Psychological Studies*, *61*(3), 267-278. https://doi.org/10.1007/s12646-016-0375-3.

Stärk, K. D. C., Kuribreña, M. A., Dauphin, G., Vokaty, S., Ward, M. P., Wieland, B., & Lindahl, J. F. (2023). One Health surveillance systems: A review of current trends and future directions. *Epidemiology and Infection*, *151*, e40. https://doi.org/10.1017/S0950268823000195.

Torgerson, P. R., Rüegg, S., Devleesschauwer, B., Abela-Ridder, B., Havelaar, A. H., Shaw, A. P. M., Rushton, J., & Speybroeck, N. (2018). zDALY: An adjusted indicator to estimate the burden of zoonotic diseases. *One Health*, *5*, 40-45. https://doi.org/10.1016/j.onehlt.2018.03.002.

Vanwambeke, S. O., Sumilo, D., Bormane, A., Lambin, E. F., & Randolph, S. E. (2019). Making vector-borne disease surveillance work: New opportunities from the SDG perspectives. *Frontiers in Public Health*, *7*, 232. https://doi.org/10.3389/fpubh.2019.00232.

Zinsstag, J., Schelling, E., Waltner-Toews, D., & Tanner, M. (2017). Roadmap to a One Health agenda 2030. *CAB Reviews*, *12*(014), 1-17. https://doi.org/10.1079/PAVSNNR201712014.

Chapter 20

Health Policy, Risk Communication, and Media Engagement

Rajesh S. Kuber[1]
and Maajid Mohi Ud Din Malik[2,*]**, PhD**
[1]Department of Radio-Diagnosis, Dr. D. Y. Patil Medical College, Hospital and Research Centre, Dr. D. Y. Patil Vidyapeeth, Pune (Deemed to be University)- Sant Tukaram Nagar, Pimpri, Pune, India
[2]Department of Radiology and Imaging Technology, Dr. D. Y. Patil School of Allied Health Sciences, Dr. D. Y. Patil Vidyapeeth, Pune (Deemed to be University), Sant Tukaram Nagar, Pimpri, Pune, India

Abstract

The implementation of One Health approaches requires sophisticated policy frameworks, strategic communication practices, and sustained media engagement to address complex health challenges at the human-animal-environment interface. This chapter examines the critical components of health policy development, risk communication principles, and media engagement strategies essential for the successful implementation of One Health. Policy development in One Health contexts must navigate multi-sectoral governance structures while maintaining scientific integrity and public trust. Risk communication strategies must address the inherent complexity of One Health issues while ensuring accessibility and cultural appropriateness across diverse stakeholder communities. Media relations and public engagement necessitate adaptable approaches that can respond to rapidly evolving health threats while fostering long-term trust and understanding. Social media platforms have transformed the health communication landscape, creating both opportunities for rapid information dissemination and challenges related to misinformation and public scepticism. Crisis communication strategies specific to One Health emergencies must coordinate responses across sectors while maintaining transparency and credibility. Building public trust emerges as a fundamental prerequisite for effective One Health implementation, requiring sustained commitment to community engagement, transparent communication, and responsive governance. These communication and policy approaches directly support Sustainable Development Goal 3 (Good Health and Well-being) by creating the enabling environment necessary for integrated health approaches to succeed across multiple domains and sectors.

---

* Corresponding Author's Email: maajid.malik@dpu.edu.in

In: Advances in the One Health Approach
Editors: Maajid Mohi Ud Din Malik, Abhay Saraf, Harshal Tukaram Pandve et al.
ISBN: 979-8-90134-202-2

Keywords: One Health policy, risk communication, media engagement, public trust, crisis communication, health governance, SDG 3

Introduction

The success of One Health initiatives depends fundamentally on effective policy frameworks, strategic communication approaches, and sustained public engagement that can bridge the complex intersections between human, animal, and environmental health domains. Contemporary health challenges, including emerging infectious diseases, antimicrobial resistance, environmental degradation, and climate-related health impacts, necessitate coordinated policy responses that transcend traditional sectoral boundaries while maintaining public support and understanding (WHO, 2025). The COVID-19 pandemic has underscored both the critical importance of effective health communication and the devastating consequences of communication failures, policy inconsistencies, and eroded public trust in health authorities.

Policy development in One Health contexts presents unique challenges in coordinating across multiple governmental agencies, professional domains, and stakeholder communities, while maintaining scientific rigour and democratic accountability. Risk communication strategies must navigate the inherent complexity of One Health issues, translating sophisticated scientific concepts into accessible public health guidance while addressing diverse cultural contexts and community needs. Media engagement has become increasingly complex in digital information environments characterised by rapid information spread, competing narratives, and heightened public scrutiny of institutional authority. The rebuilding of public trust in health institutions emerges as a critical foundation for all other One Health communication and policy objectives, requiring sustained commitment to transparency, community engagement, and responsive governance that demonstrates tangible benefits for public Health and wellbeing.

20.1. One Health Policy Development and Implementation

One Health policy development requires sophisticated coordination mechanisms that can align diverse sectoral interests, regulatory frameworks, and institutional cultures while maintaining the integrated approach that distinguishes One Health from traditional health policy domains. The complexity of policy development in One Health contexts emerges from the need to reconcile different legal authorities, professional standards, and organisational priorities that govern human Health, veterinary medicine, environmental protection, and agricultural systems (WHO, 2025). Effective One Health policies must establish clear governance structures that facilitate collaboration while maintaining accountability to various regulatory systems and professional bodies, which may have competed or conflicting mandates.

The implementation of One Health Joint Plan of Action frameworks at national levels requires careful adaptation to local political, economic, and social contexts while maintaining alignment with international standards and commitments. Recent systematic reviews of One Health implementation have identified three critical pathways that must be addressed in policy development: policy, legislation, advocacy, and financing (Pathway 1); organisational development, implementation, and sectoral integration (Pathway 2); and data, evidence, and knowledge systems (Pathway 3) (Rüegg et al., 2025). The majority of documented One Health implementations have incorporated governance and policy frameworks, but significant gaps remain in sustainable financing mechanisms and comprehensive monitoring and evaluation systems.

Policy formulation processes must accommodate the inherently interdisciplinary nature of One Health challenges while ensuring that policy recommendations are grounded in robust scientific evidence and responsive to community needs and priorities. The establishment of One Health coordination units at national levels, such as the United States One Health Coordination Unit launched in 2024, provides institutional mechanisms for sustained policy development and implementation across federal agencies (CDC, 2025). These coordination structures must strike a balance between the need for technical expertise and the requirements for democratic accountability and public engagement, ensuring that One Health policies reflect both scientific evidence and public values.

Legislative frameworks for One Health implementation must address jurisdictional challenges that arise when health threats cross traditional regulatory boundaries between human Health, veterinary medicine, and environmental protection agencies. European Union approaches to One Health governance provide examples of how supranational policy frameworks can create enabling environments for integrated approaches while respecting national sovereignty and local implementation capacity (European Parliament, 2024). However, effective policy implementation requires more than legislative frameworks; it demands sustained commitment to capacity building, resource allocation, and institutional culture change that can sustain collaborative approaches over extended time periods.

The integration of One Health principles into broader policy frameworks, including climate policy, agricultural policy, and urban planning, represents a critical frontier for policy development that extends beyond traditional health sector boundaries. Mission-oriented policy approaches offer promising frameworks for organising One Health initiatives around specific, time-bound objectives that can coordinate diverse actors and resources toward shared goals (World Economic Forum, 2025). These approaches require careful attention to political economy considerations, including how different stakeholder groups are affected by policy changes and how potential conflicts of interest can be managed to maintain policy legitimacy and effectiveness. Table 20.1 shows one health policy implementation framework.

20.2. Risk Communication Principles and Practices

Risk communication in One Health contexts requires sophisticated approaches that can address the inherent complexity and uncertainty of health threats that span multiple domains while ensuring that information is accessible, actionable, and culturally appropriate for diverse stakeholder communities. The principles of effective risk communication, established through decades of research in environmental Health and emergency management, must be adapted to address the unique characteristics of One Health challenges, including their multi-factorial causation, extended temporal scales, and impacts that may affect different populations and species in other ways (CDC, 2025). Crisis and Emergency Risk Communication (CERC) frameworks offer evidence-based approaches for communicating about health risks; however, their application to One Health contexts necessitates careful consideration of how different stakeholder groups perceive and respond to information about complex, interconnected health systems.

The development of clear, accurate, and helpful risk messages represents a fundamental challenge in One Health communication due to the scientific complexity of many One Health issues and the diverse knowledge systems and cultural frameworks that different communities use to understand health risks. Effective risk communication must strike a balance between scientific accuracy and accessibility, ensuring that technical information is translated into actionable guidance without oversimplifying complex relationships or creating false certainty about uncertain outcomes. The COVID-19 pandemic highlighted both the importance of clear risk communication and the consequences of communication failures, including inconsistent messaging, political interference in scientific communication, and inadequate consideration of community concerns and values (Ho et al., 2024).

Community engagement emerges as a critical component of effective One Health risk communication, requiring approaches that go beyond traditional public information campaigns to create meaningful opportunities for dialogue, feedback, and collaborative problem-solving. Risk communication research has consistently demonstrated that effective communication is bidirectional, involving not only the transmission of information from experts to communities but also the integration of community knowledge, concerns, and priorities into risk assessment and management processes (WHO, 2025). This is particularly important in One Health contexts where local communities may have extensive knowledge about human-animal-environment interactions that are essential for understanding and addressing health risks.

Cultural competence and equity considerations must be integrated into all aspects of One Health risk communication, recognising that different communities may have varying relationships with animals, other environmental exposures, and differing levels of trust in health authorities and scientific institutions. Recent research on equity-informed social media risk communication has identified key principles for effective communication with marginalised and vulnerable populations, including the importance of community partnerships, culturally appropriate messaging, and attention to social determinants that may affect communities' ability to respond to health information (Tang et al., 2024). These approaches require sustained investment in relationship-building and capacity development that extends well beyond individual communication campaigns or crisis responses.

The integration of traditional and digital communication channels presents both opportunities and challenges for One Health risk communication. While social media platforms and digital technologies enable the rapid dissemination of information and interactive engagement with diverse audiences, they also create new challenges related to misinformation, echo chambers, and the amplification of fear and mistrust. Effective risk communication strategies must develop coherent approaches across multiple communication channels while adapting messages and formats to the specific characteristics and limitations of different media platforms and audience preferences.

Table 20.1. One Health policy implementation framework

Policy Level	Key Components	Implementation Mechanisms	Success Indicators
National	Political commitment, legal frameworks, and financing mechanisms	One Health coordination units, inter-agency agreements, and dedicated budgets	Policy coherence scores, resource allocation metrics, and institutional collaboration rates
Subnational	Regional coordination, local adaptation, community engagement	Regional One Health networks, local implementation plans, stakeholder partnerships	Community participation levels, local capacity indicators, and cross-sectoral project outcomes
International	Global standards, technical cooperation, and knowledge sharing	Quadripartite collaboration, international frameworks, research networks	Policy harmonisation metrics, knowledge transfer indicators, and global preparedness assessments
Sectoral	Professional integration, regulatory alignment, and capacity building	Joint training programs, shared protocols, integrated surveillance systems	Professional competency measures, regulatory coherence scores, and system integration indicators

20.3. Media Relations and Public Engagement

Media relations in One Health contexts require a sophisticated understanding of how different media outlets, journalists, and communication platforms approach complex scientific and policy issues, particularly when those issues involve uncertainty, controversy, or rapidly evolving situations. The relationship between health authorities and media organisations has become increasingly important as traditional gatekeeping functions of journalism have been supplemented by direct communication through social media and other digital platforms, creating both opportunities for more direct public engagement and challenges related to maintaining accuracy and credibility in rapidly evolving information environments (CDC, 2025). Effective media relations strategies must strike a balance between the need for timely information sharing and the requirements for scientific accuracy, while also acknowledging that media coverage significantly influences public understanding and response to health issues.

The development of proactive media engagement strategies enables One Health organisations to establish credible relationships with journalists and media outlets before crises arise, laying the foundation for trust and understanding that can support more effective communication during emergencies. Media training for One Health professionals must address the unique challenges of communicating about complex, interdisciplinary issues while maintaining scientific accuracy and avoiding oversimplification of nuanced relationships between human, animal, and environmental health factors. This includes developing skills for explaining uncertainty and evolving knowledge, addressing misinformation and misconceptions, and communicating across cultural and linguistic barriers that may affect media coverage and public understanding.

Public engagement strategies in One Health must extend beyond traditional media relations to encompass diverse forms of community interaction, stakeholder consultation, and participatory communication that can build sustained relationships with affected communities and interest groups. The Johns Hopkins Centre for Health Security has developed comprehensive frameworks for building trust and improving public health communication that emphasise the importance of knowing your audience, engaging communities as partners, and developing sustained relationships that extend beyond individual communication campaigns (Potter et al., 2025). These approaches require significant investment in community engagement infrastructure and ongoing relationship maintenance, which can be challenging to sustain within traditional media relations budgets and timelines.

The coordination of media relations across multiple One Health sectors presents unique challenges due to the different communication cultures, professional norms, and institutional priorities that characterise human Health, veterinary medicine, environmental protection, and agricultural organisations. Effective coordination requires the development of shared messaging frameworks, communication protocols, and media training programs that can ensure consistency while respecting the distinct expertise and responsibilities of different organisations. This coordination becomes particularly critical during crises when inconsistent or contradictory messages from other sectors can undermine public trust and complicate response efforts.

Digital media platforms have fundamentally transformed the landscape of public engagement, creating new opportunities for interactive communication, community participation, and real-time feedback while also introducing challenges related to information quality, audience fragmentation, and the rapid spread of misinformation. Organisations must develop strategic approaches to digital media engagement that leverage the participatory potential of these platforms while maintaining professional standards for accuracy, transparency, and responsiveness to community concerns (Shi et al., 2024). This includes developing capacity for rapid response to misinformation, strategic use of multimedia content, and sustained engagement with online communities that may have different characteristics and communication preferences than traditional media audiences.

20.4. Social Media and Health Communication

Social media platforms have fundamentally transformed health communication landscapes by enabling rapid information dissemination, facilitating community engagement, and creating new opportunities for public participation in health discourse while simultaneously introducing significant challenges related to misinformation, polarisation, and the erosion of traditional information gatekeeping mechanisms. The COVID-19 pandemic highlighted both the tremendous potential and substantial risks associated with social media health communication, demonstrating how these platforms can enable the rapid sharing of lifesaving information while also facilitating the spread of dangerous misinformation that undermines public health measures and contributes to preventable illness and death (Ho et al., 2024). One Health organisations must develop sophisticated social media strategies that leverage the participatory and interactive potential of these platforms while maintaining scientific accuracy and building trust, rather than undermining, in health institutions.

The development of effective social media content for One Health communication requires careful attention to platform-specific characteristics, audience preferences, and communication formats that can effectively convey complex scientific information within the constraints of different social media environments. Research on organisational social media use during health crises has identified key factors that influence the effectiveness of social media communication, including message clarity, visual design, cultural appropriateness, and the integration of social media content with broader communication strategies that span multiple channels and platforms (Shi et al., 2024). Successful social media strategies must balance the need for rapid response and real-time engagement with requirements for accuracy verification, legal review, and coordination with other communication activities.

Community engagement through social media platforms offers unprecedented opportunities for bidirectional communication between health organisations and affected communities, enabling real-time feedback, participatory problem-solving, and the integration of community knowledge and perspectives into health planning and response activities. However, meaningful community engagement through social media requires sustained investment in relationship-building, cultural competence, and responsive communication practices that go beyond broadcasting information to creating genuine opportunities for dialogue and collaboration. This is particularly important for One Health communication, where community knowledge about human-animal-environment interactions may be essential for understanding and addressing health risks but may not be captured through traditional scientific or surveillance systems.

Table 20.2. Social media strategy framework for One Health communication

Platform Type	Strengths	Challenges	Best Practices	Success Metrics
Twitter/X	Real-time updates, professional networks, rapid response	Character limits, information overload, and polarisation	Threaded explanations, visual summaries, expert engagement	Retweet rates, engagement quality, and reach metrics
Facebook	Community building, detailed content, targeted demographics	Algorithm changes, ageing user base, privacy concerns	Community pages, event promotion, and discussion facilitation	Community growth, discussion quality, and event attendance
Instagram	Visual storytelling, younger demographics, and educational content	Visual requirements, story limitations, and platform competition	Infographics, behind-the-scenes content, story highlights	Story views, save rates, profile visits
LinkedIn	Professional audiences, policy makers, and institutional communication	Limited reach, formal tone requirements, business focus	Thought leadership, professional updates, policy insights	Professional engagement, connection requests, and article views
YouTube	Long-form content, educational videos, demonstration capacity	Production requirements, algorithm competition, time investment	Educational series, expert interviews, and visual explanations	View duration, subscriber growth, and comment quality

The management of misinformation and disinformation represents one of the most significant challenges facing One Health organisations in social media environments, where false or misleading information can spread rapidly. It may be deliberately amplified by actors seeking to undermine public health measures or the credibility of institutions. Practical approaches to countering misinformation require proactive strategies that include prebunking (providing accurate information before misinformation emerges), rapid response capabilities for addressing false claims, and sustained efforts to build media literacy and critical thinking skills that enable communities to evaluate health information independently. Research has shown that the most effective approaches to countering misinformation combine the provision of accurate information with attention to the underlying concerns and values that may make communities susceptible to false or misleading claims.

The measurement and evaluation of social media health communication present unique challenges due to the complexity of social media environments, the difficulty of attributing health outcomes to specific communication activities, and the rapidly evolving nature of platform algorithms and user behaviour patterns. Effective evaluation strategies must combine quantitative metrics (such as reach, engagement, and sharing patterns) with qualitative assessments of content quality, audience response, and alignment with communication objectives. This includes developing methods for tracking the accuracy and spread of health information, assessing the effectiveness of different message formats and strategies, and understanding how social media communication interacts with other communication channels and health system components to influence health outcomes and public trust. Table 20.2 shows a social media strategy framework for one health communication.

20.5. Crisis Communication Strategies

Crisis communication in One Health contexts must address the unique challenges of coordinating responses across multiple sectors, managing uncertainty and evolving information, and maintaining public trust and credibility while providing timely, accurate guidance during rapidly evolving health emergencies. The interconnected nature of One Health crises necessitates the coordination of communication strategies across human Health, veterinary medicine, environmental protection, and other relevant sectors, while ensuring consistency and avoiding conflicting messages that could undermine public confidence or complicate response efforts (CDC, 2025). Effective crisis communication requires pre-established coordination mechanisms, shared communication protocols, and transparent decision-making processes that can function effectively under the pressure and time constraints that characterise emergency responses.

The development of crisis communication plans for One Health emergencies must account for the potential for health threats to emerge from any domain within the human-animal-environment interface and to spread rapidly across sectors in ways that may not be immediately apparent or predictable. Crisis and Emergency Risk Communication (CERC) frameworks provide evidence-based approaches for crisis communication that emphasise the importance of being first, correct, and credible in emergency communication while acknowledging the reality that information may be incomplete or evolving during the early stages of health emergencies. The application of CERC principles to One Health contexts requires particular attention to the complexity of explaining multi-factorial causation, uncertain transmission pathways, and response measures that may affect different sectors or populations in various ways.

Stakeholder coordination represents a critical component of effective One Health crisis communication, requiring mechanisms to ensure that all relevant organisations and sectors are informed about communication strategies, messaging decisions, and evolving information, while maintaining unified public-facing communication that does not create confusion or contradiction. The establishment of joint information systems, shared communication protocols, and unified command structures can help ensure coordination while respecting the distinct expertise and responsibilities of different organisations. However, effective coordination also requires sustained relationship-building and trust development among participating organisations that must be established before crises emerge.

Risk perception management during One Health crises must address the reality that public understanding and response to health threats are influenced not only by objective risk assessments but also by cultural values, prior experiences, trust in institutions, and social and economic factors that may affect communities' ability to respond to health guidance. Effective crisis communication strategies must acknowledge and address community concerns and values while providing accurate information about health risks and protective measures. This includes recognising that different communities may be differentially affected by One Health crises and may require different communication approaches, resources, and support systems to respond effectively.

The integration of traditional and digital communication channels during One Health crises requires sophisticated coordination to ensure message consistency while adapting content and format to the characteristics and limitations of different communication platforms. Social media platforms enable rapid information dissemination and real-time public engagement, but also create new challenges related to misinformation, information overload, and the potential for panic or inappropriate response to incomplete or misunderstood information. Crisis communication strategies must include capabilities for rapid response to misinformation, proactive engagement with key stakeholders and influencers, and sustained monitoring of public response and information needs throughout the crisis response period.

20.6. Building Public Trust and Understanding

Building and maintaining public trust emerges as a fundamental prerequisite for effective One Health implementation, requiring sustained commitment to transparency, accountability, competence, and responsiveness that extends well beyond individual communication campaigns or crisis responses to encompass all aspects of institutional behaviour and public engagement. Trust in public health institutions has experienced significant erosion in recent years, with survey data showing dramatic declines in public confidence in health authorities, scientific institutions, and government agencies responsible for protecting public Health (SteelFisher et al., 2024). The rebuilding of public trust requires comprehensive approaches that address not only communication practices but also institutional policies, community engagement processes, and demonstrated competence in protecting and promoting public Health.

Research on public trust in health institutions has identified several key factors that influence trust levels, including perceptions of institutional competence, transparency in decision-making processes, consistency between stated values and actual practices, and responsiveness to community concerns and needs. The 2024 Edelman Trust Barometer Special Report on Trust and Health found that healthcare providers remain the most trusted voices on health issues, while all health institutions have experienced significant declines in public trust, with friends and family now trusted as much as scientists and medical experts for health information (Edelman, 2024). These findings suggest that trust-building strategies must leverage trusted relationships and communication channels while working to rebuild institutional credibility through demonstrated competence and transparency.

Community engagement represents a critical pathway for trust-building, requiring genuine partnership approaches rather than traditional public information or consultation models that may be perceived as tokenistic or manipulative. Effective community engagement in One Health contexts requires acknowledging and respecting community knowledge systems, values, and priorities, while creating meaningful opportunities for community participation in health planning, implementation, and evaluation processes. The Commonwealth Fund's research on restoring trust in public Health through local health coalitions has demonstrated the importance of listening to and acting on what communities identify as their health priorities, including addressing upstream factors like transportation, housing, and economic security that may have a greater immediate impact on community wellbeing than traditional public health interventions (Commonwealth Fund, 2023).

Transparency and accountability mechanisms must be embedded throughout One Health organisations and programs to demonstrate commitment to ethical practice, evidence-based decision-making, and responsiveness to public concerns and input. This includes establishing transparent processes for community input and feedback, regular reporting on program performance and outcomes, acknowledging mistakes and limitations, and providing visible responses to community concerns and suggestions. The Johns Hopkins Centre for Health Security's checklist for building trust emphasises the importance of setting clear expectations for public health responses and communication, establishing robust feedback mechanisms, and demonstrating a consistent commitment to community engagement and service (Potter et al., 2025).

The demonstration of tangible benefits and positive outcomes represents an essential component of trust-building, requiring One Health organisations to articulate and measure their contributions to community health and wellbeing in ways that are visible and meaningful to the affected communities. This includes developing performance indicators and communication strategies that highlight not only disease prevention and response activities but also broader contributions to economic development, environmental quality, social cohesion, and other factors that communities value. Trust-building is inherently a long-term process that requires sustained commitment and consistent performance over extended periods, making it essential for One Health organisations to develop sustainable approaches to community engagement and relationship maintenance that can persist through leadership changes, funding fluctuations, and other organisational challenges.

Conclusion

The practical implementation of One Health approaches depends fundamentally on sophisticated policy frameworks, strategic communication practices, and sustained public engagement that can address the complex challenges of coordinating across multiple sectors while maintaining scientific credibility and public trust. Policy development in One Health contexts requires institutional mechanisms that facilitate collaboration while maintaining accountability to different regulatory systems and professional standards. Recent examples, such as the United States' One Health Coordination Unit and European Union governance frameworks, provide models for institutional coordination and policy implementation. Risk communication strategies must strike a balance between scientific accuracy and accessibility, while ensuring cultural appropriateness and community responsiveness. This is achieved by drawing on established Crisis and Emergency Risk Communication frameworks and adapting them to the unique characteristics of One Health challenges.

Media relations and public engagement have become increasingly complex in digital information environments that enable rapid information dissemination while also creating new challenges related to misinformation, polarisation, and the fragmentation of traditional information gatekeeping mechanisms. Social media platforms offer unprecedented opportunities for community engagement and participatory communication while simultaneously requiring sophisticated strategies for managing misinformation and maintaining scientific accuracy in rapidly evolving information environments. Crisis communication strategies must coordinate across multiple sectors while managing uncertainty and maintaining public trust, requiring pre-established coordination mechanisms and shared communication protocols that can function effectively under emergency conditions.

The rebuilding and maintenance of public trust emerges as the fundamental foundation for all other One Health communication and policy objectives, requiring a sustained commitment to transparency, community engagement, demonstrated competence, and responsive governance that extends well beyond individual communication campaigns to encompass all aspects of institutional behaviour and public engagement. Research consistently indicates that trust-building is a long-term process that requires consistent performance, genuine community partnership, and visible demonstration of benefits that align with community priorities and values. The integration of these communication and policy approaches directly supports Sustainable Development Goal 3 by creating the enabling environment necessary for integrated health approaches to succeed across multiple domains and sectors.

Future directions in One Health communication and policy must address the evolving challenges of digital information environments while strengthening institutional capacity for community engagement, cross-sectoral coordination, and adaptive management in contexts of uncertainty and rapid change. This includes continued development of evidence-based approaches to countering misinformation, innovative methods for engaging diverse communities in health planning and decision-making, and institutional mechanisms that can sustain collaborative approaches across political and organisational changes. The lessons learned from recent health crises, including the COVID-19 pandemic, provide valuable insights for strengthening One Health communication and policy frameworks while also highlighting the critical importance of sustained investment in public health communication infrastructure and community engagement capacity.

Acknowledgments

The authors would like to extend our appreciation to those who offered helpful commentary during the drafting process of this manuscript. We also acknowledge the role Nova Science Publishers played in enabling the work described herein.

References

CDC. (2025). *2025-2029 National One Health Framework to Address Zoonotic Diseases and Advance Public Health Preparedness in the United States*. Centres for Disease Control and Prevention. https://www.cdc.gov/one-health/media/pdfs/2025/01/354391-A-NOHF-ZOONOSES-508_FINAL.pdf.

CDC. (2025). Crisis & Emergency Risk Communication (CERC). *Centres for Disease Control and Prevention*. https://www.cdc.gov/cerc/php/about/index.html.

Commonwealth Fund. (2023). Restoring trust in public Health: Lessons from local health coalitions. *The Commonwealth Fund*. https://www.commonwealthfund.org/publications/2023/feb/restoring-trust-public-health.

Edelman. (2024). *2024 Edelman Trust Barometer - Special Report: Trust and Health*. https://www.edelman.com/trust/2024/trust-barometer/special-report-health.

European Parliament. (2024). *Achieving Sustainable Development Goal 3 (SDG 3)*. European Parliamentary Research Service. https://www.europarl.europa.eu/RegData/etudes/BRIE/2024/762380/EPRS_BRI(2024)762380_EN.pdf.

Ho, S. S., Chuah, A. S. F., Ho, V. S., Rosenthal, S., Kim, H. K., & Soh, S. S. H. (2024). Crisis and emergency risk communication and emotional appeals in COVID-19 public health messaging: Quantitative content analysis. *Journal of Medical Internet Research*, *26*, e56854. https://doi.org/10.2196/56854.

Potter, C., Nagar, A., Fink, E., Carias, C., Sell, T. K., Brooke, C., Ravi, S. J., & Inglesby, T. V. (2025). *Checklist to Build Trust, Improve Public Health Communication, and Anticipate Rumors During Public Health Emergencies*. Johns Hopkins Center for Health Security. https://centerforhealthsecurity.org/sites/default/files/2025-05/2025-05-Checklist.pdf.

Rüegg, S. R., Buttler, A., Morand, S., Cooke, I., Pautasso, M., Frossard, E., et al. (2025). One Health implementation: A systematic scoping review using the Quadripartite One Health Joint Plan of Action. *One Health*, *20*, 100686. https://doi.org/10.1016/j.onehlt.2025.100686.

Shi, W., Yeung, T., & Dmello, J. (2024). Organisational use of social media during a global health crisis. *Frontiers in Communication*, *9*, 1421165. https://doi.org/10.3389/fcomm.2024.1421165.

SteelFisher, G. K., Findling, M. G., Caporello, H. L., Boyea, A., Espino, J., & Sutton, M. (2024). Trust and 2024 public priorities for the CDC and state health departments. *JAMA Health Forum*, *5*(5), e240862. https://doi.org/10.1001/jamahealthforum.2024.0862.

Tang, E. C., Chen, W., Jabbour, S., Novotny, T. E., Saba, M., Abdalla, S., et al. (2024). Equity-informed social media COVID-19 risk communication strategies: A scoping review. *BMJ Open*, *14*(8), e085630. https://doi.org/10.1136/bmjopen-2024-085630.

WHO. (2025). *A unified call for One Health: Driving implementation, science, policy and investment for global Impact*. World Health Organization. https://www.who.int/news/item/27-03-2025-a-unified-call-for-one-health-driving-implementation-science-policy-and-investment-for-global-impact.

World Economic Forum. (2025). How the World Health Organization's 'One Health' framework can benefit from mission-oriented policy. *World Economic Forum*. https://www.weforum.org/stories/2025/08/how-the-world-health-organization-s-one-health-framework-can-benefit-from-mission-oriented-policy/.

About the Editors

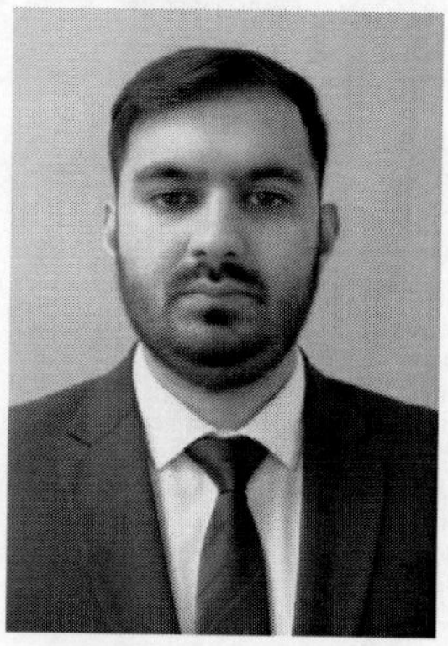

Dr. Maajid Mohi Ud Din Malik (MSc., PhD)
Assistant Professor and Head of Department, Dr. D. Y. Patil School of Allied Health Sciences, Dr. D. Y. Patil Vidyapeeth, Pune (Deemed to be University), Sant Tukaram Nagar, Pimpri, Pune, India, 411018

Dr. Maajid Mohi-Ud-Din Malik is a prominent figure in the field of Radiology and Imaging Technology, currently serving as an Assistant Professor and Head of Department at the prestigious Dr. D. Y. Patil School of Allied Health Sciences in Pune, India. His academic journey, marked by excellence and dedication, includes a PhD in Radiology and Imaging Technology from Singhania University (2020-2023), an MSc. in Radiation Imaging Technology from NIMS University (2017-2019), and a BSc. in Medical Imaging Technology from Swami Vivekanand Subharti University, establishing a solid foundation for his expertise in medical imaging sciences.

Dr. Malik's professional trajectory showcases a remarkable blend of clinical practice and academic excellence. His career began as a Clinical Radiographer at MMAMB Hospital (2016-2017), where he honed his practical skills in various radiographic procedures and patient care. He then transitioned to academia, serving at the College of Paramedical Sciences, Adesh University (2019-2023), followed by positions at GD Goenka University's School of Medical and Allied Sciences, and is currently at the Dr. D. Y. Patil School of Allied Health Sciences. Throughout these roles, he has demonstrated exceptional ability in curriculum development, student mentoring, and research supervision.

As a prolific researcher and author, Dr. Malik has made substantial contributions to the field of medical imaging, authoring over 25 scholarly books and publishing more than 38 research articles in prestigious international journals. His research interests span a wide range of topics, with particular focus on radiation safety and diagnostic imaging protocols. His doctoral research, focusing on dose length product estimation in CT scanning, has contributed significantly to radiation safety protocols in clinical practice. He currently serves as the Editor-in-Chief of two professional journals: the Journal of Advanced Research Perspectives and Radiology Hub, further cementing his position as a thought leader in the field.

Dr. Malik's innovative spirit is evident in his patents for a Controlled Sanitizer Dispensing Device and a Portable Device for Measuring Nerve Damage Due to Diabetic Neuropathy. His commitment to advancing medical technology and improving patient care has earned him recognition including the "Kashmir's Most Influential Author 2022" award by Auyk Media and The International Achievers Award 2024 by Gyan Uday Foundation. He maintains active membership in professional organizations, serving as a life member of the Indian Society of Radiological Technologists (ISRT) and holding editorial board positions in multiple international journals.

In the classroom, Dr. Malik is known for his innovative teaching methodologies and student-centric approach. He excels in integrating technology with traditional teaching methods, developing comprehensive curriculum materials, and providing mentorship to aspiring medical imaging professionals. His teaching philosophy emphasizes practical application alongside theoretical knowledge, preparing students for the evolving challenges of healthcare technology. His expertise extends beyond traditional academics to include leadership in departmental initiatives, research project supervision, and academic program development.

Dr. Malik's impact on the field is further evidenced by his extensive participation in professional conferences and faculty development programs. He regularly presents his research findings at international conferences and contributes to academic discussions on advancing medical imaging education. His work is recognized through various academic platforms, with his research being tracked through Scopus (ID: 59223060200) and ORCID (0000-0003-1743-1520). This combination of clinical experience, academic excellence, research productivity, and innovative thinking makes Dr. Malik a distinguished figure in the field of medical imaging and radiography education.

Looking toward the future, Dr. Malik continues to push the boundaries of medical imaging education and research. His ongoing work focuses on advancing imaging technologies, improving educational methodologies, and contributing to the broader field of healthcare through innovative research and publication. His dedication to excellence in both research and education, combined with his extensive portfolio of achievements, positions him as a valuable contributor to the advancement of medical imaging sciences and education.

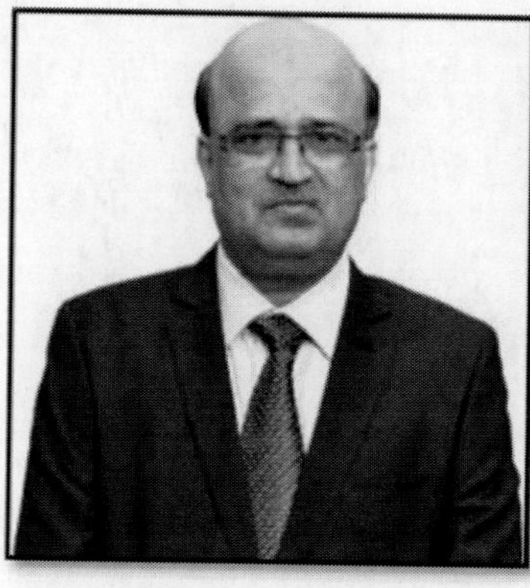

Dr. Abhay Saraf
MBBS, MD, PGDHM, FIAPSM
Director, Dr. D. Y. Patil School of Allied Health Sciences
Dr. D. Y. Patil Vidyapeeth, Pune (Deemed to be University)
Sant Tukaram Nagar, Pimpri, Pune, India -411018

Dr. Abhay Saraf has more than three decades of rich experience with Government of India, WHO, UNICEF, Public Health Foundation of India, Symbiosis International University & IQVIA in various leadership roles. Being passionate about capacity building, Dr. Saraf has developed, and launched more than 30 education programmes in various domains in the area of public health, clinical and allied health sciences domain.

He has also successfully led planning and implementation of nationwide Certificate Course on Evidence Based Diabetes Management, Gestational Diabetes Mellitus, Contraception in Clinical Practice and Immunization Practice, covering more than 20 states, 80 cities and facilitated training of around 8000 PMPs across entire country in partnerships with DMDEA, FOGSI, IAP, CHF, UNFPA and UNICEF.

A recipient of accolades and awards from various agencies, professional organizations and the government for outstanding work in the field of training, operational research, IEC, service delivery and program management. Dr. Saraf has also led numerous projects with various state governments in India and international organizations and academic institutions like MEASURE Evaluation, University of North Carolina, USAID, University College of London, and The Nossal Institute for Global Health, Australia (AUSAID), UNFPA, FOGSI, CHF, DMDEA, IAP, World Bank, DFID, Janssen & Janssen and UNICEF for technical partnerships in various states across the country nationally and internationally.

Dr. Saraf has extensively travelled and spoken at national and international fora and conferences and has guided post-graduate and PhD students.

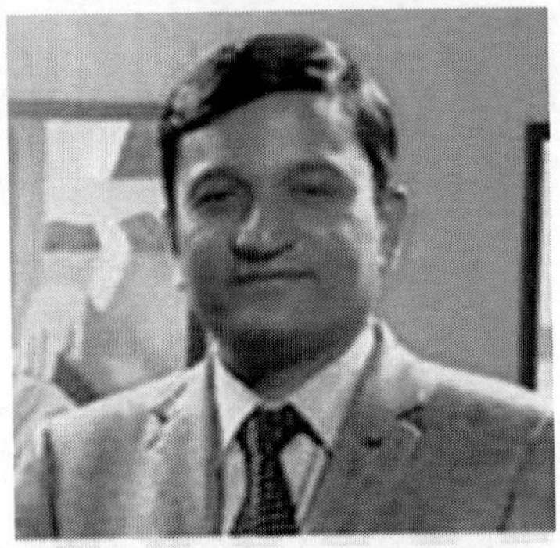

Dr. Harshal T. Pandve
M.B.B.S., MD (PSM), Adv. Trg. in Health Research MIPHA MISID
Head of Department at PCMC's Yashwantrao Chavan Memorial Hospital and Postgraduate Medical Institute (YCMH-PGI)
Pimpri Pune, India -411018

Dr. Harshal Tukaram Pandve is a distinguished medical professional and researcher currently serving as Professor and Head of Department at PCMC's Yashwantrao Chavan Memorial Hospital & Postgraduate Medical Institute (YCMH-PGI) in Pimpri, Pune. He holds an M.B.B.S. and MD. in Preventive and Social Medicine (PSM), along with advanced training in Health Research.

With an impressive academic career spanning nearly two decades, Dr. Pandve previously served as Professor and Head at ESIC Medical College, Hyderabad. His research portfolio includes 131 publications covering critical areas of public health, including epidemiology, infectious diseases (HIV and tuberculosis), climate change and health, environmental health, and medical education. His expertise extends to research methodology, qualitative analysis, and climate change adaptation strategies.

Dr. Pandve's contributions to medical science have earned him significant recognition, including being listed in the Marquis Who's Who in the World Directory as a "Distinguished Medical Researcher" in 2013. He has enhanced his academic credentials through specialized training programs, including an Advanced Certificate Course in Health Sciences Education Technology from Maharashtra University of Health Sciences, a two-week Advanced Health Research Methodology Course at St. Johns Medical College in collaboration with the National Institute of Health (USA) and McMaster University (Canada), and training in Stress and Conflict Management for Health Professionals at the National Institute of Health and Family Welfare, New Delhi.

Currently, Dr. Pandve serves on the editorial and reviewer boards of numerous reputed medical journals, contributing his expertise to advance medical research and public health knowledge. His multidisciplinary approach combines clinical medicine with social sciences and environmental health, positioning him as a leading voice in preventive medicine and public health research in India.

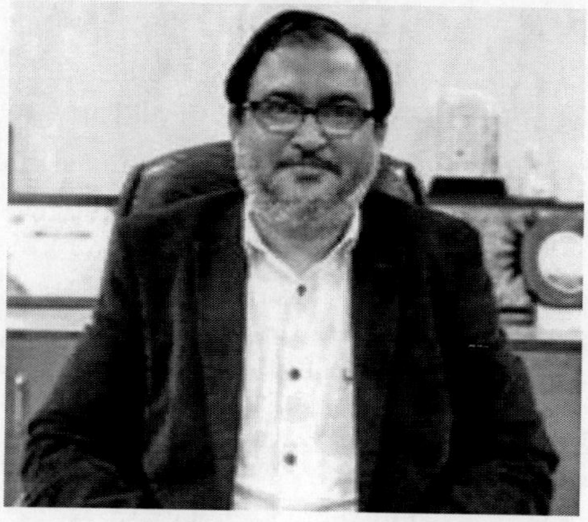

Dr. Quazi Syed Zahiruddin
M.B.B.S., MD., PhD
Executive Director,
Directorate of Research and Innovations,
Datta Meghe Institute of Higher Education and Research (DMIHER),
Sawangi, Wardha, Maharashtra, India- 442107

Dr. Syed Zahiruddin Quazi, the Executive Director of the Directorate of Research & Innovation at the Datta Meghe Institute of Higher Education and Research (DMIHER), is a distinguished figure spearheading clinical research and innovation across all the affiliate institutions of DMIHER, with a robust background in health technology, early childhood development, nutrition, maternal and child health. Recently, Dr. Quazi has expanded his expertise in Clinical Translation Research and Complex Health Interventions, particularly in biomedical engineering, with a notable focus on Tissue Engineering and Regenerative Medicine.

His leadership has orchestrated successful pilot clinical studies on groundbreaking ventures like customized implants, bone scaffolds, and cranial grafts. Collaborating with esteemed institutions such as IISc Bengaluru, IIT Kharagpur, IIT Kanpur, and VNIT Nagpur, Dr. Quazi has demonstrated a remarkable ability to foster interdisciplinary collaboration, securing INR 310+ Million R&D funding from national and international agencies such as Grand Challenge Canada, World Health Organization, AusAID, ICMR, DST, PHRI, Imprint, and Core Research Grant - SERB, DRDO, BIRAC and ICSSR

With over 250+ peer-reviewed publications in esteemed journals such as Lancet, Nature, PloS, BMJ etc. With significant editorial contributions in the Q1 ranking Science Citation Index Expanded (SCIE) journals, Dr. Quazi is listed in the Stanford/Elsevier's Top 2% Scientist Rankings.

Dr. Quazi's impact transcends academia. He has been pivotal in shaping policy frameworks and drafting key models for organizations like the WHO South-East Asia Region. Prof. Quazi is committed to indigenous product innovation, working with teachers to enhance students' employability in the translational research sector and contributing to thought leadership and policymaking at various levels. Dr. Quazi's commitment extends beyond research; he actively mentors a multidisciplinary team, fostering a culture of innovation and excellence.

Dr. Quazi possesses deep disciplinary knowledge and expertise within one or more of the domains of the translational science spectrum. Under his guidance and supervision, DMIHER is recognized by the ICMR as a part of the Indian Clinical Trial and Education Network (INTENT). His vision and expertise are poised to accelerate the translation of cutting-edge technologies like 3D bio-printed tissue-engineered products from the lab to the clinic, ultimately advancing healthcare delivery and improving patient outcomes. He plays a role in expediting the integration of cutting-edge medical technologies into real-world clinical applications.

Index

W

Z

More books by *Maajid Mohi Ud Din Malik* can be found at:
https://novapublishers.com/writer/maajid-mohi-ud-din-malik-phd/

More books by *Abhay Saraf* can be found at:
https://novapublishers.com/writer/abhay-saraf-md-pgdhm-fiapsm/